HANDBOOK OF OSTEOPATHIC TECHNIQUE

Third edition

Laurie Hartman DO

Associate Professor of Osteopathic Technique,
British School of Osteopathy

First published in 1983 by:
NMK Publishers
Second edition published in 1985 by:
Hutchinson
Third edition published in 1997 by:
Chapman & Hall
Reprinted in 1998 by:
Stanley Thornes (Publishers) Ltd

Reprinted in 2001 by:
Nelson Thornes Ltd
Delta Place
27 Bath Road
CHELTENHAM
GL53 7TH
United Kingdom

01 02 03 04 05 / 10 9 8 7 6 5 4

A catalogue record for this book is available from the British Library

ISBN 0 7487 3722 7

Page make-up by Photoprint

Printed and bound in Great Britain by The Bath Press

CONTENTS

FOREWORD

Laurie Hartman has been practising as an osteopath, and teaching osteopathy since 1964. He first published his *Handbook of Osteopathic Technique* in 1983, and it has since become accepted as the leading text in its field. It has been widely read by members not only of the osteopathic profession, but also many other professions world-wide.

During that time Laurie Hartman has travelled more and more widely to teach, helping undergraduates and postgraduates to refine existing skills and to widen their technical repertoires. He continues to be much in demand wherever people wish to learn and practise manual therapeutic techniques at a high level of skill. Having worked with him frequently since 1984 I have observed how Laurie's approach has continued to evolve, his enthusiasm for osteopathy has remained undimmed, and that his desire to help others achieve their full potential is far from exhausted. Furthermore, he has retained the determination and the ability to go on learning himself; he is a powerful advocate for osteopathy, and a marvellous example to those who would practise it.

This new and revised edition of his book is an excellent development of the earlier work, and an appropriate testimony to one of the leading technicians of his, or any other, generation. Laurie has included a greater number of techniques, many of them 'specimens' that he has 'collected' during his worldwide teaching. He has also expanded the text, incorporating sections on different approaches to technique, their backgrounds and clinical application. The reworking and augmenting of the photographic contents will greatly assist the reader in analysing techniques on a step by step basis. The expanded sections on technique selection, modification and application will enable readers to benefit from Laurie's huge experience of clinical practice and teaching, and the new format will assist in its use as a genuine working text from which everyone can learn something.

I am very pleased to have been invited to write this foreword, and have been privileged to work with someone who is quite simply unique. It is not easy to be a good teacher of osteopathic technique, and it is particularly difficult to produce a textbook that is genuinely useful to students of a wide range of backgrounds and levels of skill. Laurie Hartman has for many years been one of the world's leading technicians and teachers, and this book confirms his ability as an author.

Clive Standen
Principal
The British School of Osteopathy

ACKNOWLEDGEMENTS

I am indebted to several people who have helped me enormously in the preparation of this third edition of Handbook of Osteopathic Technique. Firstly, my wife, Susan, who not only did a great deal of the typing, but made numerous constructive suggestions as to better ways of expressing many of the ideas. She also modelled for the photographs, which required much fortitude. The photographs were ably and sympathetically taken by Emmy Anderson. My friend, colleague, and fellow teacher of osteopathic technique Clive Standen currently the Principal of the British School of Osteopathy in London helped me a great deal with constructive criticisms of the text, and Steven Lusty helped model the two-man techniques.

I cannot list all the colleagues who over the years have been inspirational in my work, but no book of osteopathic technique written in England can be complete without a mention of one of my chief mentors, the late Clem Middleton. He gave me much encouragement in the preparation of the first edition in 1983 and was the instigator of the current classifications of technique and the initial inspiration behind the idea of multiple components.

My publishers Chapman & Hall have been most helpful at every stage, and although it is invidious to single out any particular individuals, I have had a lot of help and encouragement from Lisa Fraley, Sally Champion and Rosemary Morris.

My thanks are due also to the many thousands of patients that I have treated since graduating in 1964 who have helped me develop my skills and be able to transmit them to others. That is not the reason why they came to an osteopath, but it has been a privilege to be able to assist in their health care and yet learn at the same time.

PREFACE TO THE THIRD EDITION

The original *Handbook of Osteopathic Technique* was published in 1983 privately by myself under the name of NMK Publishers. The NMK represents the first initials of my three children Nicola, Matthew and Katie. Since that time I have learnt a great deal about the business of publishing, and I am happy to leave this side of the work in the capable hands of Chapman & Hall.

Before the first edition was published I had already been lecturing at the British School of Osteopathy (BSO) since graduating in 1964. I had been teaching internationally since 1970, and in the years since the first edition, I have been travelling world-wide teaching the art of manipulative skill as practised by osteopaths trained at the BSO. I have taught at courses of between 1 and 5 days, and with groups of practitioners and students of osteopathy, chiropractic, physiotherapy and medicine. During this time there have been many advances in methods of teaching manipulative skills, and many forms of technical approach have become more widely integrated into the armamentarium of practitioners. As I have had the opportunity to work with varied groups, my personal methods have changed and adapted.

In some places there has been a distinct shift in interest towards the many forms of indirect technique. There are many reasons for this desire to integrate other methods than a traditional structural approach. Conventional structural manipulation is often seen to be too harsh. There are increasing fears of litigation. It seems too difficult or too lengthy to acquire the skills. Other methods genuinely seem to offer advantages in certain cases, or suit certain operator body types better. Recent times have seen an increasing percentage of female osteopathic students, and some of the early methods of long and powerful leverages are not very suitable for the smaller, lighter practitioners.

This book remains mostly dedicated to conventional, traditional structural technique. Nevertheless, it aims to integrate the thinking behind many of the other methods of approach to make the structural methods more delicate, gentler, and less uncomfortable for the patient.

Not wishing to be sexist, but only to give clarity and consistency to descriptions, the operator will always be described as male in the text. Therefore, for he, read she, if appropriate.

As increasing understanding of the mechanics of manipulative methods emerges, different categories of technique are better understood. These can be integrated in a more efficient way into treatment regimens either as separate entities, or as I have tried to do, as modifications or combinations of existing methods. This is not a new thing; Paul Kimberley DO in the USA proposed a version of this method of what he called 'combined technique' very many years ago.

I have renewed all the photographs, but the system of arrow notation remains the same. The arrows are designed to give some indication of general directions of force only. The text section has been enlarged to include more detail about methods other than pure structural technique. Various comments from colleagues and students have led me to include many more illustrations of soft tissue technique positions and holds.

As before, the use of video to illustrate the positions and holds has been found a useful tool, and video tapes relating to this book with page numbers constantly on screen are available.

I remain open to constructive criticism or comment that will enhance further editions of this work.

Laurie Hartman

HOW TO USE THIS BOOK

This book is divided into two main sections. The first gives a basic understanding of technique, with some mention of many of the different approaches available. There is some information on using non-structural or indirect technique. Structural technique remains the principal method taught and used in most schools of osteopathy in the UK, and this book remains primarily a work on structural technique.

The main body of the work is the photographs that are divided by regions of the body rather than methods of approach. The arrows on the photographs relate to a general direction of the forces rather than an exact specific path as it is impossible in the static photograph to show a moving procedure. In some cases a series of photographs should aid clarity, and in others the hands are away from the body to show the hold more clearly. It is suggested that the sections relating to classifications of technique and the modifying factors be read first to avoid problems of terminology.

The main emphasis in the teaching of manipulative technique at the BSO is on the lowest possible use of force, with the maximum of specificity. This skill is not easy to acquire. It can be likened to learning to play a musical instrument. A great deal of practice is necessary, many errors will occur, and a gradual learning curve with many disappointments along the way is normal. Some of the positions shown may, initially, not appear to be effective for the purpose intended. It is only when the use of multiple components in technique is fully understood and used efficiently that the effectiveness will improve.

Body tissues are like a spring in that they will tend to creep away from torsion or stress. Most of the holds illustrated in this book require the operator to take control, in a comfortable way, to prevent escape from the specifically applied useful tension. This enables completion of the technique in a position which, at first, seems to be impossible as the part appears not to be isolated in the more normal way of conventional manipulation. Once this skill is achieved in 'barrier control' or 'tension sense', then this uniquely non-traumatic system can be used to its best advantage.

There are very few operators who will find all techniques equally useful in all cases. As patients vary, so do operators, and due to differences in length of arms, height, strength, weight, and many other factors, some techniques will not be as good for some as for others. Nevertheless, with the wide variety of methods available this should not be a problem. The modifying factors again can be used to fit each technique specifically to each patient and operator. The patient's age, general state of health, mental state and degree of pain will clearly modify the approach to be used.

It is not the function of this book to enter into aspects of diagnosis and the actual choice of technique for specific conditions but purely to aim at cataloguing a range of approaches available. Some tips will be given, however, for optimum usage of the techniques shown. The actual choice of technique in a given case must depend on the diagnosis and indications and contra-indications specific to that patient.

There is a section devoted specifically to diagnosis that may help to clarify this aspect, but the reader is directed elsewhere for fuller information.

Thrust techniques when poorly applied are potentially dangerous in certain cases and it is suggested that no attempt be made to use these without the benefit of personal instruction. Those experienced in this particular category of technique and the ability to perceive joint motion barrier objectives may be able to acquire some new useful holds from careful study of the photographs.

There are specialist texts relating to many of the indirect techniques that are not fully described and pictured in this work and the reader is referred to the bibliography for more complete details on these.

The anatomical terminology used throughout is standard. The terms relating to flexion and extension refer to forward bending and backward bending respectively rather than the notation used by Fryette relating to embryonic curves. Certain vectors of force will be described which may only require very small amplitude. These are distinctly a minimal part of the technique, but in combination with other forces become an essential integral part. Some techniques will prove to be ineffectual if these very small amplitudes of the secondary components are not included. They could be termed tertiary rather than secondary components.

If this book is being used for student learning purposes it may be found that the best effect can be gained by students working in groups of threes. One is the 'patient', one the operator, and one a constructively critical observer who can comment on the fine details of positioning and posture. In this way the observer will also be learning how to see if a technique is likely to be effective as the comments from the 'patient' should confirm his adjustment and fine tuning. It takes a little practice to become an observer capable of 'seeing' good technique, but it is a skill well worth acquiring. Many students are surprised at how their tutors can 'fine tune' the position adopted to make it more effective merely by looking at it and making very small adjustments to the position or forces being used. Without an observer it has been found that the use of a large mirror can be of help and the availability of a video camera for instant playback is also useful.

Those practising manipulative therapies have a unique advantage over many other professions in that it is possible to give subjective feedback from the receiving end of techniques and treatment. If the subject merely acts as a silent model, much useful information is being lost as to the 'feel' of a technique from the receiving end. It may seem somewhat intimidating to be on the receiving end of this sort of comment. Nevertheless, students who work together and who trust each other will soon realize the benefit gained in developing the palpatory cues that match the subjective sensations of the patient. The three students can interchange so that it is possible to get immediate comment from people of different morphologies. In this way it is possible to develop more rapidly an understanding of the modifying factors as related to different patient body types. It is also a good idea to work with a variety of fellow students as the comments will be subtly different and each will be able to help the other in slightly different ways. In this manner it should be possible to develop an awareness of the best pressures and forces that are effective and yet cause the least amount of discomfort and trauma. This type of palpatory awareness is essential if low force skills are to be cultivated.

Very few techniques feel right until they have been practised many times until the hold and position is natural and almost automatic. The time taken to 'set up' the technique is critical. Many techniques will be quite uncomfortable if the position is held for more than a few seconds. Unfortunately, the time necessary to get into the correct position may invoke so much discomfort that the patient may not be able to relax, and then more force is necessary to overcome this increasing resistance. One solution to this is to practise getting into the position many times just short of a point of tissue tension. Once this part of the technique is automatic, then move on to the whole procedure rather than just the hold and the building of a barrier sense.

The traditional term **osteopathic lesion** has been largely superseded by the term **somatic dysfunction**. Although this is not strictly synonymous, it is in accord with the World Health Organization International classification of diseases. When the original definition of an osteopathic lesion was coined by Andrew Taylor Still the concept of the possibility of a dysfunction in the musculo-skeletal system without the presence of disease was revolutionary. It has taken many years for the medical profession to accept that it is possible to have altered function in the spine or peripheral joints. It has taken even longer to accept that these dysfunctions can often be treated successfully by manual methods. Many different professions are using manual techniques in treatment of these conditions, and their models of the cause, type of approach necessary and underlying principles vary slightly.

Osteopathic concepts originally looked on joint lesions in relation to positions of displacement. Techniques were designed to be corrections or adjustments to this perceived malpositioning. As more understanding of the physiology, patho-physiology and pathology has developed, so the thinking in relation to the lesion has changed. In 1959 Alan Stoddard, in his *Manual of Osteopathic Technique*, defined the condition. 'An osteopathic spinal lesion is a condition of impaired mobility in an intervertebral joint in which there may or may not be altered positional relations of adjacent vertebrae. When altered position is present, it is always within the normal range of movement of that joint.' He went on to state that although the definition was limited, it related specifically to the condition that best

responds to manipulation. This definition, and the follow-on statements relating to it remain relevant today, and form the basis of the approach used by most osteopathic manipulative practitioners.

Some schools of thought still relate to dysfunctions by their position of fixation. Some are more interested in their inability to move in certain directions. Some are more concerned with the relative hypermobility of adjacent segments required to compensate for the restricted areas. The site of maximum tenderness and symptoms is often found to be the relatively hypermobile area and is thus notoriously unreliable in diagnosis. Local dysfunction, if of recent origin, may be tender and sensitive, but quickly subsides to a low level of irritability, leaving the compensating areas to become increasingly sensitive. There is, therefore, a time-frame to the tenderness and this must be considered in diagnosis and assessment.

It is important to distinguish between a primary and a secondary dysfunction. Old osteopathic terminology described primary and secondary lesions in relation to their character and postural relationship. A secondary lesion was one that had undergone certain changes in the tissues, making it necessary to perform two stage corrections. This was not only a very complex way of looking at the problems, but was taught differently by different teachers according to their own personal model of understanding. In attempting to simplify matters without totally losing the basic thinking, the BSO has adopted a notation based on what is thought to be a logical physiological and anatomical basis.

A lesion may be primary or secondary. A

primary dysfunction can be due to trauma, either as a single incident or as a result of a series of micro-traumata. If the strains are due to the presence of some dysfunction elsewhere in the body, then we have a secondary lesion or dysfunction. There is, therefore, a primary lesion at one or more sites with a palpable dysfunction elsewhere that has been dependent on the primary for its production. Sometimes the primary has resolved naturally or due to the intervention of treatment. If the homeostatic mechanisms are capable of restoration of normality in the secondary dysfunction, then it will spontaneously correct. If they are not, due to weakness, muscular imbalance or habit, what was a secondary lesion becomes a self-maintaining entity of dysfunction in its own right. The secondary dysfunction is really then an adaptation to some intrinsic fault in the structure. An adaptation that cannot fully balance will go on to become a compensation. Adaptation is a normal physiological response to stress. It is only unsuccessful adaptation processes that lead to the need for compensation.

There is much debate as to what converts an adaptation to a compensation. Some think that it is due to patterns 'learnt' by muscles. This can lead to perverted function that eventually leads to physiological modifications that become patho-physiological and eventually pathological or at least partly irreversible. This entails the alteration of the material properties of the collagenous and elastic tissues that make up the tendons, ligaments, fascia and other soft tissue structures surrounding an articular unit. Some of these changes are not capable of spontaneous resolution once they have passed a certain stage. It is before this point that manual techniques have the most use in restoration of normal function. If muscle or fascia is too short due to compensatory mechanisms, there will be a tendency for reduced movement in adjacent joints coming under the control of these soft tissues. The bones and joints are only able to function as well as permitted by the soft tissues attached

to and overlying them. Joints work best in the middle of their range, and the reduced movement will be accompanied by times when the joints will inevitably meet their ends of range too easily and strains will develop.

Not all somatic dysfunction states are at end of range, but qualitative changes occurring in capsules and ligaments tend to make a joint with restricted mobility much more susceptible to mechanical problems. If the demands of body mechanics are for flexibility, there will be a tendency for compensatory hypermobility in some areas with its attendant symptomatology. Hypermobile joints tend to have a characteristic chronic aching on being asked to maintain a static position, and are likely to have recurrent acute locking episodes as well. The chronic aching is often due to sustained muscle hypertonia in an attempt to stabilize the area. Muscle is not designed for this sustained contraction and will change somewhat according to these stresses. Adaptive changes in the muscles required to maintain this state include partial fibrosis and changes in the fascial and myofascial tissues to become 'stringy' or 'ropy'. The so-called fibrositis and persistent muscular irritability need little description.

There is another type of secondary lesioning that is due to altered neurology from the presence of perverted viscero-somatic reflexes emanating from a dysfunctional or diseased viscus. The nature of the palpable findings in these cases will be somewhat different from the simpler mechanical dysfunctions. The tissues have a characteristic 'doughy' nature, and the palpable joint dysfunction that follows the soft tissue irritability will have a more 'springy' nature. If the condition is maintained for long enough, however, there may be adaptive changes in the somatic tissues that will not restore to normal spontaneously when the primary irritation from the nervous system has gone. The other characteristic that is different about this type of secondary lesioning is that it tends to have an indurated feel. Normal mechanical dysfunction tends to bulge out with muscle contraction producing a palpable swelling of the belly of the muscle. The muscles affected by the secondary dysfunction related to a visceral condition are often flatter muscles that tend to pull in rather than bulge out when they contract. It is very easy to miss the presence of this phenomenon. Any patient who has the misfortune to have a serious visceral condition, if examined before, during and after, will show evidence of this. It is a finding that may only become evident in retrospect, but this hindsight will enable the experience to be used to recognize the situation the next time it happens.

Asymmetry is the rule when dealing with the human structure. Nevertheless, asymmetry that is dysfunctional is significant as it is often a source of symptoms or a stressor to the system to produce symptoms elsewhere. It is often difficult to define what is relevant in the objective findings. Quality of any disturbance is seen to have far greater significance than quantity. Imbalance of action around a moving part has to be examined with the part in motion. Static examination is an essential part of testing, but moving analysis using active, passive and possibly resisted movements is necessary.

The aims of treatment can be directed to symptoms, signs, a balance between the two, or simply the restoration of function. It could be directed to helping the patient's structure become more able to adapt itself to the environment. It is assumed in this respect, that a structure that is working harmoniously is more efficient and is less likely to be a source of symptoms. A simple statement to encapsulate this is that function governs comfort.

The criteria on which a manipulative prescription is based and the choice of technique to be used are governed by the diagnosis or pre-treatment assessment. In conventional medicine, diagnosis relates to the discovery of disease and this leads automatically to a choice of treatment methods. The approach to treatment will vary slightly according to the knowledge, philosophy and system of the practitioner, but will usually fit in with established guidelines. Diagnosis in osteopathy is similar, in that it relates to the discovery of disease in much the same way as orthodox medicine, but then should lead the practitioner along a choice of several different paths. The first path is the choice whether to treat or not, and as to whether the case is suitable for osteopathic intervention. For a case to be suitable there must be some evidence of mechanical dysfunction present that can be changed or improved by physical treatment. If it is not suitable, possibly due to the presence of serious disease that would be better attended by another discipline, the practitioner must have enough knowledge about the condition to be able to refer the patient to a suitable authority. This would avoid wasting the patient's time and money on fruitless physical treatment. He must understand the contra-indications to treatment, and have enough knowledge of pathology to be able to make a reasoned judgement as to possible dangers. His knowledge and competence to decline to treat must be sufficient to avoid being negligent, yet must be tempered by a sense of realism. He must decide whether there are any possible benefits from his therapy.

If a case is deemed suitable for osteopathic treatment, a realistic assessment of the likely outcome or prognosis is essential as a safety measure. A prognosis of a good outcome that is not backed up by the results of treatment is clearly a wrong prognosis, and although the chosen path may prove to be the correct one, the time-scale may be wrong. The next path is into a decision as to the best choice of treatment techniques, and the order in which they are to be carried out. The choice of techniques to be used is governed by the examination findings at the time, and the pre-treatment assessment at each occasion. There are no absolutes; as with all systems different practitioners will have varied approaches according to a multitude of criteria. Choice of approach will depend on the understanding of the requirements of the case, and on the ability of the practitioner to carry out the chosen procedure. It would be foolish to believe that every practitioner is capable of equal skill in each technique. The wise practitioner will maximize his strengths, but will constantly be endeavouring to overcome his weaknesses and add to his strengths.

There will be a short-term and long-term aim to treatment, and it is essential to involve the patient in the diagnosis decision and the reasoning for the approach chosen. Some patients only want a 'quick fix' and then get back to work without a thought for the long-term situation. Some really want to achieve a longer-lasting result, and are prepared to perform any necessary exercise routine and maintenance treatment schedule. They are the 'customer', and have the right to choose. If a therapist feels that a chosen way is not to his liking, he then has to decide whether to obey the patient's wishes or to decline to treat and pass the patient on to someone else who is prepared to follow the patient's choice. It is the practitioner's duty to point out the pitfalls of any choice, but he must ultimately bow to the wishes of the patient. In practice most patients will realize the desire of the practitioner to help them in the best way, and will choose the method directed. However, there is the constant problem of the financial constraints placed upon any patient required to undergo private treatment, and the practitioner must be realistic in his prescription if it may entail long-term treatment.

The diagnostic process, in a medical sense, requires standard clinical methods skills and understanding of symptoms, signs and the normal course of disease processes. In an osteopathic sense there is the broader orthopaedic type of assessment and there is the osteopathic thinking, based almost entirely on applied anatomy. Orthopaedic and neurological testing are essential to discover warnings and precautions and must precede osteopathic examination. Once a particular case has had pathological entities excluded, and has been deemed suitable for osteopathic care, then the true osteopathic diagnosis will begin.

Osteopathic treatment and the techniques used can be either general as a form of 'tuning' the mechanical structures, or specific to a particular complaint. General treatment is a classical osteopathic approach taught at many schools of osteopathy, and should not be an excuse for lack of diagnosis. It should be performed for a specific reason and although it does not depend on specific individual structural diagnosis, it must, nevertheless, depend on palpatory findings.

Specific or regional treatment is based on a history, examination and palpation of the perceived dysfunction and techniques are chosen that have the best chance of restoration of function in a mechanical sense. Some operators have a model of improvement of circulation, some of releasing stiffness and tightness. Some are mainly interested in relief of pain. Whatever the chief reason for

the treatment and the techniques used in that treatment, there must be a choice of methods, frequency, duration and intensity so that the treatment techniques fit the dysfunction.

The first requirement of the diagnostic process in the mechanical sense is to find the tissue causing the symptoms. The next requirement is to assess the fault in that tissue or tissues. The reason for that breakdown is relevant as are the predisposing and maintaining factors. In other words 'why did this particular person get this particular problem at this particular time? Diagnosis in this sense requires a knowledge of the normal behaviour of tissues and the type of symptoms that can be produced when they are stressed. It is very important to discover aggravating and relieving factors so that the precise tissue or structure can be discovered. Patho-physiology is the study of tissues that are dysfunctional, but not yet in a state of true disease. Ultimately we are looking for what has been called 'the manipulable lesion'. The three processes of history, examination and palpation should ideally lead to the same conclusions. Separate operators performing the three parts of the overall assessment should be able to make an independent decision based on their findings with each method. In practice, naturally, one operator is usually responsible for the whole operation, but attempting to make an assessment on one aspect only is a very good exercise in thorough analysis.

As an example of this, consider a patient who presents with lower back ache with some radiation into his right thigh posteriorly as far as the knee. He has no sensory phenomena of pins and needles or numbness and has not noticed any weakness. He states that it has come on for no particular reason but on close questioning he had been rather vigorous in cleaning his car the day before. He is right-handed. He admits to having had similar discomfort after ten pin bowling. He is relieved by lying down, although he feels stiff afterwards. Walking seems to ease the pain, but if he walks for more than 20 minutes, the pain starts to increase, particularly if he is carrying anything. He finds the discomfort increases when he sits for a prolonged period and has noticed that it is difficult to tie his right shoelace. He has slight increase of pain when coughing or sneezing and gets a stab of pain if he tries to bend too far. He notices that when he first stands after sitting he is slightly sidebent to the left, but that this disappears after a minute or so. His job involves walking a lot, but he finds that if he has to stand still, he gets a lot of lower back aching. He has had some lower back discomfort before, but it has always been on the left side and has never travelled into the lower extremity. These episodes are increasing in frequency and often disable him for a few days at a time. His medical history is uneventful, but he has had minor meniscal dysfunction with the right knee and his left foot seems to be enlarged slightly. He has noticed that he often catches his left heel in his right trouser turn-up.

After taking the history the patient is asked to undress to his underpants and the examination begins. He is asked to stand and we observe his posture and carriage of weight from behind, in front and from the side. He appears to be reasonably symmetrical but stands with a slight bend in his right leg at the knee. When he is asked to stand with the legs straight he appears to have his left iliac crest lower than the right. The waist fold is slightly deeper on the right than the left. His right shoulder is slightly lower than the left. He has very slight varicose veins evident on the left calf. Active movements into flexion show some guarding in the lumbar area and he supports his weight on his thighs as he returns from flexion. Sidebending to the left is full, but attempts to sidebend to the right cause increase of discomfort. Extension causes no problems but he is rather stiff. Rotation is slightly fuller to the right than the left. If he is asked to let one knee sag so that he bears most of his weight on one leg, the right side of the pelvis drops far easier than the left.

In a sitting position he tends to slump and to support his weight on his hands placed behind him. In supine lying, the passive hip rotation on the left is much more limited than the right although the right is the symptomatic side. Hyperextension in the right knee is much more limited than in the left. Passive movement testing of the sacro-iliac joints in this position shows that the left side is much more rigid than the right. In a sidelying position passive movement testing shows that the lumbo-sacral segment is very restricted and tends to sidebend to the left with ease but not to the right. Neurological testing is normal as are the pulses in the lower extremities.

At first sight this may seem a confusing jumble of unconnected facts and irrelevant findings. However, from all this it is possible to make some assumptions and come to a reasoned working hypothesis as to the cause of the presenting syndrome. This working hypothesis also leads to an understanding of the case and a strategy for treatment, management and choice of techniques. If we look at the relevance of all these factors, several things become evident. Every one of these symptoms gives another clue to the overall diagnosis. His tissues are telling a story; we must decipher and unravel the relevance of each of these factors. The conclusion from the history should accord with the findings on examination and palpation.

Some aspects of the pattern of the problem seem to relate to a mild degree of disc degeneration and subsequent right-sided facet syndrome. If we treat the case from this simple viewpoint we are going to have a measure of success with the short-term pattern, but the recurrences will have to be dealt with as a repeated crisis management. Some patients are happy to do this, but if the underlying cause of the problem can be sorted out, they are often much happier.

The analysis of each finding follows:

1. The nature of the pain is much more typical of a referred pain syndrome rather than a true nerve root pressure.

2. A right-handed person cleaning a car does a lot of sidebending to the right, thus compressing the right side of the spine and possibly causing facet apposition on the right.
3. Ten pin bowling involves lifting and quite severe rotation to the left; a back that cannot rotate so well to the left may be strained.
4. Pain relieved by rest but that feels stiff afterwards is typical of discal irritability with subsequent muscle guarding.
5. Pain eased by walking that increases with prolonged walking indicates that the spine does not like sidebending and rotation.
6. The increase of pain with carrying weight when walking implicates the disc again.
7. Prolonged sitting increases irritability in the posterior structures due to the increased stretch on the posterior aspect of the disc, ligaments and muscles.
8. Difficulty in tying the right shoelace points to a restriction of right sidebending combined with flexion.
9. The cough reflex is indicative of some discal involvement due to the increase of intra-abdominal pressure.
10. Pain on bending too far is indicative of overstretch of the posterior tissues.
11. A symptom of being sidebent on first standing up after sitting is indicative of discal irritability or facet joint swelling producing a protective posture. That it subsides after a few moments indicates that the inflammatory element is not too severe.
12. Pain on prolonged standing and postural 'nystagmus' can be indicative of poor proprioceptive control of muscle and is common in ligamentous overstretch and early disc degeneration.
13. The movement of the pain from one side to the other could be due to many causes; in this case it appears that a simple facet syndrome has been converted to a disc pattern as the compression on the short leg side has become an overstretch of the soft tissues on the other side.
14. The repetitive nature of the previous episodes on the other side and the rapid resolution, point to simple facet dysfunction and joint strains. The transfer of the pain to the other side and the tendency for it to move more distally indicate possible discal irritability.
15. The meniscal dysfunction in the right knee might be unconnected, but could indicate a tendency to leave that knee in slight flexion when standing, thus predisposing to knee strains.
16. The enlargement of the left foot may be incidental, but if he tends to stand with greater weight-bearing on the left leg than the right, the foot will spread and enlarge.
17. The catching of the heel of one foot in the turn-up of the other leg is sometimes indicative of a short leg.

The findings on examination should help in the assessment:

1. He tends to stand with more weight on the left leg. This could indicate a short leg on the left and a compensation of weight transfer to the short leg.
2. His increase of waist fold on the right on symmetrical standing indicates a short leg on the left.
3. The lower right shoulder indicates a mild left convex lateral scoliosis which is in accord with the short leg theory and compensation to this.
4. The varicose veins on the left calf only are indicative of increased weight-bearing on that side and poorer venous return.
5. The guarding in flexion is typical of mild disc or facet syndrome.
6. The supporting of the weight on the thighs is typical of a discal irritability and can indicate nuclear movement and antalgic protection of the area.
7. The limited and painful sidebending to the right might indicate a facet syndrome,

or could be due to lateral displacement of nuclear material in a disc.

8. The stiffness on extension is often due to reluctance to compress the posterior elements of the disc and posterior ligaments.
9. The easier rotation to the right accords with the mild scoliosis produced by the left leg standing habit and tendency of the spine to rotate away from the side-bending under prolonged stress.
10. The knee drop test, where he is asked to let the weight drop onto one leg at a time, is much easier to the left, indicating a tendency to stand with greater weight-bearing on the left, confirming the short leg and distorted posture theory once again.
11. The need to slump when sitting is indicative of poor control of postural muscle. The need to support the weight on the hands is indicative of discal irritability.
12. The restricted hip rotation on the left is indicative of increased weight-bearing on that side, further confirming the one-sided standing habit.
13. The lack of hyperextension of the right knee is indicative that this knee is often allowed to flex slightly. This follows the same theory of one-sided standing.
14. The rigidity in the left sacro-iliac is further confirmation of the one-sided posture producing a riding up and stiffening of the sacro-iliac.
15. The restriction of the lumbo-sacral joint on passive movement testing accords with the mixed facet/disc syndrome.
16. The easier sidebending to the left helps confirm the postural habit and subsequent disc damage.

In summary we have a patient who has a difference in leg length, his left leg being shorter than the right. He tends to stand with more weight on the left leg than the right and has had repeated episodes of left-sided facet syndrome. His right knee has been kept slightly flexed for so long that it has been predisposed to meniscal dysfunction and lack of hyperextension. The lumbo-sacral disc has stood the onslaught of all this for some time, but has now become mildly degenerate, and there are signs of a mild discal irritability or even herniation. The final straw of the car washing and severe right sidebending have jammed the facet of the lumbo-sacral segment on the right and the disc at that level has reacted to the compromised movement possibility and has become symptomatic.

How can we relate these findings and conclusions to possible treatment and choice of techniques? Each different discipline of practitioner will naturally have varied ideas on how to deal with any particular case. There will be different opinions as to the relevance of the findings and even as to their existence at all. A physician might be inclined to deal with this case with rest, mild anti-inflammatory medication and advice as to posture and activity. A surgeon might advise the patient to see a physiotherapist for traction for the disc and exercises for the muscles. A psychologist would be interested in what the stresses are on the patient that have caused his back to become dysfunctional at this particular time. How would an osteopath deal with it?

The short-term management would be similar to the other disciplines as the needs of the case are for restoration of function, reduction of pain and reassurance. Assuming that there were no other contra-indications, the patient might be treated as follows.

1. Short-term crisis management of acute pain.
2. Mid-term improvement of function for resolution of the presenting syndrome.
3. Long-term treatment and education for prevention of recurrences.

The short-term crisis management might be advice to use hot or cold packs or alternation of these. Gentle soft tissue, cross-fibre kneading of the area to relax some of the spasm could be performed with the patient side-lying. This position would be better than prone as it would avoid excessive extension that might occur in the prone position. Supine articulation to both sacro-iliacs might follow. If the pain is not too severe, leg tug high velocity thrust (HVT) to the left sacro-iliac to mobilize it and help 'de-stress' the right could be useful. Sidelying flexion articulation to the lower lumbar area to increase drainage and free movement could be used. It would be helpful to the patient to explain why the injury had occurred and to discuss the possible longer-term management.

The mid-term approach would be to try to restore full function to the lumbo-sacral segment with specific HVT directed to the facet joints. Minimal lever approaches would be used to avoid torsioning the disc. The HVT would be performed mostly into compression. Providing the patient could extend without excessive pain, a vertical adjustment would be helpful to reduce pressure on the disc and to gap the facets in traction. One-legged standing habits often lead to a compression factor in the facet joints and vertical adjustment is particularly useful for this. Firmer articulation of the left hip and sacro-iliac would be used as time progresses to increase mobility there. The lack of extension of the right knee would need to be addressed, using accessory movement articulation into medial and lateral gapping and traction. Further advice about posture and exercises to stretch the tight left side and possibly strengthen the lumbar erector spinae might be necessary.

The long-term approach would be to extend the treatment interval as the symptoms improve and give natural healing a chance to settle the disc. The posture would be re-emphasized to ensure that the patient was standing more symmetrically. An assessment would need to be made as to whether a heel lift was indicated.

So, we can see that a whole lot of seemingly irrelevant and confusing findings can be integrated into an assessment, a diagnosis, a prognosis and a choice of techniques to be used in treatment.

The original classification of osteopathic techniques was evolved at the turn of the twentieth century and was divided into the general terms of soft tissue, articulation and thrust. While these were useful, they were limited and caused some problems. They were restricted in terms of dialogue between practitioners, or in ability to communicate the exact purpose of the technique being performed. Various attempts were made to reclassify the different approaches, and in the early 1970s a team of teachers at the BSO formed a new classification list. Although these have been modified slightly since that time, they remain broadly the same today. Other systems of classification exist, but I have chosen to keep to the BSO system in this work. When something is classified, it is unfortunately limited by that very classification. Despite this, it is clearly necessary to have some form of definition of the actual procedures used so that teaching can be systematized. It must be realized however, that any classification causes some problems, and will not necessarily be in accord with the particular approach of an individual practitioner.

For these reasons, the classifications that have been defined have been designed in an attempt to state what is actually being applied rather than what is trying to be achieved. In conventional medical practice it is relatively easy to define a particular medication, and the dosage. This is far less simple in manual medical systems. If one practitioner says he has performed a particular procedure, who is to define the efficiency and effectiveness of this statement? This is not to say that we should not be trying to rationalize what we are doing. It is only too easy to say that it is an art, and therefore cannot be classified. It was felt, therefore, that we should make our classification for perceived result instead of application.

The classification being used today is broadly divided into three main groupings. There is inevitably some overlap, and some particular methods are used far less often than others. Nevertheless, they are defined so that they can be described in a way to make communication easier. Education of students is also much more efficient with a structured classification, although they quickly realize that no classification covers every eventuality. The three groupings are: (i) rhythmic techniques, (ii) thrust techniques, and (iii) low velocity stress techniques.

RHYTHMIC TECHNIQUES

These are techniques where the use of rhythm is fundamental to the procedure. They are repetitive in nature but are not simply the same movement repeatedly; they are varied by all the usual modifying factors. All osteopathic technique is varied according to the response from the tissues and structures being worked. According to the perception of the mechanism of a particular technique, so it will vary in rate, rhythm, direction, force, duration and number of repetitions. There will also be variations in all the other factors possible to produce the optimum result in the particular circumstances. In many ways the control and variables in osteopathic technique are dependent on palpatory awareness as much as perceptual diagnostic factors. Palpatory skill will naturally vary between different individuals, but the main objective of all forms of manual therapy is to improve function. Improvement of function is designed to increase comfort, reduce pain and restore normality to parts of the neuro-musculo-skeletal system that are found to be working at less than their optimum efficiency. This will vary according to the demands of the individual and their environment.

Osteopathy has been variously defined over the years, but one definition of Littlejohn, a student of A.T. Still, and the founder of the BSO, was, 'Osteopathy is the science of adjustment.' There are many philosophical arguments relating to this statement, but the objective of technique is to allow the optimum ability for the body homeostatic mechanisms to perform this 'adjustment'. Rhythmic techniques, by their nature are designed to slowly re-establish movement, circulatory flow, and drainage, and to remove blockages in function in the somatic structures.

Rhythmic techniques can be used as treatment by themselves or as preparatory procedures for other categories of technique. The choice of when to apply a given technique in a treatment session naturally depends on the purpose of the technique and the desired effect. Traditionally rhythmic techniques are used to loosen tissues so that high velocity techniques can be applied more easily. This relegates them to a position of secondary procedures, which is unfortunate. They are powerful in their own right and should have a much more important role than simply padding out a treatment while preparing for more spectacular techniques. Suitably applied rhythmic technique can be a whole treatment in itself, and forms the mainstay of most osteopathic treatment sessions.

For the sake of reasonable brevity the descriptions of each technique will not repeatedly state the various modifications possible.

The reader is referred to the section relating to modifying factors and asked to consider each of these as applied to each technique classification.

A rhythmic technique is divided into eight categories.

1. Kneading
2. Stretching
3. Articulation
4. Effleurage
5. Inhibition
6. Springing
7. Traction
8. Vibration

KNEADING

Kneading can be defined as a rhythmic squeezing and massaging of muscles and other soft tissues to relax them by reducing fluid congestion and tonic irritability. The mechanism by which this produces a result is open to question. Some say that the effect is one of reflex balancing. Some think that the result comes from fluid interchange and lymphatic drainage. There is also a powerful psychological and soporific effect. The technique is applied in a slow and careful way to produce the best result. The best rhythm and tempo for any given case will only be found by adjusting the common pattern slightly to suit the particular patient. The amount of pressure applied, and the duration of the technique will also vary according to the result obtained.

Many different applicators can be used. The most common way is to use all or part of the heel of the hand or sometimes the pads of the fingers. The technique can be a pushing or a pulling, and the hands often work in opposite directions so that the amplitude of each is reduced according to the quantity applied by the other. The direction is usually across the fibres of the muscle, but can be diagonal or even longitudinal in some cases. The most critical element is the finite use of time when the pressure has been applied. If a muscle is simply kneaded repeatedly without attention to the duration of pressure, some change will be produced. If the kneading force is applied, and then held for a few seconds, the muscle will be felt to relax and 'melt'. This sensation can be likened to a hot knife through cold butter. The initial pressure produces little change, and then the knife sinks in and is felt to work its way through the butter as it melts ahead of the blade.

Kneading should not be painful, but a sense of pressure is inevitable. Good handling to produce the best patient cooperation and relaxation is very important. The operator should be aware of any discomfort being produced and modify the pressure accordingly to be at a balanced point just short of pain. The dividing line between discomfort, pain and effective pressure is often difficult to judge, and constructive comments from a fellow student or practitioner are useful. The depth of the pressure should be governed as much by body weight as by the force applied with the hand. The sense of relaxation is gained by the operator's proprioceptive mechanisms becoming aware of the collapsing tension rather than any tactile sensory input. The operator should slightly tense his hand and arm to effectively enhance this proprioceptive awareness. Very slight isometric tension used in this way gives a much better feedback of tissue response.

STRETCHING

Stretching can be defined as a separation of both ends of a muscle or soft tissue structure from each other to lengthen it. The purpose is to attempt to improve function and allow better mobility in the structures being worked as well as the articular structures that they may limit by their excessive tension. Stretching can be applied with a very short lever to influence specific intra-articular or segmental structures. It can be applied using a long lever to influence the extra-articular structures over a larger area.

Good handling is critical to ensure maximum cooperation and relaxation, and the technique is applied just short of pain, but at the border of discomfort to produce the best result. The duration of stretch applied will vary in each case according to the response from the tissues, but should be long enough to allow change to take place. If stretching is applied and released too quickly, a stretch response will be induced, and an opposite effect from that desired will take place.

If a stretch is maintained, there should be a sense of collapsing tension, and a sense of 'give' from the structures as they relax and lengthen. The direction of stretch is often felt to change as this takes place and the operator may find the path changing quite a lot at the end of the technique. If this happens, the technique may become a myofascial type of release, but this is quite acceptable and shows an awareness of tissue adaptation during treatment.

Stretching techniques should be released slowly to avoid reactive tension in the tissues from the stretch. Rhythm and tempo are also variables that need to be constantly adjusted to suit the patient.

ARTICULATION

This old osteopathic term has been retained and relates to the use of repetitive passive movement, usually employing a lever and fulcrum. The use of the lever allows the effect to be enforced without the application of high levels of force. The main difference between articulation and simple passive movement is that the operator should be constantly sensing the response from the tissues under his hand. He is then able to measure the requirements and intensity of pressure according to what he is feeling.

Articulation can be performed over a wide arc or over a very small amplitude of movement according to the requirements of the case. An example of a wide arc would be taking a shoulder from part abduction to full abduction. An example of a small amplitude would be articulation of a lumbar segment from almost full flexion to its complete range.

Many practitioners will add a small emphasis of movement at the end of range. This very small 'bounce' can be a useful way of producing more rapid change in tissues as well as allowing a more accurate assessment of their reactivity.

Articulation can be in single directions of movement or use multiple vectors of force. If multiple vectors are used, it is easier to approach a motion barrier which is not at the end of true range and is, therefore, more under operator control. Working at this manufactured barrier would seem to be inefficient, but will be found to produce the fastest change in mobility of the 'actual' barrier when subsequently tested. The movement does not produce the same discomfort as capsular stretch, but will, nevertheless, influence joint receptor mechanisms in a very efficient way. The chief governing factor in this type of articulation is good operator control. This can only come from a firm yet comfortable grip that takes command of the part in such a way as to promote confidence. Although the vectors of force can be described individually, they are best applied in a combined way to absorb the free play and slack in the tissues. This prevents the natural tendency of the tissues to escape from the induced tension state.

EFFLEURAGE

Effleurage has been borrowed from the armamentarium of the massage practitioner. There are several situations when a rhythmically applied movement of light force and slow rate is necessary. It is usually used on the superficial tissues to produce a 'drainage' effect on lymphatic channels. In traditional massage, the central area is cleared first to make room for the fluid, and then the effleurage is applied from peripheral to central. It is often used over areas where congestion is greatest to produce a circulatory response to aid decongestion. It

may be applied to be counter-irritant. Effleurage can be used as a light introduction to gentle kneading techniques that increase in intensity as the tissues relax and congestion decreases.

Most osteopaths do not use lubricants when performing technique as their use can make satisfactory grips difficult. A common exception to this is when effleurage is applied, as some form of skin oil or massage cream can help prevent soreness and may make the technique easier to perform. Several proprietary types are available with a variety of claimed therapeutic properties. If it is desired to have a light lubricant effect, a fine talcum powder may suffice.

INHIBITION

Inhibition is the one exception to the rule of stating what is being applied instead of stating the perceived effect of a technique. The term is retained as it is an historical osteopathic classification. In practice it consists of pressure applied for fairly long periods. The pressure is slowly applied and maintained for up to a minute or so and then slowly released. It is usually applied over a small area or point. The rhythm is always slow and needs a constant feedback from tissue response and reaction. It is applied with increasing pressure as the patient exhales, and is maintained until suitable change is perceived. An example would be pressure with the pad of the thumb over the lower attachment of the levator scapulae in a case of acute torticollis.

Considering recent research, inhibition may have its effect on tissue fluid interchange rather than by balancing the afferent and efferent outflow as was previously thought. This does not negate the benefit of the technique, but simply explains in a different way what we can feel with our hands.

Excessive pressure will have the opposite effect in that irritation can be produced. Clearly this is undesirable and good palpatory awareness should avoid this problem.

If 'stimulation' as distinct from irritation is desired, a faster oscillation will be required, but active contraction techniques are probably more valuable than manual procedures.

SPRINGING

Springing refers to repetitive graduated pressure over a bony point. It is sometimes combined with very short leverages. Springing is usually slowly applied and released using the proprioceptive response from the applicator and the operator's arm to sense the optimum pressure. It can be used as a diagnostic procedure over spinous processes to assess their reactivity, tenderness and resistance.

The direction of force in springing is often into accessory ranges of movement. A given joint may be maintained in a certain position by operator control, and then springing is applied in another direction to improve quality of movement. It is usually applied against the resistance of the table so that operator body weight can be employed more easily. It is usually performed from a point approaching end-of-range up to end-of-range rather than through a long amplitude. Springing is, in effect, very short lever articulation.

TRACTION

Rhythmic traction is manually applied traction performed to a point or area with some release and repeated several times. When applied to a point, the operator attempts to block adjacent joints from movement, and then using a suitable grip, tries to separate the target joint surfaces with the traction. When applied to an area, a comfortable grip is gained, and then the traction is applied until the area is felt to be affected. The amplitude is an important element as the traction must reach the target tissue or area. Rhythmic traction of this sort is usually applied from a point of some stretch to a further point rather than from no stretch to full stretch. The tissues are only partly released from the stretch before being tractioned again. The effect will be one of drainage and circulatory interchange as well as opening of intervertebral foraminae to attempt to release nerve root pressure.

Manual rhythmic traction is unlikely to be as strong as mechanical traction, but will be much more easy to control as the operator has a constant feedback from the structures. Some operators use straps to assist in these techniques, and some find mechanical traction apparatus beneficial if more sustained traction is necessary. Many modern mechanical traction tables have an intermittent setting designed to mimic the manual rhythmic traction. The main advantages of the mechanical traction table are that it is possible to use more power than can be applied by hand and that the table does not tire as does a human operator.

VIBRATION

Some practitioners use manual vibration techniques over hollow organs or sinuses in an attempt to increase drainage and enhance circulatory flow. Vibration is difficult to sustain for long periods, but when used, is usually applied at a fairly fast rate for several short intervals in a treatment session. Considerable muscle control of the operator's arms is required, and the oscillation is performed by rapid alteration of muscle tension or by fast light tapping.

THRUST TECHNIQUES

Thrust techniques can be defined as techniques using a single application of force using high velocity and low amplitude. The objective of the technique is to direct forces to a specific point, area or structure. It is not usually necessary to perform thrust techniques at the end of a range of movement. By combining many components, a barrier is formed which is at a cumulative end-of-range rather than at an anatomical end of range. If sufficient speed can be attained, the inertia of the tissues can form enough resistance to permit efficient thrust procedures. They will reach a target tissue or structure without reaching the end of range of the joint. This is much less potentially traumatic and uncomfortable, and allows a chance to use this category of technique in a wider range of patients. It is accepted that not all practitioners can achieve this ideal of ultra rapid acceleration and very controlled braking force. Inevitably some thrust techniques will be of a lower or intermediate velocity, but the aim of minimal amplitude remains consistent. A force short of adequate joint separation is not going to be traumatic; an excessive force or amplitude is potentially dangerous.

Thrust techniques are usually performed parallel or at right angles to the plane of the joint and in a direction designed to break joint fixation in the most efficient way. The barrier to motion in a well-positioned thrust technique has a characteristic feel of potential or dynamic tension. It is necessary to balance all the available components of a particular thrust technique to achieve the 'best' barrier, which is not necessarily the maximum barrier.

Original osteopathic thinking was traditionally designed to 'reverse' the path of a lesion. Diagnosis was concerned with discovering the pathway of the lesion, and thus the correct path of 'correction'. Although this is an attractive concept it has become accepted that many cases do not require this type of analysis. A simple breaking of fixation in the direction of optimum barrier is sufficient to improve range and quality, and positional correction is often unnecessary and excessively complex. Attempts to classify fixations by directions of lesion can be extremely limiting, particularly for students whose palpatory awareness is not able to perceive the fine differences. There are certainly some cases where specific directions play a part, but these are relatively rare, and results are just as good if this element is largely ignored. This approach angers some traditionalists. It is interesting, however, that their detailed

analysis and decision of lesion correction direction will be found to give the same path of optimum barrier sense achieved with far less effort by the methods described here.

The palpatory cues of barrier sense are less likely to give the operator a wrong message than a conceptional model of lesion correction analysis. This means that traditional descriptions of a rotation lesion or a sidebending lesion are becoming less common in schools adopting this principle. There may be a description of a segment that is reluctant to rotate or sidebend, but this information can be immediately introduced into the choice of vectors of force most likely to break fixation. If an accurate palpatory assessment is not possible in a static or dynamic examination, the patient can be placed in a thrust position, and the vectors and components adjusted to find the optimum barrier. The resistance to particular movement pathways will then become more evident as much of the joint play will have been absorbed, and the best path can be chosen. This places greater emphasis on good operator control and balance of available components, and is not an excuse for poorly applied technique skill. If anything, it requires greater skill, as the decision about the best pathway to produce the release will change slightly as the patient is moved into the technique position.

Neither is this an excuse for merely 'popping' joints. The purpose of any technique is improvement or restoration of normal function, not simply the completion of the technique. Re-assessment of function, range and quality is the critical element.

Traditional 'manipulation' is performed at the end-of-range, and then by the application of overpressure beyond the point of control of the patient. Well-controlled osteopathic thrust technique is not usually performed in this way. The act of inducing multiple components produces a point of useful tension that is short of the end of anatomical range. The thrust is performed in a chosen direction while the secondary components are maintained by operator control to make the barrier available. The same amplitude of the primary lever applied without the secondary components would not be effective. It is, therefore, the understanding and control of these secondary components which make this osteopathic approach different from manipulation as it is usually defined.

Current classification divides thrust techniques into five broad headings.

1. Combined lever and thrust
2. Combined lever and thrust using momentum
3. Minimal lever and thrust
4. Non lever and thrust
5. Non lever and thrust using momentum

COMBINED LEVER AND THRUST

This variation uses a thrust applied at or near the dysfunction or lesion, with or without application of exaggeration of the leverage. As an alternative a thrust could be applied at or near the extremity of a lever remote from the lesion. A static fulcrum may be created by pressure or fixation at or near the lesion. A combination approach is also possible. As an example of these different types consider:

1. Thrust at the lesion point. A typical cervical thrust technique using sidebending to one side and rotation to the other. This could be performed in a variety of patient positions: supine, sidelying or sitting.
2. Thrust at the extremity of a lever arm. An example of this might be a supine mid-thoracic thrust where the operator's hand is placed under the patient's body and the thrust is applied to the arms crossed in a variety of ways over the chest.
3. Combination thrust at a lesion point and at the extremity of a lever arm. An example of this variation would be a sitting mid-thoracic, knee in the back technique. It would be performed with the operator's hands clasped around the patient's wrists, and a simultaneous push with the knee is

performed coincident with a pull on the wrists.

In many techniques it may be difficult to separate the exact principles, and this is not a problem if everything is going according to plan. If, however, the technique is not producing the desired result, analysis according to basic principles may reveal the reason and, therefore, possibly the solution.

COMBINED LEVER AND THRUST USING MOMENTUM

This category of thrust technique is, in reality, a subdivision of the previous one described above. The momentum component is introduced for several reasons. Some patients may find the position for a combined lever and thrust technique can be threatening and uncomfortable and the use of momentum helps to avoid this. Some operators find that it is difficult to accelerate sufficiently rapidly from a static position to achieve enough controlled power to cause facet gapping. Momentum will aid these cases as it is much easier to overcome the inertia of the tissues if a gentle oscillatory movement is used in the primary lever direction. Care must be taken to avoid the natural tendency to use momentum in more than one parameter of lever direction. If this is allowed, it is far too easy to take the part into a compound lever position which is beyond that desired. The momentum must be used in the accumulation of optimum lever position and not used to emphasize several levers at once.

Momentum can be used while the part is held in a near optimum position by rolling the body back and forth. This allows the fine tuning to take place on the move, and the final sense of best barrier can be palpated more easily. An example of this might be a typical lumbar roll type of thrust manipulation. The patient is positioned for the thrust, and then gently rocked back and forth while maintaining the lever components almost consistent. This is not an increase and decrease of levers, more a rolling of the body while the levers are held. At the optimum point in the rolling, the lower component can be rotated toward the operator in the usual way more easily as the body is already moving in this direction.

The use of momentum also enables increased force to be applied when absolutely necessary. The barrier can be accumulated in the usual way, and the momentum introduced as an increase of acceleration in the chosen direction. This often proves to be of greater efficiency for small operators, particularly when working on large patients. Naturally, due consideration must be paid to precautions against applying an excessive leverage in such a case.

Although thrust technique is normally performed in straight lines, there are no straight lines in the body, and momentum inevitably induces some curving aspect to the force. This may help to find the optimum direction for any given thrust.

MINIMAL LEVER AND THRUST

Minimal lever and thrust can be further divided into two broad subdivisions. There is the true minimal lever and thrust where the part is positioned in as little lever position as is possible, and an extremely rapid thrust is performed. This is designed to break fixation before other tissues deform under the pressure and requires very rapid application and braking by the operator. This type of thrust method is probably the most difficult to perform, and many operators find it difficult to acquire the particular skill necessary to make this method effective.

There is also the more common method of minimal lever and thrust which employs multiple components in an attempt to limit the amplitude of each. The more components used, the less range will be necessary and the final thrust position can become closer to the midline. This is desirable because it is far more comfortable, and should become poten-

tially less traumatic. It is necessary to be aware of the various components available and to apply them systematically while testing the primary lever direction to sense the accumulation of compound barrier. If the primary lever is not felt to accumulate to a suitable barrier, more components can be introduced, or slightly greater amplitude introduced to those already in use. The primary lever should then be felt to become firmer and the resistance more crisp and available to the thrusting hand. Although this can be thought of in terms of minimal lever, it is rather maximal number of levers, but minimal quantity of each. It is important to leave some free play available so that the various components can be balanced against each other in the best combination for the patient, the operator and the technique.

Acquisition of skill in this category of thrust technique is well worth the considerable effort required. Results are often faster, with less discomfort during and after treatment, and tissue reactions and possible trauma are considerably reduced. Thrust technique that gaps facet joints without straining surrounding tissues is much more comfortable, and in the presence of local tissue shortening may be the only way that they can be reached. To be effective, treatment consists of a combination of approaches, not only thrust techniques, and suitable mobilizing using other categories of technique will be necessary to get a good and lasting result. Using this type of thrust technique it is also possible to manipulate many cases where conventional full lever techniques might be impossible. An example might be a case where there is a disc prolapse. If full rotatory thrust is applied there is considerable danger of further impinging a nerve root, or of allowing further extrusion of disc material. Minimal lever technique might allow the facet joints to be gapped as the disc is not torsioned anywhere near as much as in full lever techniques. Releasing the facets might be a useful way of helping to promote faster healing. Caution is clearly necessary, as although the technique may then be possible, is it a desirable procedure?

NON LEVER AND THRUST

Non lever and thrust technique is a type of thrust where the operator applies a force to a bony point aiming to break fixation in a facet or joint structure. Some preliminary compression may substitute for the use of levers, and high speed is often necessary to overcome the resistance of the facet before the force is dissipated through other tissues. This type of approach is more commonly used by chiropractors, but many osteopaths find it of use in some cases. An example might be a prone thoracic thrust technique where the operator uses the hands applied to opposite sides of the same or adjacent vertebrae. The thrust is made directly toward the table or into a sidebending or rotation direction according to the needs of the case.

NON LEVER AND THRUST USING MOMENTUM

A thrust using non lever forces and using momentum recognizes that some operators find momentum aids the discovery of the optimum sense of barrier in their patient. The technique is the same as any other non lever thrust, except that oscillatory momentum is induced in the direction of the final thrust. At the optimum moment, the thrust can be applied as an emphasis of one of these oscillations.

LOW VELOCITY STRESS TECHNIQUES

The term low velocity stress technique may be unfamiliar to many practitioners. The terms muscle energy technique, functional technique, strain and counter-strain technique, myofascial technique, harmonic technique, specific adjusting technique, gentle therapeutic manipulation, neuro-muscular technique and

cranio-sacral technique may be more acceptable.

The BSO classifications embrace all these methods under the broad heading of low velocity stress technique. The four subdivisions of these techniques are:

1. Using sustained leverage
2. Using sustained traction
3. Using sustained pressure
4. Using sustained articulation

The common factor is the maintenance of a sustained position, pressure or movement and the waiting for a response from the tissues. They are all slowly applied using sense of optimum relaxation and change for the better in tissue function. They are reactive techniques rather than direct action techniques and the reader is referred to the section relating to indirect technique for fuller details.

USING SUSTAINED LEVERAGE

An example of a low velocity stress technique using sustained leverage might be a gently held combined lever and thrust position where the operator waits for a sense of tissue release and collapsing of barrier. Sometimes the barrier will be felt to ease in one direction, and further barriers can be addressed in slightly different directions. This can be likened to peeling away the layers of the dysfunction.

Examples from the categories of indirect techniques might be functional technique or some types of muscle energy technique.

USING SUSTAINED TRACTION

An example of low velocity stress technique using sustained traction might be a 'disengagement' of a capsulitis in an acute shoulder. A firm traction might well irritate the tissues, but using a careful hold and maintaining a very light traction until tissue release is felt might be more appropriate.

Examples from the categories of indirect technique might be some of the holds used in myofascial technique.

USING SUSTAINED PRESSURE

An example of low velocity stress technique using sustained pressure might be pressure applied over a muscle and fascial area until a sense of release is perceived. Although this overlaps with inhibition from the section relating to rhythmic technique, there are subtle differences. Pressure is usually lighter than that used in inhibition, and the force can be directed at bony structure instead of purely soft tissue structures.

Examples from the categories of indirect technique might be some of the holds used in strain and counter-strain technique.

USING SUSTAINED ARTICULATION

Low velocity stress technique using sustained articulation is really a conglomerate of the previous subcategories and might include many of the cranio-sacral techniques. Some functional techniques also fall into this heading, as does harmonic technique.

CONTRA-INDICATIONS AND PRECAUTIONS

All systems of medical treatment have contra-indications to their use, or the timing and dosage of their use. There is more than one way of looking at contra-indications to osteopathic technique and treatment. Although there are some deficiencies in the system, this book will continue using the notation of the description of absolute and relative contra-indications. It provides some useful guidelines that are not too difficult to follow.

Some authorities feel that the manipulative prescription must be guided only by which type of manipulative technique is suitable and possible for the case. The idea is that no case is beyond the aid of osteopathic treatment. The choice of technique will be made with due consideration for all the factors presenting. Procedures will be used which cannot be expected to produce any damage, whatever the condition. In this way, treatment of even a terminally ill patient can be undertaken. If there is any small benefit gained, even for a very short time, this can be justified. I have some sympathy for this type of thinking, but feel that it is inappropriate for a student to be expected to work in this way. For this reason the considerations of absolute and relative contra-indications remain in use.

As in all skills it is possible to develop a sixth sense for warnings and precautions. If an experienced operator puts his hands on a patient, there will often be an immediate awareness of a disturbed tissue state when there is any reason for caution. This sixth sense is a combination of learning and experience. Many hidden cues are being used that cannot even be identified on a conscious level. It can become a very reliable method of deciding to stop and re-consider in a given case. This must be in addition to reasoning and normal caution, but must not become a substitute. It is far better to be too cautious and to be wrong, than to be not cautious enough, and be wrong! Hindsight gives 20/20 vision, but this is no comfort to a patient hurt or, worse, permanently or even fatally damaged. Until this sixth sense has been developed over a considerable passage of time, some rules are advisable.

Absolute contra-indications relate to situations where certain techniques should not be used. It would be rare, however, for no treatment at all to be possible. **Relative contra-indications** relate to certain cases that require special caution for an identified reason as to the choice of technique. As experience grows, some techniques previously considered unwise may become possible with suitable precautions for the case.

Thrust techniques are virtually outside the active control of the patient and joints may be taken to their limit of anatomical movement where ligaments and capsules are put at risk of damage. This means that contra-indications to thrust technique will generally be more specific than for other types of technique. However, strong articulation, springing, or very firm soft tissue kneading are powerful in their own right and also require caution. Adhesions around joint structures are often stronger than the normal tissues and force applied may damage normal tissues before adhesions are broken. In the presence of adhesions, force is often increased in an attempt to break them down and the risk factor increases proportionately. Generally, the shortest amplitude possible consistent with the production of the desired result is to be encouraged. Even the highest velocity, if combined with ultra-short amplitude can be made relatively safe. Naturally, this is a skill-dependent factor that requires time to develop and not every practitioner is going to be able to acquire this skill.

The increasing use of the category of minimal leverage technique helps to reduce risk and many cases previously incapable of being thrust can be treated in this way. Caution is still necessary, however, as forces generated can still damage vulnerable tissues.

A decision must be made as to whether a given case is treatable at all and if it is, which techniques are most likely to help deal with the presenting problem. If a case is deemed to be untreatable using any category of technique, suitable consideration must be given to methods of referral and the patient must be informed why this decision is being made. If this is not done, there is a danger of them going to another manipulator who may not recognize the contra-indication, treat the patient and cause them damage.

A case which is not going to be helped by treatment is contra-indicated, not because harm will be done, but because no good can be done. In the presence of a seemingly 'hopeless' case where many other therapies have been used, there may be a case for some 'trial' treatment. It is a good idea to make a 'contract' with the patient to try a few treatments and if there is no good result, to review and reconsider. There is then less of a problem about treating apparently hopeless cases.

There is a school of thought that feels that the use of high levels of traction can render all manipulative procedures 'safe'. They feel that as joint surfaces are separated and foraminae opened, the chance of nerve or blood vessel damage and impingement is reduced. In my view it is dangerous to place absolute reliance on this. In some cases, particularly when using violent techniques, this may be true. Traction, in its many guises, is a valid and useful method of treatment, but to use it to render safe an otherwise unsafe procedure seems an inadvisable approach. Excessive reliance on any absolute rule such as this is responsible for a rigid approach with no possibility of variation for different circumstances. The osteopathic approach is to make constant subtle changes according to the needs of the tissues at the time they are being worked.

ABSOLUTE CONTRA-INDICATIONS

Situations where a particular technique is absolutely contra-indicated include those in which there is the possibility of tissue damage if the technique is performed. It is better to think of tissues rather than conditions, as there may be conditions that are unknown and that are, therefore, not diagnosed. If tissues are the main consideration, applied anatomy and physiology are the guiding factors.

As an example of this, consider a patient who complains of increasing back pain the longer he is upright. He gets some relief when lying down, but is much worse when carrying any weight. He has increased pain when descending in an elevator as it draws to a stop and finds that even lifting an arm out in front of him causes back pain. This pattern of symptoms is typical of a weight-bearing structure giving pain on increased loading. The two main weight-bearing structures in the lower lumbar spine are the discs and the vertebral bodies. Disc disease is not in itself a contra-indication to treatment, but will alter the choice of technique. Vertebral body damage is clearly a condition where treatment must be withheld until a clear diagnosis has been established. If there is bony weakness due to a secondary cancerous deposit, any technique putting forces through that segment would be unwise. Many other scenarios could be described to illustrate tissue analysis but applied anatomy and knowledge of tissue behaviour in health and disease is the key.

The most dangerous conditions are those that could weaken structures and so could possibly lead to a fatality or at best a severe injury. The greatest liability to this possibility is in the upper cervical region where inherent weakness in the vertebral ligamentous supporting structures may lead to nerve or vessel damage if unsuitable forces are applied. The vertebro-basilar system is particularly vulnerable to damage if excessive torsion is used. The results of this could be catastrophic and some tests exist to assess the possibility of potential trauma. No tests are an absolute safety screen, but may help to eliminate the most obvious cases from having ill-advised techniques and treatment. There is no excuse for insufficient diagnostic care and lack of precautions that could amount effectively to negligence. Every precaution that is necessary must be taken before undertaking any treatment to vulnerable areas.

The tests most often quoted as useful screening in the upper cervical spine follow:

1. EXTENSION TEST

Have the patient seated and slowly bring his head and neck into extension. Then sidebend and rotate it to one side and then the other. Any evidence of nystagmus, dizziness or dysarthria should cause the operator to abandon all attempts at thrust techniques and should lead to an investigation of the reasons for the symptoms. These are classical symptoms of postural hypotension which is indicative of compromised vertebro-basilar circulation.

2. HAUTANT'S TEST

Have the patient seated and ask him to stretch both arms out in front at shoulder height. Have him close his eyes and then extend the neck and sidebend and rotate it to either side. If one arm sinks and pronates,

this is a sign of impaired circulation in the vertebro-basilar system.

3. DE KLEJN'S TEST

Have the patient lie supine with the neck in maximum extension. Slowly increase the extension and add sidebending and rotation to see if there is an increase of symptoms as described in the extension test.

4. FLEXION TEST

If extreme cervical flexion produces symptoms of paraesthesia, particularly in the lower limbs, the possibility of a cervical bar must be considered. A spondylotic bar can occur in patients of a generally younger age group than may be expected. This simple test is a useful diagnostic screen for this condition. Clearly any vigorous cervical manipulation would be unwise in the presence of this symptom.

Absolute contra-indications would include any case where there is evidence of severe nerve or cord compression. Where there are cauda equina signs or evidence of neuropraxia, further investigation is essential.

Lack of diagnosis, or even of a reasonable working hypothesis, is also an absolute contra-indication. It is very easy to fall into the trap of treating by recipes without even thinking about the possible implications of the techniques chosen and treatment in general. As the human body is so ready to accept the benefit of manual treatment, many practitioners are tempted to take the easy path of treating first and diagnosing afterwards, if at all. Most times they will get away with it, but eventually hidden pathology or anomaly will catch them out. Some sort of working system is seen to be essential to avoid this tendency.

Extreme pain or resistance should be another warning that must be heeded. There must be a re-evaluation of the signs and symptoms if this is met. It should never be necessary to force against pain or resistance. Find another way, or another day. The few occasions when manipulative therapy has been responsible for injury are mostly those where the practitioner has continued in the presence of substantial resistance from the patient. The patient's tissues know best and if they are giving a message, take notice of it. The less the experience of the operator, the greater the need to consider the absolute contra-indications in the light of pain or resistance. With increasing experience it may be possible to allow some of the absolute category to move toward the relative contra-indication category.

RELATIVE CONTRA-INDICATIONS

Under this heading could be included a complete list of pathologies that may affect bone, disc, ligament, etc. Any patient who has a pathological condition may also, incidentally, have mechanical dysfunction in the musculo-skeletal system. As long as the object of the technique is to deal with the mechanical disorder and suitable care is taken to protect the patient's welfare, contra-indications may be considered relative in that case. The main reason for grading osteopathic techniques into their various different varieties and different modifications is that it should be possible to make a prescription of a particular approach to technique that would suit a given patient. A combined leverage and thrust technique using a long leverage in an 80-year-old with a stiff neck would clearly be unwise. This does not mean that a very light and delicate minimal leverage thrust technique or muscle energy technique could not be carried out in such a case.

Relating the technique to the physique, age, general health and state of the tissues at the time is part of the diagnostic process. It should form part of the pre-technique assessment in each case.

ADVERSE REACTIONS

Adverse reactions to treatment could be due to a hypersensitive patient, an undiscovered pathological state or excessive force or dosage in the previous treatment. An excessively emphasized history and histrionic reactions may be purely due to fear and distress or low pain threshold. Any of these mean that choice of technique must be modified accordingly. If suitable care is taken to grade the treatment from the lightest possible forces and only increase force according to the needs of the case, then the chance of adverse reaction and over-treatment is minimal.

Despite the most meticulous care, a severe reaction to treatment in general, or particular techniques, can occasionally occur. There are many ways of reducing the effects of adverse reactions. Some practitioners advise rest and heat. Some advise analgesics or anti-inflammatory medications. Some will apply gentle effleurage techniques and yet others will carefully repeat the treatment plan previously applied. My personal approach is to examine the patient thoroughly using examination procedures which are basically treatment manoeuvres and try to find the reason for the reaction. If there is an area of inflammation and congestion, then apply gentle techniques from the indirect categories to settle the situation down. I generally then ask the patient to report in a couple of days by telephone or in person. The mere fact of making contact and discussing the situation seems to defuse the situation and restore the patient's confidence.

DOSAGE AND TIMING

Dosage and timing is important in considering relative contra-indications. A severe reaction may settle in a day or so to a situation of a considerable improvement in signs and symptoms. If the same patient were to be seen during that phase of soreness from treatment, the practitioner might have wrongly assumed that he had approached the earlier treatment wrongly. For this reason, daily treatment is generally to be discouraged. If the operator is prepared to perform only minimal treatment on each occasion and is ready to accept the possibility of an accumulating adverse reaction, then this may be acceptable. There may be reasons of urgency due to impending travel, sporting event or important life event that make daily treatment essential. From experience, I would say that absolute specificity is necessary in these cases. Short, purposeful treatment, aimed at one specific target tissue on each visit, seems to produce the best result without excessive reaction.

DISCS

The vexed question of whether to manipulate in the presence of evidence of disc herniation or prolapse will be the subject of discussion as long as manual therapy is in use. The use of magnetic resonance imaging (MRI) has shown that many cases with disc disease have been manipulated with great success. Had the MRI been performed earlier and a decision taken not to manipulate, the patient may not have had such a good result! Once again each case is individual and all factors must be considered in coming to a conclusion about the best approach. In the author's experience, providing there are no signs of extreme nerve pressure, either before treatment, or when applying the technique positions slowly, then disc prolapse is a sign for caution, not abandonment. Powerful rotatory techniques in the presence of radiological evidence of large osteophytes are best avoided for fear of nerve impingement. Forced flexion techniques are unwise where there is evidence of disc prolapse in the lumbar spine as increase of prolapse can occur.

INFLAMMATION

A joint that is acutely inflamed is best left to rest for a while until treatment is com-menced. Over-zealous attempts to force a joint to become fully functional in this situation will often lead to extreme reactions. Inflammation due to ankylosing spondylitis or Reiter's disease is a situation where excessive active treatment is best avoided. Gentle settling techniques can be of use to reduce the irritability enough so more powerful procedures can be used later. The timing and selection of when to treat can only be gained by thought, consideration and experience.

ILLNESS

Although the original purpose of osteopathic treatment was for the treatment of systemic disease through the medium of the musculo-skeletal system, osteopathic medicine of this type is not as widely used as osteopathic treatment for mechanical dysfunction syndromes. This may not be the choice of work for many practitioners, but is governed by self-selection of patients. Cases where there is evidence of systemic disease can be treated either as a complement to conventional medical care, or as an alternative. If a patient is unwell systemically and is seeking treatment for the systemic disorder there will be a difference in approach from the same patient asking for treatment for a mechanical disorder. A patient who has influenza, for example, may not get much help from treatment for their low back condition as their muscles and connective tissues may not be able to take the benefit of the treatment. The general illness will be making the system weak and normal mechanical treatment will often be wasted. It will tire the patient and the tissues will often be reactive and ultrasensitive. This would then be a reasonable contra-indication to treatment at that time. Some diabetics may find their insulin balance disturbed by osteopathic treatment. Providing they are warned to keep a close check on their glucose levels, this should not be a problem.

PREGNANCY

During pregnancy, any technique that might jeopardize the health of the mother or developing infant must be avoided. The chief danger, of producing a spontaneous abortion, occurs in the first trimester. The possibility of producing a miscarriage with properly applied osteopathic care is so slight as to be almost discounted; nevertheless, in a patient with a history of spontaneous abortion care is essential. Statistically, the highest incidence of miscarriage is in the 12th and 16th weeks of pregnancy. These are times when treatment is best withheld in such a case. This is not because it could cause a miscarriage, but more because there is the possibility of being accused of producing it. Treatment during the later stages of pregnancy will necessitate techniques modified somewhat from normal methods. Hormonal relaxation in tissues makes most osteopathic procedures easier to complete and light techniques can be most effective. With sufficient care a patient can be treated right through her pregnancy, and in certain cases osteopathic care has even been given during parturition itself with benefit. The BSO has an expectant mothers clinic that undertakes extensive work on pregnant women with excellent results.

ARTERIAL CALCIFICATION

Calcification of the abdominal aorta is not in itself a total contra-indication to treatment, but clearly must dictate choice of technique. Caution is essential and extreme rotatory techniques best avoided. In general, patients with this condition will be of an age where this type of technique is unwise anyway. Calcification of the aorta in a younger patient may be due to extreme hypertension and this must be taken into consideration in the choice of technique.

SPONDYLOLISIS AND SPONDYLOLISTHESIS

The existence of spondylolisis or spondylolisthesis is not in itself a reason to withhold treatment. If the symptoms are directly referable to the spondylolisthesis and there are cord signs, then osteopathic techniques directed to the segment are best avoided as there is the possibility of causing further damage. However, many cases have the condition as an artefact that has no bearing on the tissues causing the symptoms. Its existence then does not preclude the use of carefully applied technique. Techniques that are specific and are applied to adjacent segments may well reduce stress on the unstable segment and can be very useful in the overall management of the case. Mobilization of an unstable spondylolisthesis is unwise and if it is due to a recent trauma, there is some evidence that complete immobilization can produce healing of this stress fracture condition. A congenital defect will not respond to temporary immobilization.

LIGAMENTOUS LAXITY

There are several situations when ligaments may be excessively lax. Inflammatory disorders such as rheumatoid arthritis not only affect peripheral joints. The ligamentous apparatus supporting the dens of the axis against the atlas can become disrupted. Any excessive force in this area could be disastrous in these cases. Long-term use of systemic steroids can produce osteoporosis, but can also have a disorganizing effect on ligamentous structures, particularly in the upper cervical spine. Therefore, once again the possibility of ligamentous laxity in the upper cervical column is present. It is impossible to state what is a 'safe' dose, but any patient taking more than 10 mg daily over a period of more than 6 months should be treated with caution. Anticoagulants have been incriminated in producing ligamentous weakening due to breaking down the fibrin matrix of the connective tissue. This seems to target the upper cervical ligaments again, so any vigorous techniques in this area must be tempered by extreme caution. Any patient who is taking anticoagulants is going to be somewhat more susceptible to micro-trauma, bleeding and slower healing in tissues, so the category of technique chosen must be of the lowest invasiveness. Patients do not take these drugs unless they have quite serious underlying pathological conditions and it is necessary to evaluate the overall approach to treatment with great care.

MEDICATION

Several perfectly normal, valid medications that patients may be taking can change the effects of manual treatment. I have already mentioned the effects of systemic steroids and anticoagulants in the section on ligamentous laxity, but other substances must be considered. Analgesics clearly modify the response to pain and although they cannot obliterate it, they can reduce it to a point where patient feedback is inaccurate. Due consideration must be made for this effect. Antidepressants will modify pain response and some patients will have apparently strange reactions to physical treatment when they are taking them. Any patient who is taking powerful medication of any kind should be questioned as to the reason for the prescription. If they are unsure of the reason, the practitioner should investigate the actions of, side-effects of and reactions to the substances so that he can be aware of the medical aspects of the case. There may be good reasons as to why the medical attendant has not given much information. Probably the most important medication that a patient may be taking is the one with which the therapist is not familiar. It should be standard procedure to investigate every medication that patients have prescribed so that important precautions can be identified. In a very short space of time the common drugs will be understood and memorized. It is also wise to know the effects of the common recreational drugs, alcohol and tobacco. Patients taking large amounts of alcohol will have different responses to pain and may become deficient in some of the B vitamins, for example. Heavy smoking has been shown to reduce spinal circulation to the extent that some practitioners have insisted that patients do not smoke for 2 hours before or after treatment. They feel that much of the benefit of treatment will be lost if the patient does smoke in this time. They also feel that bringing the subject to the patient's notice in such a graphic way can help trigger a thought process in those who want to stop to help them along the path. Every practitioner will have to consider whether their conscience allows them to work in this rather moralistic way; nevertheless, the ill-effects of smoking on spinal health are becoming more evident as further research takes place.

SCOLIOSIS

Mild degrees of scoliosis are common but extreme scoliosis requires modified techniques. If an organic scoliosis is reasonably stable, it would be unwise to attempt to 'correct' it. Vertebral bodies will have changed shape and there will often be calcification of ligaments and fascial attachments. There will often be osteophytic outgrowths and severe torsional techniques may cause problems of nerve impingement. Vigorous techniques are generally not indicated.

SPONDYLOSIS AND SPONDYLARTHROSIS

The presence of these common ageing processes are not reasons to withhold treatment, but the thoughtful operator will naturally modify approaches according to the degree of degeneration. Some categories of technique will be perfectly acceptable and others not. Expect the worst reaction, and then if you are wrong it will not be too disastrous.

MALIGNANCY

In any patient who has had a past history of malignancy, the most thorough and searching examination should be carried out. It is essential to have an accurate diagnosis of the tissue causing symptoms. If the tissue symptom is of a mechanical nature, then there is no reason why treatment cannot be carried out. Symptoms that might originate from secondary malignancies may well appear to respond in the short term to physical treatment, but the benefit will only be temporary and is probably due to circulatory and psychological factors.

VERTIGO

Some types of vertigo can be helped substantially by physical treatment, particularly to the neck and upper thoracic area. Some types can be aggravated. Meniere's disease and postural hypotension can be irritated by over-vigorous and rapid techniques. Both may well be helped, however, by appropriate techniques for the situation. Both cases may prefer to be treated sitting up rather than fully recumbent.

PSYCHOLOGY

Psychological dependence on physical treatment is not uncommon and providing the operator has assured himself that the patient does have a true physical cause for his symptoms, then treatment can be valid. It must be said, nevertheless, that this type of patient becomes an expert in emphasizing minor physical disturbances. The less experienced practitioner may well find themselves treating such a patient who has been the rounds of others. Any patient who has seen several other practitioners should be looked on with extreme caution. It is easy to assume that the other practitioner has missed something obvious. They may have done, but it is far more likely that they have done the

obvious thing and as this has not produced the result, the patient has moved on to someone else. Every practitioner wants to give the patient a good result; if drawn in to a situation where the patient is very importunate for treatment, it can be very difficult to resist. Several treatments later, if there is no result, it can be very difficult to extricate oneself from the situation unless a 'contract' has been established in the first place. This is the type of case where it is wise to establish an agreement to a re-examination after a predetermined number of treatments. If the desired changes have not taken place, it is best to avoid further treatment until further investigations or a second opinion have been sought.

FEEL

If something just does not feel right, then this is a good reason to perform more thorough investigation or examination. The sixth sense of this combination of learned facts, experience and temporarily forgotten aspects can be very reliable. If something just feels wrong, stop and reconsider. If signs and symptoms do not match, this is the time to think again. There may be hidden pathology or anomaly. There may be psychological factors, or the patient may be overemphasizing their problem for some other reason. It is clearly necessary to find out more accurately what is going on.

The whole subject of contra-indications is dependent on accurate assessment of the cause and nature of the presenting condition. If an accurate diagnosis has been made, the contra-indications should be obvious. Slow, deliberate technique while getting feedback from the tissues is probably the guide that most practitioners rely on. It is not a finite science, but rather an application of science, art and reasoning.

Although the teaching at most osteopathic training establishments world-wide has been predominantly structural in approach, there is a considerable interest, and validity, in many of the more newly developed methods. Indirect methods are generally less invasive in application, although they may be no less effective in action. They require just as long to perfect as direct methods, but give the student or practitioner who is not experienced in direct technique an ability to treat the patient immediately in a generally safe and comfortable way.

Indirect methods should not be an excuse for inefficiency in technique. They should be a supplement and complement to primary methods, and add a dimension to treatment that cannot be gained as easily with structural approaches. There are some cases that will only respond to some of the indirect techniques, but these are rare, and conventional structural technique remains the mainstay of osteopathic practice for most practitioners.

Increasingly, as knowledge of these methods spreads, they are being integrated with the more common structural methods as adjuncts, as supplements, or as a substitute in some situations. Most experienced practitioners unconsciously use a combination of approaches. No single method has all the answers to all mechanical dysfunction problems in the neuro-musculo-skeletal system.

The reasons for the development of indirect technique are interesting and varied according to location. In some countries it has been due to a backlash against the powerful manipulative methods in common usage, and is seen to be more holistic and cooperative rather than being confrontational. In some

quarters it has been due to the ever increasing fears of litigation when 'manipulation' is performed and an articular sound is heard. This can lead to accusations of possible harm and wrong results. That a well-constructed treatment based on good technique using structural methods should not be painful or traumatic is clearly not considered by individuals who use powerful and uncomfortable methods. There may be many reasons why practitioners continue to use such approaches. They may not have been trained sufficiently in gentle and effective technique, or have not been able to acquire the skills adequately. They may feel that firm force is an essential requirement, or that it is what the patient expects. In my view, excessively high force is generally a sign of weakness in approach. Force conceals weakness. This is not to say that force is not necessary, but simply to state that the minimum force capable of producing the required result should be the aim of the thinking, caring practitioner.

The various categories of indirect technique therefore have many uses and possible advantages. In this section the description of these methods is not designed to be a full exposition, but simply an introduction. Experienced practitioners of these various methods may be somewhat irritated by my attempts to simplify and abbreviate the systems, but this simplification is the whole purpose of this section. The reader is referred to the bibliography for more details of literature relating to each of the various types of technique and treatment. There are many other methods in use, and this list is not as comprehensive as some might like; however, I have tried to include the main methods in wide use by osteopathic practitioners. Although no method 'belongs' to any system, some approaches are more commonly practised by other manual therapists such as chiropractors and physiotherapists. I have tried to remain essentially osteopathic and to try to reflect the main methods in use in Great Britain rather than that in world-wide. From my travels and observation elsewhere, I suspect that the British situation closely resembles most other countries. There may be regional and national differences that are due largely to the lack of availability of technique teachers.

I have tried not to be judgemental in my comments, but only to speak as a structural osteopath who has eclectically incorporated many other methods into my armamentarium as I have found them useful. There are some methods that I rarely use, but I may incorporate some of their principles, if not the techniques themselves. The various methods are listed alphabetically.

CRANIO-SACRAL TECHNIQUE

Cranio-sacral technique was first described by William Garner Sutherland DO. He was a student of Andrew Taylor Still, so clearly got some of his knowledge from the fountainhead of osteopathy. He postulated the possibility of movement between the cranial sutures and bones and that they could become dysfunctional. He put forward the idea that these dysfunctions were amenable to manual manipulative methods. The technique rapidly grew to include some basic concepts. These were:

1. The existence of an inherent motility of the central nervous system.
2. An inherent motility and pulsatile nature of the cerebro-spinal fluid.
3. The existence of reciprocal tension membranes, namely the meninges, particularly the falx cerebelli and the tentorium.
4. The mobility of the cranial bones around articular axes.
5. The mobility of the sacrum between the ilia.

With the combination of these principles, and a range of holds and techniques, the cranio-sacral system and dysfunctions in movement patterns can be addressed. The head is held in a variety of predetermined holds, and the practitioner 'tunes in' to the cranial rhythmic impulse (CRI). This rhythmic impulse is described as being an ebb and flow of approximately 10–12 cycles per minute. He may find disturbed movement or flow. If this is the case he can apply gentle forces to stimulate the potency of the system and the fluid drive to perform any correction deemed necessary. The sacrum can similarly be treated with holds that allow it to float on the fluid drive and free itself, guided by the practitioner. The dural attachments to the sacrum can be freed to allow better function at the upper end of the system in the cranium. As time has passed, the concept has been developed to make it applicable to most structures of the body via the CRI. The impulse is best located in the cranium, but can be felt to a greater or lesser extent all over the body. Treatment using this principle can be applied to many structures remote from the head. For this reason, many practitioners now like to refer to treatment of the involuntary mechanism, rather than cranial osteopathy.

Although cranio-sacral techniques were at one time the exclusive province of osteopaths, they are now (like most techniques) being used increasingly by other manual therapists. However, the fuller implications of cranial work with whole body health seem only to have been considered in detail by osteopaths. Osteopaths using cranio-sacral techniques often treat many conditions other than local head symptoms and many good results are produced. There is substantial interest, and increasing evidence of the particular benefits in neonates and small children, although the techniques can be used with efficacy in all age groups. Of all the systems of indirect technique, cranio-sacral methods are probably the one approach used by some practitioners as an exclusive treatment technique. This shows the effective nature of the approach. If it did not produce good results, they would not be able to sustain a private practice with its sole usage.

FUNCTIONAL TECHNIQUE

Functional technique was evolved by Bowles and Hoover, DOs in the USA in the first half of the twentieth century. It has been extensively developed by Professor William Johnson DO, in Michigan. It is a system of osteopathic technique based on the premise that segmental dysfunction is palpable as an increasing resistance to motion demand in certain directions in a lesioned segment. This has been called the bind sensation. Any dysfunction will have certain pathways of 'ease', where resistance to movement is felt to progressively collapse. The 'bind' states can be treated by finding a pathway of least resistance in the segment. If all directions and pathways of 'ease' can be found this should allow 'quietening' of proprioceptive feedback and 're-setting' of Gamma gain in tendon and joint receptors.

The dysfunction can be detected by a variety of methods including palpatory awareness of limitation of movement quality rather than range of motion. He then assesses the responses to find which ones bind, and which ones ease. Whereas conventional manipulation challenges barriers to 'break' them down, functional technique eases the segment into a multiple movement pathway of accumulating ease. This aims to aid relaxation of the adnexial tissues and produce more harmonious mobility. It is based on the concept that afferent feedback to the spinal cord is disturbed in a dysfunctional segment. The proprioceptive mechanisms are maintaining this disturbance, and by passing the segment into a pathway of ease, the afferents will quieten. This should lead to a reduction of efferent firing. The sum effect of this is to cause a new setting of the afferent to efferent balance, and a more harmonious movement pattern. Although the physiological explanation is open to ques-

tion considering more up-to-date thinking, the validity and effectiveness of the method is not in doubt.

Holds have been developed for treatment of most articular structures. Although the principles of moving away from a barrier are opposite to conventional structural technique, they can be integrated with other treatment techniques very easily to form a combined system. The system is guided purely by palpatory feedback from the tissues and is, therefore, dependent on good palpatory skill. Conventional manipulative skill gives the practitioner the ability to perceive accumulating barriers. Functional technique requires the skill to palpate disintegrating barriers. This may take some conversion of thinking and awareness, but most can acquire it fairly quickly with suitable instruction.

GENTLE THERAPEUTIC MANIPULATION

Gentle therapeutic manipulation (GTM) is a system of active patient movement guided by the practitioner in specific directions and in specific order. The active movement of the patient is monitored by gentle pressure in particular directions over the dysfunctional area by the operators' fingertips. It was first demonstrated in Great Britain by John Spence DO, in 1994. The system originated in New Zealand, and like many of these indirect approaches, evolved from a combination of other methods.

Immediate change in perceived muscle tension and fascial irritability is apparent after successful treatment using this method. Relatively little is known of this method in Europe so far, but interest is growing as results are seen. It is commonly combined with specific advice as to ice packs and specific exercise as a follow-up to treatment. Although it employs hardly any applied force, there may be tissue reaction due to the changes produced. The rationale is thought to be of joint and tissue release by way of guided pathways of active movement producing a return to more normal harmonious patterns.

HARMONIC TECHNIQUE

Harmonic technique is a system of approach that uses a harmonic pressure against different areas of the body, and allows a natural recoil to take place. It is a re-discovery of some of osteopathy's oldest methods. The early pioneers of osteopathic technique used harmonic oscillating movement as part of their treatment. It became less used as time went by and more linear methods became popular. Although most schools of osteopathy taught some form of rhythmic technique, it was not generally taught as a system in itself. E. Lederman DO re-discovered, classified and re-introduced harmonic methods, and has extensively researched the physiological effects of this, and other methods of manipulative approach.

The patient allows the part being worked to be pushed, pulled or moved in a specific direction, and the natural recoil and rebound of the tissues return it to neutral. This action is repeated in a harmonic fashion until an oscillation is taking place where the operator is acting as a catalyst. The best balanced harmonic rhythm is when the effort on the behalf of the practitioner becomes least. The operator starts the oscillation and changes speed until this dynamic balance is found. The rate of oscillation will vary according to which part of the body is being worked and length of the lever. The technique is continued until a sense of relaxation is perceived in the area being worked. Holds have been developed for most body areas, and the technique can be used as a treatment in itself, or as a preliminary to other categories of technique if desired. It is seen as most useful where the rhythmic pattern of movement of a part has been lost. An example might be as in a severe arthrosis of the hip. Conventional stretching will clearly make some change, but a gentle rolling of the thigh, allowing the

natural recoil to return the thigh to neutral, would be a typical harmonic technique. The range of movement might change only slightly, but the quality of movement should improve markedly if the correct harmonic has been found. There will also be circulatory changes stimulated by better relaxation and fluid interchange.

The technique is not merely an oscillation back and forth. There are certain directions that are essential for the system to produce the best results, and amplitude is also important.

There are several possible explanations for the effect of harmonic technique. There are evidently neurological, hydraulic, mechanical and psychological reasons why it works.

MUSCLE ENERGY TECHNIQUE

Muscle energy technique (MET) was first described by Fred Mitchell Sr. DO, in Michigan USA in 1958, and was developed extensively by his son Fred Mitchell Jr. Much further development has taken place under Ed Stiles DO, also of Michigan. It is a system of therapeutic approach that relies on diagnosis of a mechanical dysfunction, and treatment with active patient resistance in certain directions against the resistance applied by the operator. The barrier to joint motion or muscle function is found and the operator holds the part against this barrier. He then gets the patient to push either away or toward the barrier depending on the required result and effect. After a few seconds, the patient is instructed to relax, and the barrier should have been found to have moved. The new motion barrier is found, and the activity repeated several times. The mechanism is perceived to be a re-balancing of the afferent to efferent feedback from the spinal cord. There are four main methods of approach: isotonic; isometric; isokinetic; isolytic.

Isotonic muscle energy technique is where the operator resists the patient's active muscle contraction and allows slight movement in the direction of muscle contraction to maintain the muscle in the same tension. The 'retraining' of muscle is perceived to change the tone and body awareness of the muscle so that it can learn a new pattern of useful contraction.

Isometric muscle energy technique is where the operator resists the patient's active muscle contraction and does not allow movement. This causes the muscle to remain at the same length throughout. This is used to either strengthen the muscle, or to allow the practitioner to use the reflex relaxation after contraction to apply a stretch. It will also produce a reflex relaxation in the antagonist muscle which can then be stretched more easily.

Isokinetic muscle energy technique is where the operator resists contraction of a muscle or group of muscles in the patient and allows a gradual lengthening of the muscle during the resistance. This is perceived to act as a re-education to the muscle to normal movement and contraction patterns.

Isolytic muscle energy technique is where the operator resists the contraction of a muscle or group of muscles in the patient and overcomes the resistance to 'breakdown' the muscle. The patient must resist with enough effort to cause the muscle to contract, but at the same time must allow the operator to overcome the resistance to the effort. The effect of this is for the muscle or muscle group being affected to lengthen under the stretch while it is contracting. This is designed to have the effect of breaking down resistance to movement caused by muscle protection and allowing greater freedom of function.

Each one is designed to have a different action on muscle and can be performed against or with a barrier. Although this concept may now be found wanting physiologically, results of recent research show that the method is in wide-spread and effective use.

MYOFASCIAL TECHNIQUE

Myofascial technique has developed relatively recently as a conglomerate of several different approaches. It has some similarity in approach to some of the cranio-sacral approaches. However, it can be applied to all areas of the body as it works on the muscle to fascia and fascia to bone and viscera interface. It may use some of the principles of muscle energy technique in that resistance is utilized. It uses perception of fascial plane tension in diagnosis and treatment procedures. There are various common methods of application.

The technique is often applied by the operator finding an area of perceived dysfunction and gently guiding it toward more harmonious working with adjacent areas. The pressure will vary, and the time taken will depend on the speed of release perceived by the operator's palpating hand. This is generally a very slow and gentle method that is perceived as relating to the neurological control of the muscle and fascial attachments. This concept relies on accurate feedback from the fascia and muscle state as to the optimum relaxation phase of the area. Control of the phase of breathing is also emphasized.

Some myofascial technique approaches use quite strong stretch along the fascial planes with either single or multiple, slowly applied stretches. Some approaches use diagonal transfascial stretches. One of the chief critical elements of myo-fascial technique success is the use of sufficient time in the hold position to allow adequate fluid interchange and soft tissue 'creep' to take place. Muscles are essentially fluid in life, and as fluid is non-compressible, some of the action is probably produced by sustained pressure allowing fluid to change its position within the fascial tubes.

The two models of approach may seem at variance, but like many other approaches will depend on many factors as to their applicability in any given case. As in most systems of approach, practitioners usually polarize to a particular method. Some may find one method easier; some may prefer the rationale of one method; some may feel one is more effective.

NEURO-MUSCULAR TECHNIQUE

Neuro-muscular technique was developed by Stanley Lieff DO and Boris Chaitow DO, English osteopaths. It employs a system of progressively searching sliding pressure designed to find dysfunctional areas and then treats them with varied directions of deeper pressures. It attempts to 'normalize' these areas by allowing improved circulation and 're-setting' of the neural control of tendons and muscles. Its main action is on connective tissues, fascia and muscle attachments. In the spinal area the practitioner uses thumb pressure on the para-vertebral gutters, directly over the facet joints and using the fingers as a fulcrum, oscillates over each level until the lesion is detected. He then sometimes uses a lubricant such as a massage oil to apply mostly longitudinal pressure repeatedly over the segment in question and one or two adjacent segments.

Neuro-muscular technique can also be applied along the whole length of the spine, concentrating on areas of dysfunction with firmer pressure. It is also sometimes used on the abdomen and limbs. There is a complete system of approach that has been documented to apply it to a wide range of conditions. Although this technique is not as widely used now as it was in the first half of the twentieth century, it has a certain following. It is now not taught in many osteopathic schools. There are some similarities with Rolfing and some other deep massage techniques. Practitioners using this method feel that it can produce longer-lasting results than some of the articular-directed techniques.

SPECIFIC ADJUSTING TECHNIQUE

Specific adjusting technique was evolved mostly by the late Parnell Bradbury DO DC who was a chiropractor and osteopath. He combined the current thinking of the two professions at the time to introduce a system of osteopathic manipulative methods that used chiropractic thinking on malpositioning and replacement. The technique is mostly a thrust approach using extremely rapid yet gentle force that is often performed just short of a facet gapping. It is designed to replace or retrace the pathway of lesioning position, and relies on specific positional diagnosis and specific directions of adjustment. The system was little known or taught for some years until being re-introduced to osteopathic education by Tom Dummer DO at the European School of Osteopathy in Maidstone. It is now being carried on by some of his pupils.

STRAIN AND COUNTER-STRAIN

Strain and counter-strain technique was first described by Lawrence Jones DO in 1981. He put forward the notion that many somatic dysfunction syndromes are accompanied by specific trigger points. These points are often very remote from the lesion and may not accord with conventional anatomical thinking, but are consistent and have a characteristic sensitivity and tenderness The technique consists of locating the trigger point relevant to the particular dysfunction and then positioning the patient in such a way as to cause the trigger point to become painless. The position is then held for some 90 seconds and the patient is then slowly returned to a normal posture. If the technique has been successful, the trigger point will have disappeared, or at least substantially reduced. The holding of the position will often be accompanied by a sense of release, heat and freedom. Testing the articular lesion should also show a return of function in terms of mobility.

The technique can be applied to any area where the trigger point has been identified, and even if it is not used as a sole method, forms a good preparation to further structural techniques. It may seem somewhat non-dynamic as the position held for 90 seconds is not in any way rhythmic, but nevertheless it is often successful in releasing specific fixations. There have been some attempts to shorten the time, and although these are not in accord with the origins of the technique, they are more acceptable to some practitioners. To allow the shortening of the time it is necessary to perform the hold with somewhat more pressure or emphasis.

The thinking behind the reasons for the existence of the trigger point and its precise location may vary with different practitioners. The perception is that the lesion is due to an aberrant pathway of movement and is maintained by muscle spasm. The part must be taken back through the lesion pathway until an antalgic position is found. The part is maintained in this position for 90 seconds, which is long enough for the proprioceptive feedback from the Gamma gain mechanisms to quieten down. The proprioceptors then re-set, and the spasm reduces, allowing normal articular patterns of movement to be restored.

The part has thus been taken back to the position in which the lesion occurred and allowed to recover slowly, guided by the operator pressure and control.

VISCERAL TECHNIQUE

The origination of visceral technique is unclear, although Barral in France is often credited with first describing it. It is a form of functional technique as applied directly to the viscera and their fascial attachments. It has many similarities to cranio-sacral technique, in that the barrier sense is used in easing perceived dysfunctions with extremely gentle forces guided by the operator's listening hand. The hand is at one and the same time a diagnostic instrument and a therapeutic tool. The resistance to motion or function is sought, and the appropriate technique used to normalize the lack of function. All viscera are perceived to have one or several axes of movement. The practitioner applies a hold to the viscera with or against the axis or axes. He very gently tests the range and quality of movement in all available planes. If necessary, he then applies a 'corrective' force against a perceived barrier, or applies an 'ease' direction of combined pathways to allow greater freedom of movement and release of excessive tethering. Barral has stated that the force applied need rarely exceed 300 grams.

Visceral technique has become very widely used in the continent of Europe, and is now being taught in the United Kingdom at undergraduate and post-graduate level. The work has been developed and documented well by several authorities, but Jean Pierre Barral from France and Stephen Sandler from the UK need special mention here for their logical descriptive texts and descriptions of the techniques. Many schools now integrate the teaching of visceral techniques with all the other approaches to the body that will have an influence on the visceral systems. This is a logical development from looking at visceral technique in isolation.

An interesting development in the field of visceral technique has been the study of the relationships between the organs and their supporting tissue as well as the adjacent somatic structures. *Grays Anatomy* and other standard textbooks refer to the folds in the peritoneum that connect organs as peritoneal ligaments. These so-called ligaments, such as the gastro-colic ligament, provide potential for organ restriction if they are thickened or fibrosed, thus potentiating the eventual dysfunction of the organ. Visceral technique taught at the British School of Osteopathy involves diagnosing and treating these visceral restrictions. Their manipulation involves holding and release techniques as well as guiding and functional techniques which make use of the fact that as structures they contain muscular elements as well as collagenous fibres. It is hoped that, by restoring a normal functional relationship between the organs and their neighbouring structures (both visceral and somatic), one can move away from dysfunction towards better health. This concept of working on viscera that are dysfunctional as opposed to pathological has been found to be both safe and efficacious.

Although these descriptions of indirect techniques are necessarily brief, they should help to give a taste of the various methods. This may give the reader sufficient interest to permit further study to be undertaken. To this end the recommended reading list should be of some use.

Any psychomotor skill can be varied by several modifying factors. From the sporting world let us use a tennis shot as an example. The direction of the feet, the bend of the knees, the size of the racquet and the twist of the wrist are modifying factors. They will be determining the success or failure of the stroke. If the player directs his feet across the direction of the ball trajectory rather than in the same direction, the stroke will have more power. If the knees are slightly bent, the recoil of the strike against the ball will direct the force into the ball, and not into the player, thus increasing the potential power of the stroke. It can be seen, therefore, that any of the modifying factors will interconnect with the others to make up the composite whole that we might call a tennis stroke. The principle of understanding the modifying factors and using them to the advantage of the activity is without question, although some are clearly more important than others.

If we relate this to osteopathic technique, several important factors come to mind. Posture and handling have been separated and warrant complete sections to themselves as they are so critical, but the others are only slightly lower in the scale of relevance.

A list of the factors that most people vary when modifying a technique follows. There are several others that will come to mind with a little thought. The exercise of doing this will be of some benefit as the effort of identifying them often reveals vital factors not previously considered.

1. Speed or velocity.
2. Duration or length of time.
3. Amplitude or distance travelled.
4. Plane or direction of force.
5. Force or quantity of effort.
6. Onset or the point at which the useful part of the technique begins.
7. Arrest or the method and point of end of a technique.
8. Compression or the use of close-packing in a technique.
9. Primary and secondary levers or the identification of the principal direction of force, and the vectors that help stabilize the part to make the primary lever more efficient.
10. Respiration or the phase of breathing when the force of the technique is to be applied.
11. Resistance or awareness of accumulating barrier sense.
12. Contact point pressure or local close-packing of tissues and pushing aside of unwanted structures.
13. Hunch or the ability to develop a sixth sense that something needs or does not need a particular approach.

SPEED OR VELOCITY

The speed at which a force is to be applied for a given technique will be dictated by the type of technique. A rhythmic technique will have a slower speed than a thrust, but will be repeated several times whereas a thrust is usually only performed once at a given site. There must be some determination of whether the speed is the same throughout the technique, or if there is an acceleration and subsequent deceleration, and the rate and amplitude of these changes. It can be seen immediately, therefore, that other modifying factors of onset, arrest and amplitude are immediately varied by the consideration of speed. A useful rule about speed is that rhythmic technique should be performed slowly enough for tissue change to be palpated during the procedure. Suitable changes can then be made to find the optimum path for tissue response. Thrust technique is usually performed at as high a velocity as possible. Once the tension has been accumulated in the target tissues minimum effort is then dissipated into other tissues, and the maximum effect of the technique is applied to the desired site. The critical thing about use of speed is that it should always be under the tight control of the operator. Do not use the patient's tissues as the brake to the force. The control must be directed by the operator using his muscles as a brake. This requires close-packing of the tissues and a thorough understanding of the vectors necessary for the successful completion of the technique.

DURATION

The duration of application of force in a given technique will vary again according to the type of the technique and the response from the tissues. A rhythmic technique will be repeated several times until a sense of change has taken place. It is easier to over-treat than to under-treat. Many students, and some practitioners, feel that they want to give the patient the maximum benefit and will work for too long in a given way on a part of the body. Too much is possibly worse than too little. A technique performed for too short a time may not produce much benefit, but it is unlikely to make the situation worse. However, a technique performed for too long may well make a pain syndrome more uncomfortable by fatiguing the tissues.

A sustained release technique will be held until a sense of release occurs. A thrust technique may be primed several times, but the actual technique will only take as long as is necessary to perform the thrust itself.

Effective technique needs less time to perform but the duration of a particular treatment session itself is not really a function of technique but is another matter completely. Every osteopath seems to have his idea of the duration of treatment necessary to produce the appropriate amount of change in the tissues and the condition. I have known variations between 5 and 60 minutes for a treatment session. My feeling is that there are different needs to every case, but due to the constraints of most practitioners' appointment systems, this is not a very practical statement. Experience should allow most practitioners gradually to reduce the time needed to work on each case in an effective way. There will naturally be an optimum for each practitioner and his set-up of consulting rooms and changing areas, etc. Patients seem to want a long treatment giving good value for money and the maximum involvement, but they do not like a long waiting list! The two are not usually mutually compatible.

AMPLITUDE

The amplitude, or distance travelled by the applicator, is governed by some of the other modifying factors. In a rhythmic technique the amplitude will tend to be fairly long unless it is a springing technique when the oscillation is very short. In a thrust technique the amplitude must be very closely controlled to give the technique as short an amplitude as possible consistent with the successful completion of the procedure. High velocity, short amplitude remains the mainstay of manipulative thrust techniques. As composite levers accumulate at a point the sense of resistance should cause the amplitude to reduce until the forces are focused accurately. This sense of resistance or barrier is critical to manipulative technique.

PLANE

The plane of force in a technique will be governed by the purpose of the technique and the direction of the tissues being worked on. In a cross-fibre kneading technique, the plane will be across the muscle. In a stretching technique, the plane will be along the muscle ligament or fascia concerned. In a thrust technique the plane will either be across the joint to gap it, or along the joint to produce a sliding force. It can be seen, therefore, that an accurate knowledge of the anatomy of the part is essential, as is a good sense of accumulating resistance to applied forces.

Unfortunately, anatomical variations are the rule not the exception, and although certain principal directions are going to be accurate within certain limits, there may be considerable variation from the expected planes in many cases. There are no straight lines anywhere in the body, and all forces should have a slightly curving vector so that they are more likely to reach the correct plane for the technique in question. An analogy might be to attempt to drop a small pebble into a funnel. The ideal would be to drop it straight down the centre. However, it would be more normal to drop it in and see it rattle around until it finds its own way down the centre by running around in ever-decreasing circles until it drops. Technique is often performed by applying forces in a particular direction and then making many small adjustments until the optimum direction can be found. If the force is applied without these minor adjustments, the quantity will often need to be very high. The correct plane has not been accessed and force is being used to overcome the resistance rather than accuracy. This is unwise, uncomfortable and potentially dangerous.

The plane of a given technique may change as the forces are applied and tissues deform in front of the applicator. This is not uncommon, and it is necessary to allow for this possibility and not be too rigid in approach so that the variation can take place guided by the tissues.

FORCE

Force is a variable that again integrates with all the others to make a technique specific, successful and accurate. High force should not be used as a substitute for accuracy. The aim should be to use as little force as possible that will achieve the desired effect. Generally it is better to generate force by good control of levers and components than to apply high levels of force to make up for inefficient technique. The higher the force, the greater the chance of injury and the greater the control necessary.

When higher force techniques are necessary, it is essential to keep the target tissue in mind so that the force is directed accurately and specifically rather than allowing forces to dissipate in the surrounding tissues. A suitable analogy is the difference between a shotgun and a rifle. The power of the shotgun will have a major effect at close range, but at any distance it will dissipate and the effect of the force will be minimal at any given point. The rifle, however, will be ineffective in hitting anything except the object in the direct line of fire, but will be extremely powerful in its effect on that object.

The part of the hand applying the force, the length of the lever, the amplitude and the sharpness of the arrest will all modify the actual force applied. Re-duplication of force will have an interesting effect according to the maintained pressure after the initial force. If a force is applied and removed the natural recoil of the tissues will allow deformation to take place at the target site and in the surrounding tissues or structures. If there is a dysfunction, with fixation and hypertonus, the fixed point may not release as the other tissues are relatively more compliant and can absorb the applied force of a technique. However, if a force is applied, released and then re-applied immediately afterwards and held, the effect will be quite different. The force will go into the tissues, and recoil out but will meet the fixed part of the operator's hand or arm. Having met this resistance the force will not be able to dissipate, and will recoil back into the tissues. If the operator holds this position for a few seconds there will be an induced oscillation of force within the structures that may allow release to take place.

It is difficult to find an analogy for this phenomenon, but imagine a ball bouncing and then your hand placed directly in the trajectory of the ball. If the ball hits your hand before the whole of its energy has been lost, it will speed up its bounce. It will also usually escape to one side as the energy has to find an outlet. Using this in technique is a little different. The patient is positioned in such a way that the only direction the tissues can go is against the hand and the force is, therefore, thrown directly back to the target site. This type of technique is often used by chiropractors in classical 'toggle–recoil' thrusts. The principles can be equally well used by osteopathic practitioners although chiropractors often use specifically designed tables with 'drop' sections to enhance the effect.

Force is also modified partly by the size of the applicator. Assume that the palm of the hand is used to transmit a force, and is, let us say, 4 inches across and 4 inches long. Assume also that the force applied is of 16 pounds pressure. Simple arithmetic will reveal that there will be an applied force of 1 pound per square inch. However, if the area of the applicator is reduced to 2 square inches, by the operator gripping in such a way that only a small part of the hand is performing the effective part of the technique, the force will have increased to 8 pounds per square inch. Despite using the same quantity of overall force, the effect will be some 8 times as powerful, and directed much more specifically to a point or area. Naturally, there will be times when a small area of contact is preferable, and others when a much larger area of contact would be more appropriate. A thrust technique using very high specificity might require great specificity

and a small applicator would be used. Therefore, within the handhold that uses the whole of the palm and fingers to produce contact, there might be an area of the hand, such as the pisiform, that performs the cardinal part of the technique. If a larger area of contact is required, such as in a kneading technique applied to a muscle group, the whole hand would be applied, and less emphasis placed on focusing to a small part of the hand. Even in this case, there might be the need to focus with the heel of the hand at the culmination of the technique so that the part of the muscle needing the pressure could be worked more efficiently.

ONSET

The onset, or point at which the effective part of the technique is to be applied, is naturally a subdivision of many of the other modifying factors. If the onset of the effective part of the technique is made too early, the force will be dissipated before the technique has had a chance to reach the target tissue. This effect can be used purposely to minimize the stress on the tissues, but if it used without realizing that is happening, naturally the benefit of the technique will be reduced. If the onset of the technique is delayed until towards the end of a movement stroke, the power will inevitably increase as there will be much less room for the tissues to deform ahead of the hand. Most categories of technique can have their effect enhanced or reduced by small variations of the onset of the effective part of the procedure. The difficult thing is sensing at what point to start the critical part of the technique.

Consider for a moment a classical lumbar roll thrust procedure. A thrust early on in an oscillating movement of the patient will have a far weaker effect than one performed at the end of a rotatory oscillation. A large patient might need the thrust applied much later in the technique than a small and frail one. However, excessive attempts to control this variable can lead to lack of confidence, and there can be a tendency to become fixed and unable to move at all. The variation of onset is happening whether on a conscious level or not; it is merely necessary to become aware of it so that it can be varied slightly when necessary.

ARREST

The point at which a technique finishes can be referred to as the arrest. This can be graduated, as in a soft tissue technique, or sharp, as in a thrust technique. There can be a sudden release of tension, a slow release of the accumulated tension, or a re-duplication of force as previously described. Each one will have a varied effect and must be considered with all other variables. The method of arrest and release from tension also needs to be considered. If the arrest is slow and then the applicator is rapidly removed from the contact point, there will be a different effect from that produced if the applicator is removed slowly. Even if this effect is psychological, it is still relevant to consider it. If a technique is arrested just short of the release of tension, and then re-applied, there will be another difference in the rate and quantity of the distortion of the tissues that will inevitably affect fluid interchange.

Although these may seem minor factors, they can make the difference between a successful technique, and one that is only partly successful. The rate of change in a target tissue is of importance in dosage of treatment and will influence the overall result. Many operators hardly pause to consider how they finish a given technique. However, even a little thought given to this variable may allow a smoother integration of one technique into another. The choreography of treatment will be that much smoother and a situation where the patient can relax will be much easier to produce. Naturally, the result is the objective,

but the vehicle to reach this result is only slightly less important.

COMPRESSION

The term compression needs some explanation. Compression is not the opposite of traction. Indeed, it can be combined with traction within the same technique. Compression can be applied in several different directions, either separately or in combination. The direction most often used is a compression into a 'close-packed' position. The act of applying compression has several interesting effects. If compression is considered simply as another vector of leverage and force it can be brought into perspective. In the same way that adding components to a composite lever will reduce the quantity of each component, compression can act to reduce lever amplitude. If you apply any technique in the usual way and then add a compression between your hands, the patient's tissues, and yours, will meet a point of resistance. This resistance, or barrier, will be that much earlier than if the compression was not used. Let us consider some examples.

Apply a cross-fibre kneading technique to the lumbar erector spinae with a patient prone as you normally would. Try adding a compression force into the table, and a compression of your chest and arm muscles by a small isometric contraction before the stroke lateral from the spine. You should find that the stroke is of a smaller amplitude as you have absorbed some of the slack with this 'pre-loading' of the tissues. This will have several effects. Firstly, the amplitude will be less; secondly, the force can be reduced according to how much compression is applied; thirdly, the sense of release in the tissues should be easier to feel. The cues should become much crisper. As another example, consider a lumbar roll type of thrust manipulation. Position the patient in the normal way and then, instead of increasing the rotation at the moment of thrust, introduce a compression force toward the table and toward yourself. The patient is, therefore, sandwiched firmly between your pelvis and the table. If you now apply the rotary force, you should find that the range or amplitude of the movement has been substantially reduced. Take this further, and start the technique with even less rotation and it should still be possible to attain a satisfactory lever position to focus to the target joint without the common discomfort induced around the patient's ribs and shoulder.

It can be seen that compression works, but what is the mechanism? There is no definitive answer to this question, but there are several possible explanations. The effect of compression may be due to squeezing the fluid within fascial tubes: the fluid is naturally non-compressible and will, therefore, become relatively solid. There will, therefore, be a reduction of range of movement as the relative mass of the part increases. This possibility relates to the hydraulic effects of fluid pressures and tensions. The effect may be due to the compression acting as a stabilizing of the part. This may be due to an increase of muscle tension that is produced in a similar way to the effect of strapping an unstable joint. It has been shown that strapping a joint acts by increasing the resting tone of the area, and by 'switching on' the proprioceptors that have ceased to function at their optimum. There may be effects due to the elimination of fascial slide that, therefore, focuses the forces to the articular structures in a more efficient way. There may be effects due to the squeezing having a psychological action by the patient becoming aware of operator control and, therefore, having a greater ability to relax and cooperate. There are several other possible explanations that make sense. Not having a logical one, I am, nevertheless, happy to recommend the continuation of the method, as it is so effective, comfortable and useful.

Some authorities insist that all manipulative techniques be applied in traction to increase safety. I would go so far as to say that compression is far more useful as it allows a substantial reduction of force and amplitude. I feel that the traction rule has many potential pitfalls. By separating joint surfaces and putting surrounding ligaments on tension, there is definitely a safety component introduced, but amplitude generally needs to be greater, and the discomfort of this negates the benefits. Any attempt to 'protect' discs and other structures using this method is laudable, but prone to a possible false sense of security. To some extent this rule developed out of the belief that all joint dysfunction syndromes were due to small disc fragments, and that traction helped to replace these. MRI and more sophisticated diagnostic methods have found this belief wanting, and the use of traction in manipulative procedures for this reason has been slowly superseded. There is no doubt that traction has its uses, but it is not a panacea.

PRIMARY AND SECONDARY LEVERS

The primary lever can be identified as the principal or executive vector of force within a particular technique. The secondary levers, or components of the composite lever, are stabilizing and enhancing vectors that allow the greatest efficiency in the primary lever direction. The primary lever in a thrust technique is usually in a sliding or a gapping direction in relation to the joint surfaces in question. Sliding forces generally need less force than gapping, and are preferable when possible. Although the inclinations of facet planes conform broadly to certain pre-defined directions, there will often be some variation. The direction of a primary lever is determined partly by a knowledge of the anatomy, but ultimately by palpatory awareness. The greater the number of secondary levers, the less is the required contribution of each one, and the nearer to the midline the part can be while the technique is performed. Clearly the nearer to the midline, the less the distortion and stress on the tissues, and the greater the comfort. With greater comfort, the patient is better able to relax, and there is less likelihood of trauma in treatment and adverse reaction afterwards.

To illustrate primary and secondary levers I will again use some examples. Flex your wrist until it can go no further without discomfort. Become aware of the quality of resistance from the tissues to this minor stress. Use the other hand to push the hand further into flexion, and become aware of the immediate increase of normal resistance and strain. Return the wrist to the resting position, and put it into a degree of ulnar deviation. While maintaining this ulnar deviation, add flexion until resistance is felt. It will be noticed that the point of resistance in flexion is at a lesser point than before, and that the quality of the resistance is different in feel from that induced before. Now try gripping around the wrist and hand with the other hand and repeating the exercise. This adds a compression vector to the overall leverage. The feel of the composite lever will be quite different on a subjective level in the wrist being levered, as well as in the hand doing the levering. This simple example illustrates the use of a composite lever with a primary force of flexion, and secondary levers of ulnar deviation and compression. The quality of the resistance felt will not only be different, but will be less uncomfortable than a simple flexion. Additionally, if you were to use it as an articulation movement repeated several times, even though the joints are not being taken to their normal articular limit, there would be an increase of range produced. This effect can be used freely in treatment and makes technique very much less uncomfortable. With practice, specificity improves also, as the variables allow the desired structure or tissue to be targeted accurately.

Another example might be a classical thrust technique in the cervical spine. The primary lever is usually rotation in an attempt to slide one facet on the affected side forward on the one below. The normal method of locking is to induce some sidebending to the affected side and to rotate to the other side. This so-called physiological locking obeys Fryette's laws and adds specificity to the technique. Using the principles just outlined you could add several other secondary levers to minimize the amplitude of the rotation. The ones most commonly used in this case would be sideshifting, compression and anterior shifting. The total of all the vectors would reach a 100% locking position, allowing the facet to be freed in the desired direction. However, the quantity of each could be reduced as the number is increased. All thrust technique requires a little free play so that the optimum plane can be found. The accumulating barrier will be felt at an earlier point than without the secondary levers, and the potential for a successful technique will be enhanced. To an outside observer, the manipulative position would not seem effective as the neck is not torsioned as in the common method of only two or three vectors. The operator would also need to be in much more control than normal as the tissues would tend to escape from the induced tension. Body tissues are like a spring, and if allowed freedom to take their own path, will usually take the easiest direction. This easy path is one that allows the minimum distortion and the maximum ability to dissipate force over a large area. If the technique is applied without the optimum tension it is unlikely to succeed, but it is also extremely unlikely to cause pain or distress.

In every technique there will be an executive or primary lever, and there will be secondary or stabilizing levers or components of the composite lever. Some complex techniques may even have what might be termed tertiary levers that come into play only rarely if suitable barrier sense cannot be achieved. Even though I have avoided terminology relating to lesion positioning, the decision about a primary lever can be taken on this basis if desired. The system of identification of lever vectors is usable in both approaches.

Even an operator who has no knowledge of this positional thinking will inevitably be using it, as the optimum position for any technique is made up of several different forces. Once the consideration of primary and secondary levers has been identified, it should be possible to return to a technique that is not working and identify what is missing. Like all the other modifying factors, lever identification must be integrated with all other aspects to make it fully useful.

RESPIRATION

The active use of respiration in technique is not new, but the identification of the different phases of breathing that can be integrated in technique to personalize each procedure to the patient may be. Naturally, it is not necessary to perform every technique at a specific phase of respiration. It would be far too easy to confuse and upset the patient with constant instructions about when to breathe! Nevertheless, there are times when the active use of breathing can be useful. Many practitioners ask their patient to take a deep breath and then to breathe out just before a thrust technique is to be performed. This is designed to produce the optimum state of relaxation in the tissues and the patient. This is sometimes useful, but if this is the only use of breathing, many other possibilities are being ignored. Exhalation certainly can produce relaxation, but in very flexible subjects this in itself can be a problem. Patients who are generally hypermobile and have a fixed area needing techniques applied, might be better addressed when they are inhaling, to produce a sense of focusing in the tissues by firming them up. During inhalation the normal physiological curves of the spine are slightly flattened, and this fact can be used in technique.

During exhalation there will be more recoil and give in the tissues and this may prove to be a disadvantage. This is particularly true in flexible subjects whose tissues may be able to dissipate the force before it reaches the target site. However, even in a flexible subject, at the end of exhalation the tissues are at the point of minimum ability to release further, so technique performed at that point can be extremely specific. If technique is performed on largely inflexible subjects who happen to be at the end of an exhalation phase, there will be much more possibility of trauma and discomfort. This will particularly be the case when working on the thoracic spine and rib cage.

RESISTANCE

The resistance to a manipulative procedure should come from the target tissue or structure. There should not be more than the minimum resistance from other structures surrounding it. Indeed, the zone of effective resistance to the force should be as small as possible to ensure that the forces reach the desired structure in the most efficient way. If progressively accumulating forces are applied in a general, coarse way, there is the distinct possibility of straining surrounding structures. The other possibility is of the force being dissipated in the other structures and not having the desired effect on the part in question. Adhesions around a dysfunctional segment will often be stronger than the surrounding normal tissues, and forces applied will distort the normal tissues and not affect the dysfunction unless the forces are accurately localized. Imagine two pieces of wood joined by a strong glue joint. Attempts to separate them with force might just as likely break the wood as the glue joint. If, however, the glue joint itself were to be struck with a hammer, there is a good chance that it would separate without as much damage to the rest of the wood, the maximum resistance to the force having been formed exactly at the joint itself.

It is difficult to acquire the skill necessary to be able to sense the optimum state of resistance in a joint or other structure while maintaining the other structures in a state of minimum tension. It is not difficult to sense an increasing barrier by being aware of excess tissue distortion and strain. This is very different from an accurately applied force using controlled forces to a target segment within a zone of minimum induced tension. Generally the closer the applicator can be applied to the structure being worked on, the better. The optimum resistance depends on the best accumulation of forces controlled by using several of the modifying factors in combination. The best sense of resistance is very dependent on the next modifying factor described, contact point pressure.

CONTACT POINT PRESSURE

The amount of pressure with the applicator, and the method of application of that pressure, are other critical variables. It is almost impossible to produce the best resistance in a joint or structure unless enough pressure has been used to remove the slack from the overlying structures. This pressure must be very carefully applied if it is not to become painful, and the part of the hand or other structure used must be considered carefully. The method of application as well as the total quantity is also important, and depending on the type of the technique, the pressure rarely remains static, but increases and decreases as the technique progresses. All techniques have a beginning and an end, and the point of onset and arrest has already been discussed, but variations in pressure will influence the other factors to a large extent as well. As an analogy, visualize attempting to break a piece of wood laid across two bricks. If the force were to be applied from a distance, considerable impact might be necessary. If, however, you were to stand on the wood and simply bounce up and down, there would be a good chance that it would break under the strain.

The total force would be similar, but the initial pressure of standing on it would bring the structure nearer to a breaking point without so much impact. Naturally, the use of contact point pressure can be excessive as well as insufficient, but like most of the other modifying factors, can be decreased as well as increased as necessary.

HUNCH

Some will say that the use of hunch or sixth sense should have no place in a scientific activity like osteopathic technique or treatment. All activities that require skill or knowledge, and rely on variable factors, are liable to so many variations that sixth sense is inevitably used. Rather than denying this, it seems to make more sense to use it constructively. This does not mean that one should rely purely on feelings and not use reasoning and logic. It is normal for this sixth sense to develop, and one can use it constructively providing it is backed up by some reasoning. When an experienced practitioner is asked why he is doing something in a particular way, the answer is often, 'because it feels like it needs it'. If we analyse this statement it is possible to see that there is a combination of learning, forgotten experiences, conscious comparisons and previous mistakes and successes. Experience can be defined as the ability to recognize common patterns. The recognition is one thing; being able to act in an appropriate way is another. Hunch is really all of these. It is necessary to guard against the trap of the 'always, never' syndrome, where the two words are used as an excuse for not thinking something through thoroughly. If a practitioner finds himself saying, 'I always . . .', he may not be flexible enough to allow the essential variations that allow the technique and the treatment to vary subtly to suit the particular case. The same is true of 'I never . . .' Providing this is used for contraindications, I have no argument with it; if it is used in other situations too often, it shows a rigidity of mind that cannot fit with good manipulative skill that is tailored to the individual patient.

It can be seen, therefore, that the modifying factors are being used whether an operator is aware of them or not. By bringing them to a level of analysis and conscious thought, it should be possible to use them constructively to tailor a given technique to the particular patient.

The term handling refers to more than just the placement of the operator's hands on the surface of the patient's body. The term should encompass all aspects of tissue sympathy from the initial contact right through to the very last touch of any treatment or technique.

The initial touch in any given technique should be smooth, gentle yet firm and impart confidence to the patient. Consideration must be given to the 'choreography' of the treatment session so that one move can be smoothly integrated with the next, in an apparently seamless way. An aspect often not sufficiently considered is the initial application of the hand. If the whole hand is applied in one action this may be uncomfortable and threatening to the patient. It is often better to apply first the fingertips, then the palm and lastly the heel of the hand. Depending on the part being worked, it may be more appropriate to use the ulnar part of the hand subsequently spreading to the palm, heel and then fingers last of all. The time for this gradual introduction of touch will vary with different operators but the thoughtful operator will use comments from a fellow student or practitioner to judge the optimum in a variety of situations. An average for most operators is about 3 seconds from initial touch to full contact. This may seem rather a long time but feedback will reveal that it is about right.

The amount of pressure in any situation will also vary. Within reason, the firmer the contact, the more confidence the patient will have and, therefore, the better they will be able to relax. However, the chief guiding factor in this contact point pressure is how much of the hand is in use. Again, a rule is to apply as much of the hand as possible within the par-

ticular technique. Subsequently the operator makes one specific part of the hand the executive applicator of force to be applied for that technique within the overall hand contact. This type of consideration seems to be needlessly detailed and complex. However, close attention to this aspect can improve patient compliance, relaxation and ultimately success in any given technique or treatment.

Handling not only refers to the use of the hands but must include all other parts of the operator's body, particularly those coming into contact with the patient. For example, where the patient's head is cradled in the hands of the operator, it is important to ensure that the patient's ears and eyes are not being obstructed by part of the operator's clothing or arms. When patients are sitting, most of the movement of their body is often performed by pressure from the operator's body rather than the hands. In this way the communication of the required position or movement is transmitted efficiently without excessive pressure on a possible painful site.

A simple rule relating to efficiency in handling is for the operator to examine carefully the position of his elbows. In most techniques, at the culmination of the procedure the elbows should be as close to his body as is practicable. To check on this element it is a good idea to assume a variety of technique positions and then see if it is possible to modify the hand and elbow positions for greater comfort and effectiveness. Comments from a cooperative fellow student will prove valuable in this respect.

Clearly it is important to avoid discomfort produced by the pulling of hair, excessive skin drag and digging in of wristwatches, rings or long fingernails. Operator's long hair should be suitably tied back, and front-fastening clinic coats avoided. It should not be necessary to mention that breath smelling of alcohol, garlic or cigarettes, and fingers stained and smelling of nicotine are unprofessional and, therefore, not acceptable.

In many techniques it may be necessary for the operator's body to be in close proximity to the patient. If this is likely to cause potential embarrassment due to the part of the body being used, then a suitably interposed pillow or rolled towel may come in useful. Female operators will, no doubt, be especially aware of the need to avoid embarrassing breast contact with the patient and may choose other techniques when necessary to overcome this problem. Patients may feel extremely vulnerable if they are aware of contact with the operator's genital area. This must be avoided.

Belts with large buckles can dig into the patient as can other items of jewellery such as necklaces and name badges and it is as well to remember this in clinical practice.

The power of touch should not be underestimated, and in emotionally unstable patients can produce strong reactions and responses. In such cases it is essential to be sympathetic and yet firm and reassuring in such a way as to show care without excessive involvement. It is very easy for the caring practitioner to fall into the trap of palliative stroking that may give this type of patient a false impression. However, neither is it acceptable to be heavy-handed in an attempt to avoid seeming excessively sympathetic.

From the point of view of patient satisfaction, some practitioners will be able to build and maintain a practice far faster than others. Some of this may be due to subliminal awareness by the patient of superior handling by one practitioner over another. Although each practitioner will develop their style of approach, some adjustments can be made; there is no better way of discovering useful modifications than giving treatment to a colleague who is empowered to make constructive criticism of the handling used. It could be very intimidating to have one's work scrutinized in this way, but if the purpose is for self-improvement it is very worthwhile. Even the finest sports personalities in the world have their coaches whose job it is to make such minor adjustments in method to improve performance. We are naturally interested in the result, but the comfort, efficiency and effectiveness of the methods are open to substantial variation and without constructive comment we are unlikely to know how to adjust them.

Care should also be taken in the use of equipment. If a hydraulic table is used, find the best way of elevating and lowering it to avoid excessive jarring. Avoid banging into the table when walking from one side to the other and move pillows with due consideration for patient comfort to avoid the head being jerked to one side.

The term handling also relates to all aspects of patient care including the operator–patient relationship. It is not suggested that excessive formality is necessary, but that a truly professional relationship will help the patient to develop trust. Patient education about the nature and purpose of different aspects of treatment is a useful part of practitionership. It is not practical to give exact descriptions of each manoeuvre. However, involving the patient in the treatment process by way of information and discussion is clearly a way of helping them to understand what is happening, and is likely to avoid misunderstandings.

Factors relevant to operator **posture** are: weight in relation to gravity; the contact with the floor or table; the position of his head; and all other aspects of weight distribution consistent with the ability to transmit forces in the best way for each technique. The term **stance** relates more to the position of the operator in relation to the table, and the proximity to the patient. Although the two are to some extent interdependent, there are differences. For example, an operator can be in a good posture from the point of view of balance and ability to control the amount of weight he is to carry, but be in a totally inappropriate placing for the technique to work well. He might have his feet pointing in such a direction that when he applies the culmination of the technique, the force dissipates away from the intended path. He is then not in sufficient contact to control the target area as his foot position prevents him directing the force in the desired direction.

If one operator tries to copy the posture of another exactly, purely by imitation, he is unlikely to make every procedure a success. The morphology of each practitioner is inevitably different. It is clearly essential to learn to control the operator's body with the forces he is to apply. This will lead to good control of the aspects of the forces needed in treatment of the patient for maximum benefit and minimum effort in technique.

The patient–operator interface, that constitutes the use of the operator's weight, balance, and grip or hold, must be efficient if it is to be effective. There are many elements of this particular modifying factor in technique that can be adjusted by some simple but subtle changes. Once the ideas and the reasons for them have been considered, it takes a little practice to make each one a natural flowing part of the technique. This effort will be amply rewarded in less long-term effort, strain, and possible physical problems for the operator, as well as increasing the effectiveness of each technique for the patient.

All techniques employ forces applied to the body of the patient. These forces can be extremely delicate and light, or can progress to quite high forces when necessary for a specific objective. Clearly the lighter the force applied, the less the potential trauma to the tissues being worked, but if heavier forces are necessary, they must be very carefully controlled to avoid excessive discomfort. After all, the main purpose of manipulative treatment is an attempt to relieve pain, not cause more!

If we analyse operator posture from the feet up there are many simple things that can alter the way techniques are applied. If the feet are placed parallel, any forces applied to the patient will require the operator to push with an equal and opposite force to avoid the tendency of his body to be pushed away from the plinth. If the feet are in an inefficient position it may be necessary to stand further from the plinth, and then be in a poorer balance position. This will require an increase of muscle tension in his body that immediately takes away some of the control of the technique. The simple expedient of having one foot slightly ahead of the other means that it is easier to generate forces that have more control and balance than if the feet are parallel.

To make one foot the front foot and the

other the rear does not necessarily require the operator to step back with one or forward with the other. All that is necessary is to swivel slightly on the balls of the feet so that the feet are pointing either to one of the top or bottom corners of the table depending on the direction necessary for the technique. In very few techniques will the feet be pointing straight across the table.

If the reader will look carefully at some of the pictures later in this book he will find that in most cases there is a front foot and a rear foot. Further study will reveal that in most cases, if a rhythmic technique is being used, the weight is being used to transfer the force to the patient through the hand on the same side as the front foot. However, if the technique is a thrust technique, then the weight is being transferred to the patient through the hand on the same side as the rear foot. This is not an absolute rule, but it applies with very few exceptions. Further study will reveal that the operator is sometimes not in contact with the table at all. At other times he has shortened the lever by leaning with some part or parts of his lower extremities against the table edge. Shortening the lever by leaning on the edge of the table is far more common in rhythmic techniques than in thrust techniques.

In most thrust techniques it is easier to accelerate rapidly and then form the sharp braking action necessary to produce the short amplitude movement if the heel of the rear foot is elevated slightly off the floor just before the thrust is applied. The subsequent contact of the heel with the floor forms a trigger for the completion of the thrust when the operator drops onto it. In most techniques the feet should be tending to point in approximately the same direction. If they are substantially different in direction there is the tendency to lock the operator's posture as the technique progresses and only to be able to move in a downwards direction.

Most techniques are easier to perform with some flow if the operator's knees are slightly bent. If one knee is kept straight, movement of the operator must pivot around that straight knee, and this will artificially limit the ability to perform the technique. Slightly bent knees also permit movement in the antero-posterior plane and up and down movement as well, thus allowing a far greater flexibility of approach. Sometimes, however, it will be found that one knee straightens at the end of a given technique. This gives the ability to firm up the technique at the last moment, and can often be a useful inclusion.

In a similar way most techniques are performed better if at least one of the operator's hips is somewhat flexed. Any technique that requires the hips to be extended will inevitably be extending the operator's back. Although there may be times when this is necessary, excessive extension repeated too often can be just as much of a problem as excessively repeated flexion. The use of a front and a rear leg allows one hip to be flexed while the other may be extended. This inevitably puts the operator's spine in a twisted posture which, when excessive, can be problematical. Nevertheless, some twist means that the technique can be performed with the operator in a firmer position to allow better transmission of forces.

The operator's own lower back is best held in as near neutral position as possible, and if it is necessary to bend over the patient, then the flexion usually comes from the hips while keeping the lower back straight. To avoid strain the small amount of twist already mentioned must not be allowed to become an excessive torsional movement to end-of-range. Single techniques such as thrust techniques should be less of a strain to perform than rhythmic techniques that may need to go on for some time, but the possibility for overstrain of the operator is always present. A single application technique performed many times in a week can become a repetitive strain if inefficient methods become a habit. If the lumbar spine is held in a neutral lordosis directly over the centre of gravity between the feet, then the position is likely to be the most efficient in the majority of cases.

The operator's middle back is best held in a neutral position without excessive strain into either flexion or extension. Some degree of torsion is possible as the muscles are capable of controlling articular stress, and this has the effect of firming up the technique. It should be noted that with the mid back the operator's own ribs play an important part in many techniques. If the operator is in firm contact with the patient's body, a slight twist in his back will bring the side of the operator's rib cage in contact more than the springy part of the sternum. This also allows the operator's arms greater freedom to move as the one foot forward posture can tend to separate them slightly from his body.

The operator's upper thoracic area is placed under considerable risk of mechanical stress as the arms are being used all the time. The mechanical leverage of arms is transmitted to the rest of the body through the shoulders and upper thoracic area. For this reason, it is clearly important to always keep the shoulders and upper thoracic area as relaxed as possible. A good rule is that if the operator can see his shoulders from the position he is in to perform the technique, they are probably too high for maximum efficiency. A small amount of isometric tension in the operator's latissimus dorsi muscles will ensure that the shoulders are pulled down far enough so that he has a better chance of increasing the compactness of his body. This will allow transmission of the force to the patient in the most efficient way. Isometric tension and breath-holding must be used with caution to avoid locking the operator's rib cage excessively.

It is perfectly understandable to want to see what one is doing in technique, but the head is a heavy object. If the operator allows his head to incline forward excessively, increased strain is being caused to the upper thoracic area. The weight of the head is being placed in front of the centre of gravity line and greater muscular effort is required to

maintain the position. This does not mean that the operator must look up at the ceiling, but that he must be aware of the need to keep his head as high as is reasonably practicable. Simply keeping the neck long is often enough. This simple aspect is enough to control almost the whole of the spinal posture of the operator.

The operator's elbows are an important part of many techniques. Most procedures are performed better, and with a greater degree of accuracy, if the operator pulls his elbows as close to his sides as is feasible. This need not be taken to extremes, but if any technique is not working as intended, a simple adjustment of posture of elbows is often all that is needed to 'fine tune' it to a better efficiency. Elbow position is a simple thing to consider in this regard. Even in techniques where it is impossible to bring the elbows close to the sides, a small isometric pull downwards and inwards of the operator's arms will have a beneficial effect of firming up the hold, and increasing the proprioceptive awareness of the operator. The slack of the operator's own joint play is also reduced if this small 'setting' of the arms is undertaken.

The hands of the operator will be applied to the patient but overstrain can be avoided by minimizing flexion or extension of the wrist. When techniques require the use of the thumb for pressure, this is best applied in as little abduction as possible. Some isometric setting of the hand will allow the 'switching on' of the joint proprioceptors in the hands and arms which will enhance the palpatory awareness of the operator considerably. This also has the effect of slightly protecting the hands from overstrain by giving a sense of graduated resistance to all forces being applied. It is sometimes easy to fall into a habit of ulnar deviation and allowing the ligaments on the radial side to be repeatedly stressed. Although this may not produce a true hypermobility, there is some indication that it may produce discomfort if frequently repeated.

Female operators may have problems, in

some techniques, with the proximity of their breasts to the patient. If the operator is required to place their chest against the patient, which may be a source of embarrassment or difficulty, then a pillow or suitable pad can be interposed. Similarly operators of both sexes will want to avoid excessive proximity of their groin area to the patient. The trust built up between practitioner and patient can easily be destroyed if these simple common sense aspects are not considered. It is easy to forget that most patients are going to be somewhat apprehensive or nervous about treatment. They may already feel vulnerable by being partly clothed, and a thoughtless operator who does not realize the implication of his proximity to the patient is at risk of problems in this regard. Tension sense, or barrier sense, is acquired not only through the hands of the operator. In many cases the friction with the patient through the operator's own chest transmits as much feel for the best time to apply a thrust as does the feeling through the hands. One is looking for interpretation of the subtle difference between tissue stress, and tissue potential for activation of force when a technique is applied. The subtle cues that come from a joint placed in a position of 'potential' are felt through the accumulation of forces sensed by the whole body of the operator.

The phase within the breathing cycle of the operator when techniques are to be performed is sometimes of importance. Some operators tend to hold their breath and strain against the fixed abdomen and thorax by this temporary Valsava manoeuvre. This has the effect of firming up the technique, but also has the undesirable effect of raising the operator's blood pressure. This is clearly best avoided. There are times when this explosive force of breath-holding is useful, but it should not be used too frequently. Some operators tend to breathe out when performing thrust techniques to help speed up the move. Although this can be useful, and avoids the tendency to hold the breath, it is better not to perform the technique at the extreme of exhalation as the operator's rib articulations are in a vulnerable position to strain.

Breathing also changes posture; on inhalation the spine lengthens and straightens slightly, and the reverse happens on exhalation. It is easier to transmit a sense of relaxation to the patient if the operator is relaxing himself. A controlled outward breath will often help to produce an optimum sense of tissue relaxation in the patient. If the operator asks the patient to breathe out at the same time, this shows how another modifying factor of patient respiration can be combined with operator posture and breathing to good effect.

The ideal test of whether a posture is balanced for any given technique is to attempt to perform the manoeuvre without a patient. This may seem very artificial, but it demonstrates balance, control of the operator's body, and the ability to perform the technique without excessively leaning on the patient. Also, the understanding of how much tension the operator needs to put into his hands is often poorly considered. If the hand is merely applied to the surface of the body and pressure is increased until mild discomfort is felt by the patient, there will be a completely different sensation than if the operator puts his own hand and arm into a slight degree of isometric tension and then repeats the same exercise. This type of dynamic tension in the operator must be practised to acquire the correct level for each technique. Some techniques require quite firm isometric tension in the operator, others very light. An example relating to other activities that may make this more easily understood, is to imagine threading a needle. Excessive tension in the hands would make this a very difficult exercise, but insufficient tension would make it equally difficult, but in a different way. Another example would be pushing a drawing pin into a resistant surface. This would clearly require a different type of tension and control to the threading of a needle with cotton.

The ability to take the grip in a firm but comfortable way, promoting confidence in the patient, and yet not causing unnecessary discomfort, is not easy to acquire, but with a helpful fellow student can be suitably developed. If any posture is causing excessive fatigue for any reason the cause must be found. Performing a technique once in isolation is not how treatment is carried out in practice. Treating many patients in a day requires the operator to master the business of minimizing strain on his structure if he is to be able to carry on the work without injury and excessive fatigue.

In any activity requiring psychomotor skill, the expert makes things look very easy. This is true in sporting or other activity such as manipulative technique. The reason that it looks so easy is that the practitioner has learned to avoid the things that make it look difficult! Most of these aspects are related to the way forces are transmitted or developed. Good control of posture and, therefore, the practitioner himself is one of the key ways that this can be done in osteopathic technique.

There is a blurred dividing line between what is technique and what is treatment, and the term **applied technique** relates to fitting the chosen technique to the patient and the situation that has presented. There are several factors that need to be considered in addition to the modifying factors already identified. Some of the previously mentioned modifying factors also need amplifying:

1. Handling
2. Positioning
3. Posture
4. Weight-taking
5. Operator relaxation
6. Holds
7. Apparatus
8. Approach
9. Planning
10. Difficult situations
11. Response to reactions
12. Category of technique
13. Interval between treatments
14. Advice and aftercare

HANDLING

In addition to the factors identified in the section devoted to handling, is the need to consider the transition of hold from one technique to another. It is not sufficient to have good handling in a technique if the transition phase involves a rough and irritating approach. Patients in acute pain, in particular, need sympathetic handling, precision and care to avoid further unnecessary pain. Patients who are nervous or embarrassed need extra care, and judicious use of gowns or other suitable covering should be considered.

POSITIONING

Positioning or moving the patient on the table must be performed slowly and purposefully, particularly if they are in acute pain. It may be necessary to perform a whole treatment with the patient in one position, and this can try the ingenuity of even the most inventive practitioner. If it is necessary to move the patient, it is often better to guide the movement, after describing what is required, rather than try to do all the work yourself. Acute pain is best controlled by the patient initiating the motion rather than the therapist. Once they have started to move, then operator assistance is useful. In this way they do not feel so threatened by being moved into a painful position and can be much more in control of their pain. Most techniques can be performed in a variety of positions. It makes sense to find the most comfortable for patient and operator providing this does not require the acute patient to move excessively. It is possible to reduce operator fatigue by alternating, say, sidelying with prone lying in subsequent patients. In this way you can use your pushing muscles in one patient, and your pulling muscles in the next. Alternating in this way can be a useful method of being inventive and adding variety to the day. It will often allow the discovery of different and useful ways of performing a particular treatment in different types of case.

POSTURE

I have already commented extensively on posture but will reiterate here the critical factors of safety for patient and operator, and effectiveness in technique by the use of efficient posture. Many operators have suffered injury from strains in treating patients. Much of this could have been avoided by more care over posture. Good posture allows the operator to reduce strain on his own structure, and to reduce the possibility of excessive force being applied unwittingly to the patient.

Small and light operators of both sexes become extremely efficient at utilizing leverage rather than weight when performing technique. When learning technique it is a good idea to have some instruction from a small operator to help to acquire this skill. Virtually every operator will meet a patient one day who is much larger than normal. It is only then that the problems that the small operators have daily, become evident. Strength is really no substitute for skill.

WEIGHT-TAKING

It is clearly wise to reduce to the absolute minimum any techniques that involve taking the patient's weight. On some occasions there is no other way, but if the table can be made to do some of the work, physical stress can be minimized. Avoid breath-holding if it is necessary to lift a patient. Learn from the weight-lifters who exhale when lifting. Obey the advice you give the patients about keeping a straight back when lifting!

OPERATOR RELAXATION

It is important to be aware of the necessity to relax when performing osteopathic technique and treatment. A state of tension not only transmits itself to the patient and their tissues, but reduces the appreciation of palpation, leverage, pressure, stretch and other sensory perception. Fatigue is also increased if the operator is tense during treatment. This is not an excuse for sloppy technique, but rather a reason for smooth and controlled movement that can become almost balletic and apparently choreographed if practised efficiently.

HOLDS

The hand placement or hold for a given technique can be varied in several different ways. The thoughtful operator should not grip excessively with the fingertips. It may be difficult to avoid excessive tension in the grip when performing a new hold for the first few times. The balance between a firm and positive hold, and one that is painful, uncomfortable or irritating, is very delicate. It is a good idea to constantly re-evaluate the approach to any particular technique; the method that has become most comfortable by frequent usage may not be the most effective for the purpose intended. Most operators restrict themselves to a relatively limited range of techniques, and can have great difficulty when called upon to perform them in a different way. This is avoided if variety is added as a regular feature.

APPARATUS

It is useful to experiment with different types of apparatus such as stools, pillows, pads and plinth types, etc. A height-adjustable plinth is extremely useful to allow the patient to be at the optimum height so that different areas can be worked without excessive bending or stretching. In a multi-practitioner setting an adjustable plinth or table is essential. A rising head-piece is useful, but failing this pillows of various sizes can be a substitute. Any plinth that is height-adjustable should have the minimum free play in the adjustment mechanism to allow forces to be transmitted to the patient and not the hydraulics of the table. If the table is too springy the force used in technique will need to be harder and sharper to overcome the bounce of the mechanism. If the only table available is a fixed height one, it is better to be too low than too high. It is far easier to lose height by spreading the legs than to stand on tiptoe and be off-balance. However, a table that is too low will be very tiring to work on. Pillows of different sizes and density are necessary, partly to prop the patient up when lying in different positions, and partly to act as fulcra for some techniques.

There are advantages and disadvantages in different widths of table. Patients generally feel more comfortable on a wider table, but as they automatically tend to lie in the middle of the table, they may be so far away that many techniques can place a strain on the operator. Table width can be 18–28 inches (46–71 centimetres). The narrow table will tend to be unstable, and will produce unease in elderly patients who may be fearful of falling. The widest will be preferred by patients but, in addition to the problem stated above, it will be impossible to place the patient astride for sitting techniques. If the patient is sitting across the table with the backs of the knees resting on the edge, they will still be a long way from the operator. Sitting techniques will require the operator to reach a long way to apply any hold, and that can place his own back at risk. All tables are a compromise. One way to get around this problem is to have a table that tapers from about a third of the way from the head end to a narrow foot end. This means that astride techniques are possible at the foot end, and that sitting across techniques can be performed toward the foot end. When the patient is lying down they will have the impression that the table is wide, as the part they can see is wider than the rest.

The padding should be dense enough to prevent the combined weight of the patient and the pressure of the technique from 'bottoming out' the foam. This is of particular importance in prone techniques where the costo-chondral junctions are at risk of damage if the table padding is too firm. If the padding is too soft, it will be difficult to absorb enough of the spring when treating, and some of the effort of technique will be lost in the padding

rather than being targeted to the desired tissue. However firm or soft the table padding, most patients prefer having a pillow under the abdomen when lying prone. This avoids excessive pressure on ribs, breasts and genitals. It also allows the lumbar spine to be taken out of excess lordosis. Excessive lordosis can produce pain if pressure is applied to the lumbar area. The padding of the plinth should extend over the sides so that the patient does not have discomfort on the inside of the arms when lying prone with the arms over the edges. Many techniques require the operator to lean against the side of the table. If it is padded this will be more comfortable.

For hygiene, the plinth is now generally covered with a plastic material, whereas cloth was often used in the past. Cloth will harbour skin debris and dust and is not really suitable, although it does have the advantage that towels or paper covers do not slide on it as they do on plastic and vinyl. If the patient is asked to lie directly on the plastic it will be sticky and unpleasant, so some covering is usually placed over it. Towelling is ideal, but will tend to slide. Fitted elasticated covers avoid this, as will those with string ties under the table, although they are rather fiddly to tighten and tie when the cover is changed. Paper cover sheets are hygienic and look good when fresh, but are expensive and create a disposal problem. They also look awful when rucked up and creased and torn after the patient has turned over a few times. Pillows should be covered with a suitable paper towel or serviette.

Some female patients wear large bras with multiple fixings. It may be preferable to ask them to remove these, and, for the sake of propriety, to provide a rear-fastening surgical type of gown.

Most practitioners wear a clean clinic coat of their preferred style. Although some operators choose to work in less formal clothes, there is some evidence that many patients prefer their practitioner to be dressed like a practitioner. They find it easier to relate to them and develop a relationship based on trust and understanding. There are a few practitioners who choose to wear a suit and tie, and although this may be acceptable for a hospital consultant, it is not really practical for a therapist who is required to get into some contorted positions on occasions! It is clearly better to avoid the use of excessive jewellery that can catch on the patient or their hair.

APPROACH

The operator should cultivate an unhurried, calm, reassuring approach to the patient. This is particularly important with new patients, the very nervous, the elderly and small children. Excessive formality should be avoided, but an over-friendly approach could be misinterpreted as flippancy or suggestiveness and this must be guarded against. The operator must appear to be calm and in control even when highly pressurized by the telephone, late patients and his own problems. Lack of confidence is sensed by the patient very quickly and is taken as a sign of weakness. However, if the patient is taken into the confidence of the operator and involved in the decision process, they often appreciate this immensely.

PLANNING

It is not a good idea to give casual, off the cuff, unplanned treatment. It is very common to be pressurized into fitting someone in to an already full schedule for 'just a quick look'. Some practitioners seem able to do this with no problems, but many will be prone to make mistakes and errors of judgement.

Empirical treatment will tend to have very mixed results. It is better to have a specific objective in mind based on a diagnosis and backed up by some idea of prognosis. The thoughtful operator should be considering the immediate and longer-term objectives of the techniques that are being used. A planned treatment avoids unnecessary re-positioning

for the patient who may be in great distress when performing rotational movements. It is often better to work toward a part that is in acute pain rather than go straight to it. Nevertheless, a thorough palpatory investigation of the site of discomfort is reassuring for the patient and can give clues about the types of techniques most likely to influence the affected tissues. Insufficient force to achieve the required result can be remedied by a re-duplication of the technique using a graduated approach until the result is obtained. Much experience is required to judge just the right degree of force in any particular case, and it is better to be ineffectual than dangerous. An ineffective technique can be repeated and altered until it is effective; a dangerous one may be disastrous. It is unwise to persevere with any technique, particularly a thrust technique, in the presence of extreme pain or resistance. Similarly, if a patient is unable to relax, there may be hidden pathology or anomaly.

DIFFICULT SITUATIONS

There are numerous difficult situations that can occur in practice, and it is not my intention here to consider any except those related to technique. Patients can be very importunate of time and energy and encourage a practitioner to perform procedures he may consider unwise. It is better to politely decline than to perform a technique one is uneasy about and then have problems due to reactions or injury. It is naturally important to avoid medico-legal complications, and in this respect the best rule is that of informed consent. It is not possible or desirable for the patient to be informed of every single procedure that is to be applied and its percentage risk factor. However, the overall likelihood of success, and a broad outline of what is going to be done, and the tacit permission to perform the treatment techniques is a necessary preliminary to treatment. In cases where a practitioner has been accused of wrongful treatment, a very common factor is lack of communication and information. The General Council & Register of Osteopaths has gone so far as having a consent form available so that patients can put in writing their agreement to treatment in what might be considered sensitive areas of the body. These aspects of treatment must be considered more and more in the light of litigation experienced by practitioners in the USA. Cases that may seem frivolous matters to Europeans are sometimes fodder for legal actions.

RESPONSE TO REACTIONS

Some discomfort after treatment is common. If this is excessive it might be termed a reaction to treatment or technique. The degree of invasiveness in the chosen technique will clearly have some influence on the frequency of reactions, but some patients will have severe reactions however careful the approach. A feedback from the patient as to reactions will give considerable guidance as to the advisability of continuing treatment or the need to make a re-assessment. Reactions out of proportion to those expected should always give cause for re-evaluation. Like any other medicine, manipulative treatment has to be given in the correct dosage. An overdose can cause adverse reactions, whereas under-treatment may be unable to produce the desired symptomatic and objective changes. It is, nevertheless, a far more common mistake to over-treat than to under-treat. If in doubt, hold back.

Due to the muscle 'memory' phenomenon it is often necessary to repeat a given procedure on subsequent occasions. It is unwise to attempt miracle treatments in one session. Making allowances for variations in fitness, resilience, sensitivity, and state of general health, different patients will react differently on various occasions. An accurate record of treatment and techniques performed is not only a legal requirement; it is wise as it gives possible clues to the cause of any adverse reaction. Providing a thorough examination has been performed, and no sinister cause for the reaction can be found, a gentler repeat of the same procedures can often reverse the effect of the reaction and provide relief from symptoms. Most patients will accept an adverse reaction if they are forewarned, but may not believe it is normal if they are told after the event.

CATEGORY OF TECHNIQUE

Choice of the best category of technique to use and the order of technique usage is based upon the requirements of the case and the duration of the problem. The least invasive approach is naturally the best, but if satisfactory results are not being obtained subjectively and objectively, that is the time that most practitioners will increase the intensity of method. However, simply using firmer methods in the absence of a good result is not necessarily wise. A good rule would be to use the gentlest procedure likely to give the desired result considering all factors in the case. As has been stated elsewhere, the effect of a technique may be out of proportion to the application of force. Some amazing results have been obtained with the gentlest of approaches when a patient has already been treated unsuccessfully by other practitioners using violent methods.

INTERVALS BETWEEN TREATMENT

The interval between treatments is often critical. The decision as to the spacing of treatment is only arrived at by a consideration of all the relevant factors relating to the chronicity, acuteness, urgency and practical factors of distance, etc. If a patient reports benefit out of all proportion to the techniques used, it is generally better to suspend treatment for a while as it is possible to reverse the situation. Even though it may mean sending the patient away with no treatment and possibly no fee, this is preferable to causing a return of the symptoms by treating them just because they have an appointment. Many conditions are uncomfortable after treatment, then feel much better, and then slowly worsen as normal life patterns take over. If treatment is undertaken in the 'good' phase it is far too easy to stir up problems. The best timing is probably just as the symptoms are starting to recur. Naturally this does not always fit in with appointment schedules, but a reasonable compromise can be found.

Maintenance treatment at extended intervals of several months has been found to reduce the frequency, intensity and duration of acute mechanical dysfunction attacks. Many practitioners undertake this sort of work, although some feel that it is not getting fully to the bottom of any particular syndrome. Being realistic, occupational, postural and degenerative states mean that it is not always possible to fully correct any dysfunction, and some maintenance makes sense. The patient must be involved in the decision to undertake this type of approach. If the patient is symptom free on a maintenance visit, it would be unwise to perform forceful techniques as symptoms could be caused. However, some say that this is the best time to be doing firmer work as the patients' tissues are unlikely to be so reactive. The decision must be individual to each case and each operator.

ADVICE AND AFTERCARE

Most patients ask for exercises. Most patients, however, do not do the exercises prescribed! Providing they are really motivated to do them, carefully designed exercises of a stretching or strengthening nature make sense. Many patients find that exercise rather than exercises is preferable. They may be persuaded to walk, swim, do yoga or dance rather than perform specific exercises. Some will assiduously follow instructions. Some will overwork themselves in an attempt to get a quicker result, and some will do nothing and feel guilty about it. Each case must be judged on its merits.

Patients are generally very keen to have advice as to prevention of recurrences and quicker results in treatment, so long as it does not involve them in any effort! Many practitioners are not aware of the respect the patient has for their advice, and it must be carefully given so as not to cause unnecessary distress by their being unable to carry out that advice. Unwise advice to change job, for example, might cause loss of respect for the operator who gives it as it may be completely impractical. Advice given with the best intentions and consideration for the patient's welfare is fine, so long as it is tempered with realism.

All techniques that work by focusing forces to a specific joint need some method of producing that specificity. The usual method is to combine levers in such a way as to produce a locking or focusing. This means that other adjacent structures are excluded from being the target for the forces and are, therefore, to some extent, protected. Excessive attempts to 'protect' them, however, are just as likely to harm, from 'over-locking' which can produce discomfort and potential trauma.

How is locking produced? The usual method in the spine is to induce some torsion with a combination of sidebending to one side and rotation to the other. This so-called 'physiological locking' is in accord with Fryette's laws, and is the mainstay of manipulative work utilizing thrust techniques. There are several other ways that a combination of levers can be produced to focus forces. Compression, in combination with much smaller quantities of the other levers, can be effective, as can the use of accelerating rhythm and oscillation.

Methods of producing this focusing have traditionally been taught using the terms 'physiological locking' and 'ligamentous locking'. The difference between these two methods is that physiological locking implies facet apposition and ligamentous locking implies progressive tissue tension. In practice both of these methods are used in combination. A thoughtful operator will use the combination of several complex leverages to position the part in an optimum placing so that only a slight emphasis of leverage will achieve a focus at the desired point.

Locking need not consist of a steady 'wind up' to a point and then the application of overpressure. This will often be very uncomfortable for the patient. If held for more than a few seconds, the discomfort will cause the barrier to increase and there can be a sense of over-locking. An absolute point where the forces come together needs to be found. If this can be done without actually applying the full necessary leverage until the last possible moment, the patient will feel more relaxed and better able to cooperate with the procedure. This can only be done if the operator is aware of the feel of the tissues as the barrier accumulates, but just short of full tension. This allows him to tease the tension point several times from slightly different angles until the optimum can be found. If the same exercise were to be performed at the absolute point of full tension and locking, the discomfort would probably be unacceptable.

If the accumulation of tension was to 80–90%, the comfort level would be acceptable. The last 10–20% or so can be added for as short a duration as possible to finish the technique. The skill necessary to work in this way requires the ability to palpate a pathway of resistance rather than an absolute position. This ability is well worth developing.

Some authorities insist on the need to lock 'down to' or 'up to' a point or segment. The intersegmental changes taking place in this sort of application of forces are somewhat complex. The situation is also governed by normal variations in anatomy and physiological function of the part. Also relevant are the distortions of anomaly and pathological processes. These will produce distorted patterns and altered quality of movements, particularly at the ends-of-range.

The physiological movements of the spine

are such that most manipulative techniques require composite levers to achieve the stabilization necessary to localize force. Most techniques can be performed with a variety of levers, and quantities of those levers. As an example, consider a technique where 30° of flexion is combined with 60° of rotation and 20° of sidebending. If the flexion is applied first, there will be a tendency to use more than the desired 30°. The technique will still work, but it will be found that the other levers have been decreased by the same amount as the flexion has been increased. Conversely, if the rotation is put in first, it tends to become an executive part of the technique as the mind is focused on maintaining the rotation as the other levers are applied. These interesting phenomena can be used to advantage by playing with the order as well as the quantity of the different components until the optimum application is found. Experienced operators usually apply any given leverage as a composite movement and are constantly varying the quantities of all the directions as the tissues yield or otherwise in each direction. Locking does not then become full leverage and overpressure. It achieves the desirable situation of being as near a neutral point as possible until the critical time when the technique is finalized as an arc of movement.

The term locking is actually a misnomer. Nothing is actually locked; rather the forces are concentrated more at one point than any other. Extreme movement in any direction followed by overpressure can stretch, deform and possibly damage tissues, particularly if combined with high applications of force. Use of locking helps to focus the localization without any lever reaching its maximum range, although the primary, or executive, lever is taken further than all the others. The commonest method in the spine is to use sidebending to one side, and rotation to the other. The addition of small quantities of flexion or extension, compression or traction, etc., will further aid the localization. The way any particular operator builds up the levers to a given technique will vary slightly from patient to patient. There will be a number of other variable factors such as table height, patient positioning on the table and different ability with either hand. Nevertheless, the principles obey certain ground rules. Any particular area of the spine can be manipulated using thrust techniques in a whole variety of positions and ways. There are certain directions that will be most effective, least traumatic, and most comfortable for operator and patient. A useful guide is that locking can be produced most effectively when consciously using movements least available in the particular segment or area. Conversely, the greater the available range, the more the variety of locking procedures that will have broadly similar efficiency.

As an example, consider the mid cervical spine. This area has a wide range of flexibility in most directions in a normal subject, and so it will usually be possible to position in most combinations of leverages. However, the lower cervical spine has less range of movement due to the variation in facet angles and other factors. The range of extension particularly is limited, and therefore manipulation using extension will produce a locking with much less amplitude of leverage than flexion.

In the upper cervical spine, the movement least available is sidebending, and therefore sidebending will produce the quickest and most efficient locking without using large ranges of movement. Naturally, if too much sidebending is used, over-locking and pain would result just as easily as if any other lever were applied excessively.

Having identified this principle it is possible to evaluate the particular directions that this theory will support in each area. Naturally each case must be considered on its merits, with regard to other factors such as age, condition, size, etc:

1. Upper cervical – emphasize sidebending, although the neck as a whole can be in

flexion or extension. Excessive extension in the upper cervical area is undesirable as there is the potential for stress on the vertebro-basilar structures.

2. Mid cervical – all positions are possible, therefore use a balance between them all, but generally emphasize rotation as it is least uncomfortable.

3. Lower cervical – use extension in addition to main leverage of rotation. Flexion is also effective, but needs a greater range than extension.

4. Upper thoracic – most ranges are limited so use whichever combination is most effective in the particular case; extension combined with a primary lever of rotation is usually the choice.

5. Mid thoracic – depending on the degree of kyphosis, usually extension combined with sidebending.

6. Thoraco-lumbar – extension produces quickest locking, although extreme flexion is effective, if more uncomfortable.

7. Mid lumbar – as this is a generally free-moving area, a neutral position emphasizing rotation produces best effects.

8. Lower lumbar – as the facet angles are so prone to variation, and the lumbo-sacral angle varies so much, it is difficult to make any useful rules. However, sidebending applied first, followed by the rotation element using flexion in the lordotic spine, and extension in the flat spine will usually be effective.

Any general principles are open to comment and criticism, but the analysis behind these ideas should allow the development of personal approaches and individual development.

When applying locking forces there are some other considerations that need clarifying. Stand with feet parallel and turn the upper body to the left. You are performing left rotation in the spine. Now stand with the upper body fixed and perform a swivelling of the feet and pelvis to the right. Despite the fact that the body is being turned to the right, you are still performing left rotation at a spinal level. This may seem self-evident, but if considered carefully can alter the approach to a particular technique and possibly make it effective where it may not be otherwise. The focusing of forces to a specific point in a comfortable way for the patient and the operator is the essence of skill in manipulative technique. If a particular combination of leverages is applied in a steadily progressive way to a point of full tension, not only will the patient be uncomfortable, but the operator is unlikely to be in an optimum position to complete the technique efficiently. However, if the build-up of the accumulating tension is sensed, and the absolute point of maximum tension is 'teased', it should be possible to accelerate through to the thrust position more efficiently. This means that the point can be approached from several different angles, and allowed to increase and decrease to find the best balance of all the components. This 'playing' with the joint is not a vague searching, but is a purposeful, considered variation of all the components and directions of force. There should be a constant search for the optimum in a position of least strain on the tissues.

In the peripheral joints similar methods can be used, but this time the focusing is best performed by using compression as a focusing force. Compression acts as a limiter of amplitude and can be useful to bring effective barrier sense nearer to the midline, thus avoiding painful torsional leverages. The other consideration that is particularly effective in the peripheral skeleton is the use of induced levers by taking both hands in opposite directions. Consider the force necessary to wring the water out of a sodden cloth if one hand was to remain still while the other did all the work. Consider how the force could be reduced by both hands working in opposite directions. Some schools of thought in the manipulative field insist that one hand be fixed, while the other does all the work. Although this seems to make sense, the effort, discomfort and strain is much more than if both hands share the work.

It does take quite a lot of time and practice to make this effective in finding this pathway of optimum potential without the guidance of full tension. The time taken to acquire this skill is well worthwhile in that it can produce quicker results, less adverse reactions to treatment, and better patient satisfaction.

If this method seems intangible at first, carry on using full leverages as with traditional train-ing and gradually refine the methods being used by introducing these principles a little at a time. It is very easy to fall back on methods, which although effective, are uncomfortable, procedural and require higher force, effort and strain for patient and operator. To quote a cliché, 'If you keep looking back, you will end up going there.' There are no absolutes in osteopathic approaches; the infinite variety of possible composite levers allows most situations to be catered for.

EXERCISES FOR DEVELOPING TECHNICAL SKILL

Any psychomotor skill can be improved and developed by suitable practice. It is not possible to practise every technique or method sufficiently to become skilled enough so that the process is automatic without a considerable quantity of time and effort. However, there are some exercises or drills that may help to shorten the learning time for students and I have included a few here. It is unfortunate that it is extremely difficult to find activities that are similar to the skills needed for osteopathic technique. There are many things that can be done to improve mechanical handling skills for dealing with inanimate objects. These do little in helping the student to appreciate the subtle differences in tissue states that exist in patients. We are dealing with living structures in real people and the psychology, age, weight, size and nature of the problem all subtly alter the approach and forces necessary. With this in mind it must be said that the best exercise is constant practice with a willing fellow student who is empowered to give constructive feedback as to handling, comfort and effectiveness.

Not all exercises or drills will be of equal benefit to all individuals. We all have our own personal model of learning and some systems of skill development will feel more natural than others. Osteopathic skills can be divided into palpatory skill and technique skill although one is not really possible without the other.

From a general viewpoint, anything that improves hand and eye coordination should be useful. Most people, at some time in their life, undertake sport of some sort or another if they are physically able. As experience and practice develops, they gradually improve their skill to a certain level dependent on the amount of time and effort used. If a student is going to be an osteopath, their whole life's work is going to be concerned with performing osteopathic treatment. It would seem to make sense therefore to practise the skills until they are efficient. For many reasons some are unwilling to do this. Although life places many demands on our time, without sufficient practice it is fair to say that a student is unlikely to become an efficient technician. The practice must, nevertheless, be of the correct methods. Bad habits, particularly regarding posture, can be very difficult to correct later.

The best sports are going to be those that the student enjoys and will, therefore, participate in regularly. Racquet sports help in coordination, but dance and contact sports are probably better for posture, balance and the psychomotor development necessary for osteopathic technique. Physical strength is not a requirement for an osteopath. However, a reasonable level of stamina and fitness is useful. A high proportion of students who become good technicians have done some training in martial arts. It seems that the discipline, fitness and body awareness have many uses in their subsequent osteopathic career. Team games seem to have less to offer in terms of the future needs of an osteopath, but that is not to say that they do not have their use in general fitness.

Here are a few specific exercises:

1. Face a partner and take up a posture with one leg forward of the other. Place a football between one of your outstretched hands and that of your partner so that it is sandwiched between you. Take turns in pushing and pulling. If you coordinate with your partner, the football will remain between your hands. If you do not coordinate, you will drop it. Responding to the subtle cues of your partner's movements will help develop coordination and response to motion. It will also help in developing the feel for 'setting' the hand in slight isometric tension which is necessary in many techniques. Reverse hands.

2. Pull a toilet roll gently until the tissue is taut. Apply a sharp tug, aiming the force at the perforations of the sheet. Avoid simply unravelling the roll. Practise moving the force to the next row of perforations while missing the nearer one. This drill improves the ability to sense tension and to direct force beyond one point to another.

3. Stand facing a partner and place one leg in front of the other. Extend one arm slightly and place the back of the hand against the back of your partner's similarly extended hand. Decide who is to be the mover and who is to be the follower. Take turns in moving the hand at different rates, and in different planes and directions. The follower must try to remain in contact at all times. This is similar to exercise 1, but uses direct contact rather than via the football. Alternate hand and leg positions.

4. Stand facing a partner with one leg in front of the other. Grip each others' wrists and gently assume a rhythm of push and pull. Attempt to pull or push your partner from his firm stance, but be aware that he is doing the same with you. Force will not work; you must use balance and transmission of energy and rapid change of direction to be effective. This will improve balance, coordination and sense of tissue resistance. Alternate legs.

5. Acquire some bubble wrap as used in protective packing. Place it on a table and use your heel of hand or pisiform to burst one bubble at a time. Draw an ink line around one bubble and try to burst the bubble within the line and no others. Examine your hand and see if you have a neat ink circle around your pisiform or only an arc of a circle. Progress to doing the same thing on your thigh so that there is normal tissue underneath the bubbles and not the firmness of the table. Progress to performing the same task on a partner's back to see how little force you can apply and yet still achieve the objective. This will develop skill and accuracy in minimum force technique.

6. Have a partner place a single hair underneath a single page of a smooth telephone book without you knowing where it is. Use light pressure and scanning of the surface with your fingers to locate the hair. See if you can do the same with the heel of the hand. Try with eyes shut or open and standing or sitting to see which is your personal best method. When you become adept at this, have your partner place the hair under several pages of the book rather than just one. See how deep you can still feel it. This improves palpatory perception and trains you in which part of the hand is best to use in palpation.

7. Perform a similar exercise to 6, but use a coin instead of a hair. Have your partner place the coin at varied depths and try to judge the depth. Have him vary the size of the coin and try to estimate the size by palpation. This palpatory exercise is similar to the previous one but it develops different aspects of your skill in estimating size and bulk.

8. Perform the magician's trick of snatching the tablecloth from under cutlery or crockery. Use unbreakable crockery at first! Once you have acquired the skill to pull

away the tablecloth without disrupting the articles on the table, try the same exercise sitting, or with varied leg positions. Try it bent over or straight to find the optimum posture necessary for the sharp pulling action. This exercise should improve your fast movement and acceleration skills.

9. Play 'red hands' with a partner. Have your partner extend his hands in front with palms facing down. Place your hands, palms upward, lightly under his so that they are just touching. Keep very slight movements going and try to extract your hands fast enough to gently slap the back of your partner's hands before he has had a chance to snatch them away. If you manage to slap him, you repeat the move until he manages to anticipate your movement and snatch his hands away so that you slap the air. When this happens, you reverse roles. Try not to snatch the hands away at every move; wait until the slapper is committed. This improves response to motion and reaction time, but will give sore hands if continued for too long!

10. Have a partner suspend a crisp banknote between finger and thumb. Place your finger and thumb on either side of it near the bottom, without touching. Have him drop the note and try to catch it before it passes through your hand. As you improve, gradually widen the gap between your finger and thumb and raise your hand nearer the top so that there is less time to react. This is another exercise in response to motion and improves your ability to move only at the right speed when necessary.

11. Learn to juggle with suitable juggling balls. This teaches you to relax and yet remain alert and responsive to moving objects. This is extremely good for coordination and hand–eye reactions.

12. Have your partner mime a simple movement. Stand in front of him and copy this movement as if you are a mirror. Gradually make the movements more complex and see if you can follow his mime. This will improve your ability to learn technique by watching and copying.

13. Sit at a table with your forearms horizontal. Relax and then try to contract your brachio-radialis muscle alone on one side. You may find that this is difficult, but with practice it should be possible to isolate this one muscle alone. When you have achieved this, move on to specifically contracting part of your forearm extensor group. To do this, lift one finger and watch and feel the muscle contract. Try different fingers. Progress to contracting specific parts of the muscle group without moving the fingers. Try to contract your biceps muscle without visibly contracting brachio-radialis. These exercises give you the ability to use your muscles in a controlled fashion. This is a very useful facility when performing thrust techniques that require accurate use of defined parts of your structure for specificity.

With a little ingenuity it should be possible to develop most daily activities into suitable practice for some aspects of technique skill. When vacuuming, swivel from foot to foot to practise weight transfer necessary in many articulation techniques. When washing a car try different directions of circling the hands to find the variety possible in addition to the most natural directions. Try placing a few pieces of fruit or vegetables in a bag and identifying each one by feel. Trace the outlines of the bones of your own wrist; see how much pressure is comfortable and how you can deflect the tendons out of the way to get to the deeper structures.

Until it is possible to develop some form of thrust meter or pressure-sensing device to objectively measure forces and directions, these simple drills should help in a small way to aid understanding, palpation and skill.

Accurate and efficient techniques for the lumbar area are extremely important. The highest percentage of patients presenting to osteopathic practitioners are suffering with low back pain, and techniques for the lumbar spine will probably be used more often than any others. The practical difficulties for a small operator in reaching a facet joint no bigger than the thumb nail, in the back of a patient weighing anything up to around 200 pounds, can be considerable. The sheer depth of the joints, the difficulty of controlling the area in many subjects, and the common complicating factor of an underlying acute or chronic disc lesion add to the problems. For treatment to be more specific, accurate mechanical diagnosis is essential. There is, therefore, a requirement for techniques designed to be efficient and feasible for the operator to perform without undue stress on his own structure.

It can be a problem to localize a force to a segment or segments while attempting to 'protect' adjacent areas that may be hyper-mobile. It is often difficult to manipulate a specific segment, but in some cases unless this is achieved, the relief from a particular pain and dysfunction syndrome will not occur. General mobilizing can be extremely helpful, but the nature of release achieved with a well-timed, accurate and specific thrust can be not only a short cut, but the only way to get full restoration of function. Although size of operator should not be a critical factor, it must be said that in some cases a larger operator will have a distinct advantage. The use of excessive force rather than accuracy, however, conceals a weakness in approach.

Cases of possible disc injury require particular care to avoid worsening the situation. An educated, aware practitioner should be conversant with neurological symptoms and signs. Extreme antalgic posture is present for a reason and consideration should be given to that reason before attempts to 'correct' the posture are made. Many pathological states in the body can manifest as low back pain and the reader is referred to literature on pathology and diagnostic screening as an essential prerequisite to treatment in this area. A patient should be fully investigated when they are clearly ill, have lost weight for no apparent reason, or have intractable pain that does not subside on rest.

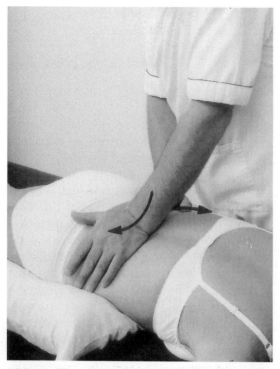

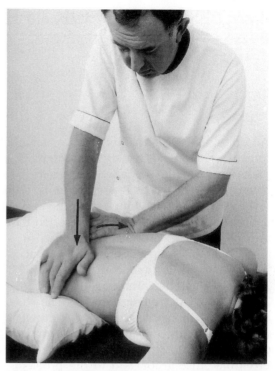

13.1 ▲ Kneading soft tissues lumbar area prone
The operator is working on the muscles on the side furthest from him. The near hand is holding back on the area to apply a small compressive force toward the table and to prevent rotation of the spine and to sense the best resistance from the tissues. Push with the active hand into the muscle belly until a sense of resistance is felt, and then maintain this position for a few moments until a sense of activation is felt. There should be a sense of 'melting' as the muscles relax, and then you can follow this sense until the muscle is gently but fully eased. The direction of the pathway may be in a curve, and it is important to allow the tissues sufficient time to guide the force direction rather than to impose on them. The pressure is then slowly released until the cycle can be repeated on an adjacent area. The whole cycle can take up to about six or seven seconds. Most operators will not use such a long cycle, but paradoxically it is often found that the slower one works, the quicker and more effective the results.

Tips: Least useful in cases where prone lying is a problem and in acute cases where there may be a tendency for the muscles to go into a greater spasm when the patient subsequently moves. **Extra considerations**: Note that a pillow is placed under the patient's abdomen to reduce excessive hyperextension of the lumbar spine.

13.2 ▲ Kneading soft tissues lumbar area prone
Perform the technique with the near hand while the other stabilizes. There is no particular advantage in which hand is used. However, it may be easier to reach right down to the sacral attachments of the erector spinae using the caudal hand rather than the cephalic one, as in technique photograph 13.1.

Tips: Least useful in cases where lying prone may be a problem. **Extra considerations**: Try asking the patient to turn the head to one and then the other side to assess which produces the most useful tension. Combining phases of breathing with the technique may be useful. The pillow is optional to increase patient comfort if necessary. Most patients find that a pillow underneath the abdomen is preferred when prone lying.

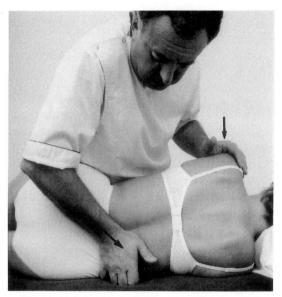

13.3 ▲ Kneading soft tissues lumbar area side-lying The patient has the knees and hips flexed to increase stability on the table. Stabilize the patient's body with your cephalic hand and apply the kneading force to the muscles nearest the table.

Tips: Most useful in cases where prone lying may be a problem. Least useful in large patients where the reach for the operator may be too great. **Extra considerations**: In acute cases this may be the only way to work on the lumbar muscles as prone lying may be impossible due to spasm. Try varied angles of hip and knee flexion. Try working on the muscles by pulling up instead of pushing down. Try performing the same procedure when standing behind the patient.

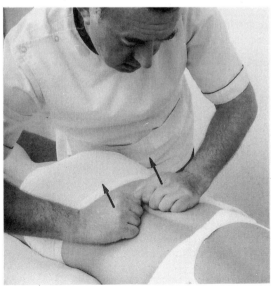

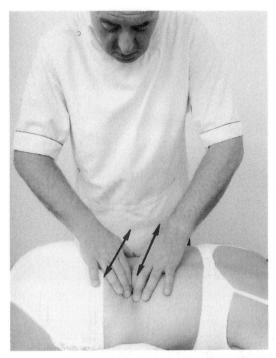

13.5 ▲ Articulation into sideshifting lumbar area prone Grip the transverse processes of the vertebra concerned with the pads, not the tips, of the fingers and thumb and use a direct sideshifting force from side to side. The oscillation can be quite firm when used carefully, and this will act as a useful test as well as a mobilizing force. As the hands are applied to adjacent vertebrae, differences in mobility can easily be felt, and this hold can be used to mobilize, or other techniques can be applied to deal with the restriction in movement.

Tips: This is a movement of the whole of the patient's body around the vertebra, and needs quite a long amplitude to be effective. Least useful in cases of antalgic sidebent posture as this movement will cause pain when working against the curve.

13.4 ◄ Stretching superficial fascia lumbar area prone Gather skin and superficial fascia over upper lumbar area, and then apply a lifting force so that a gapping is produced. In some cases this can be made into a thrust, and the fascia will separate with a vacuum gapping sound.

Tips: Most useful in cases of tightness in the superficial fascia which can be a factor in maintenance of pain syndromes. Least useful where the skin is very tender.

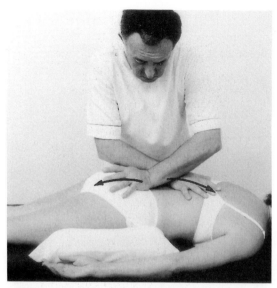

13.6 ▲ Harmonic technique lumbar area prone
Fix the sacrum in some traction towards the patient's feet and fix the thoraco-lumbar area towards the head. The harmonic technique is performed by a rhythmic oscillation of the patient's whole body in a caudal and cephalic direction. See earlier section relating to harmonic technique.

Tips: The range of mobility available in a longitudinal plane is going to be smaller than in a rotary plane, but is, nevertheless, often useful in re-establishing rhythm and mobility. Least useful in cases where prone lying is a problem. **Extra considerations**: It is also possible to perform rotary harmonic technique if the tension is maintained between the hands, and the whole body oscillated into rotation. The pillow under the abdomen often makes the position more comfortable for the patient.

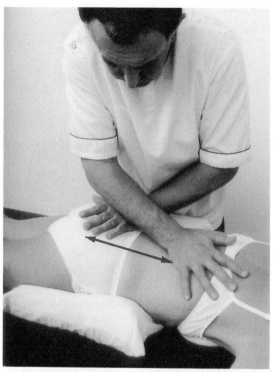

13.7 ▲ Sacral springing and traction prone Flex the sacrum as far as is comfortable, and fix the thoraco-lumbar area with the other hand. Aid the flexion of the sacrum with the elbow of the one hand by pressing the other hand into the table.

Tips: Try adding various amounts of rotary movement of the pelvis or the body as a preliminary before the sacral flexion. This can enable forces to be directed to either side of the lumbo-sacral joint rather than simply flexing the sacrum. Most useful in cases of very tight lumbar fascia where this position removes some of the soft tissue tension and allows the force to reach the facet joints. Least useful in cases where prone lying is a problem.

13.8 ◄ Harmonic technique pelvis and lumbar spine supine Take up any slack in the tissues of the pelvis by pressing firmly into the table with both hands. Perform the oscillation with alternating pressure towards the table with the heel of each hand on the anterior superior spines. This induces a rotatory movement in the lumbar spine. See earlier section relating to harmonic technique.

Tips: Try using varied amounts of traction as an additional movement. Most useful in fairly small patients where the stretch to reach is not too far. Least useful in large patients, or for small operators where the reach is a problem.

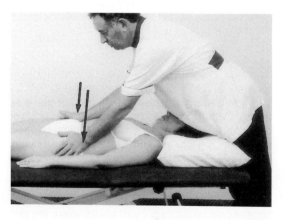

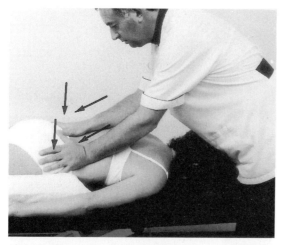

13.9 ▲ Harmonic technique lumbar spine and pelvis prone Apply pressure above the crests of the ilia and a variable traction force towards the patient's feet. A harmonic oscillation is induced into rotation, sidebending and traction. See earlier section relating to harmonic technique.

Tips: Least useful where prone lying would be a problem.

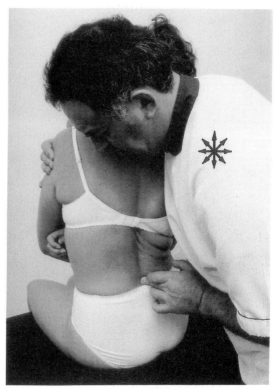

13.11 ▲ Functional technique typical hold The operator is controlling all possible vectors of patient movement while monitoring the sense of ease and bind at a particular segment. The controlling hand is directing the body towards accumulating ease at the target segment. See earlier section relating to functional technique.

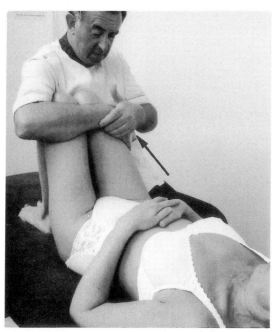

13.10 ◄ Traction supine Fix the patient's legs against your chest and push gently downwards so that the feet are fixed to the table. Lean back to produce a traction force in the lumbar spine. This hold can also be used in a harmonic fashion.

Tips: Most useful where a gentle traction force is required. **Extra considerations**: Try varying the angles of hip and knee flexion to focus the force to different areas.

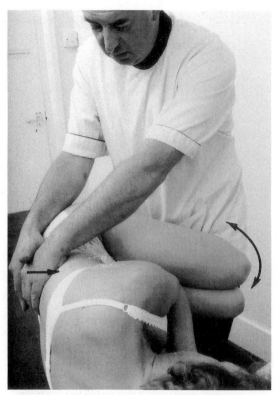

3.12 ▲ Articulation into flexion sidelying Flex the patient's hips until a sense of gapping is felt at the target segment. Rock from foot to foot and turn this diagnostic procedure into an articulation with an increase of pressure with either hand to localize the force.

Tips: Most useful in almost all cases of lumbar vertebral dysfunction. Least useful in extremely large patients or in the presence of any disorder preventing hip flexion. **Extra considerations**: Try using one hand to pull the pelvis into more flexion or the other hand to hold back above the target vertebra or both.

13.14 ▶ Articulation into flexion supine Sit on the table and hold over one or more spinous or transverse processes. Flex the hips with the other hand. Hold the patient's legs against your chest so that as you rock back and forth, the force causes a flexion movement of the lumbar area.

Tips: Least useful if there is any hip disorder preventing flexion. **Extra considerations**: Try using varied degrees of sidebending or rotation at the same time to enhance localization.

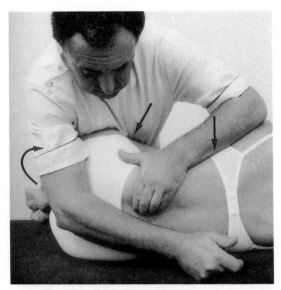

13.13 ▲ Articulation into reinforced flexion Pull the sacrum directly toward you while bracing the ribs towards the table. The upper hand fixes above the target segment while you pull the sacrum into flexion.

Tips: Try varied amounts of compression of the thighs toward the table and adding elements of sidebending or rotation to the flexion, to focus on particular parts of the segment. Most useful where a strong localized force is required. Least useful where the patient is very large and the reach around them would be too great.

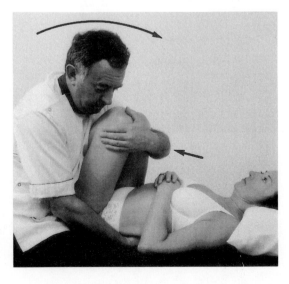

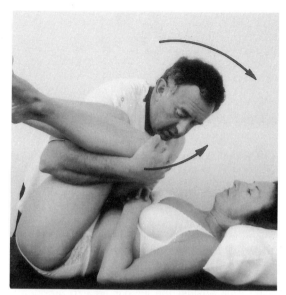

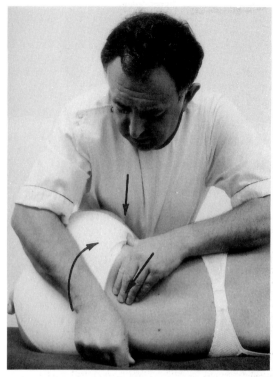

13.15 ▲ **Articulation supine** Stand at the side of the table and fix over one or more of the spinous or transverse processes. Cross the patient's thighs and apply a flexion and sidebending force as you lean forward. This hold makes it easy to introduce some element of sidebending to the primary movement of flexion.

Tips: Least useful in any patient with hip mobility restriction. Most useful in very flexible subjects where the position automatically absorbs some of the excess movement. **Extra considerations**: Try using a fisted hand to form a stronger fulcrum in suitable cases.

13.17 ▲ **Articulation into sidebending sidelying** Compress toward yourself, and down into the table. Sidebend the pelvis away from the table with the caudal hand as the other hand pushes down on the spinous processes.

Tips: Most useful where very localized articulation is necessary, and in cases where a firm lever through the hips may be undesirable.

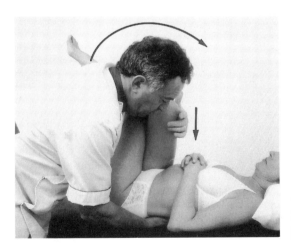

13.16 ◄ **Articulation supine** (alternative view) The hold is as in photograph 13.15, but shows hand placement from the other side.

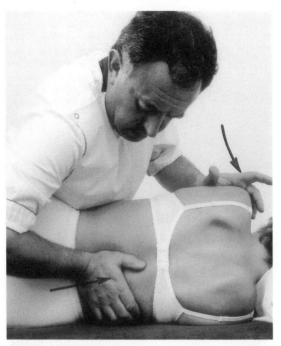

13.18 ▲ Articulation into extension sidelying
Fix the patient's shoulder girdle to the table with a
compressive force and apply a direct posterior to
anterior force over the lumbar spine.

Tips: Most useful where a very localized force is
required. Least useful in large subjects where a
small operator may find it difficult to develop
sufficient leverage. **Extra considerations**: Try
varying the initial patient position on the table to
find the optimum in each case.

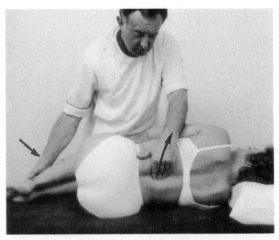

13.19 ▲ Articulation into extension sidelying
Fix the patient's knees against your thigh, and fix
the patient's feet to the table with your caudal
hand. Pull against the lumbar area to produce a
direct force into extension.

Tips: Least useful in very stiff subjects who
would be very difficult to move with this hold as it
would require great strength in the pulling hand to
overcome the stiffness. **Extra considerations**: As
extension is elicited from above, try asking the
patient to extend the head and upper back to
enhance the action of the technique.

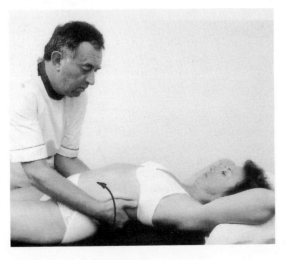

13.20 ◄ Articulation into extension supine Pull
upward on the transverse processes on both sides.
The patient has interlaced the hands behind her
head to enhance the extension force.

Tips: Most useful in small subjects and children,
and when directing the force into the upper lumbar
area. **Extra considerations**: Try extending and
then adding an oscillatory rotation force as an
additional vector.

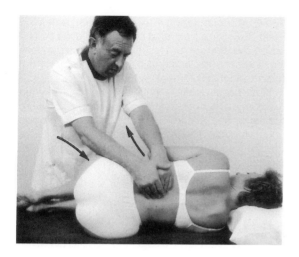

13.21 ◄ Articulation into extension sidelying
Overlap the hands and pull directly on the area to introduce extension. The patient's knees are directly fixed by your thigh to form a counter-force. Keep the patient's hips at 90°.

Tips: Most useful where a fairly strong force is desired. **Extra considerations**: Try introducing an element of sidebending or rotation to assist the primary movement.

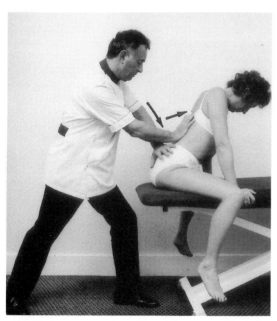

13.22 ▲ Articulation into extension sitting Take up the slack of the area with crossed hands and as the patient is rocked back and forth an extension force is produced. By placing the cephalic hand on either side of the area, a rotation or sidebending force can also be introduced. The patient is astride the table to stabilize the pelvis.

Tips: Least useful in elderly patients or those where the astride position may be a problem. **Extra considerations**: Try asking the patient to move the hands further forward to change the angle of approach to the area.

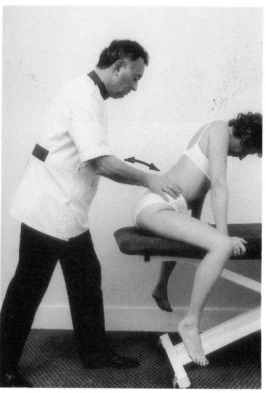

13.23 ▲ Articulation into extension sitting Apply thumb pressure to the paravertebral area of the segment to be mobilized. The patient is asked to hold the edge of the table and then you can push against the area rhythmically to introduce the extension force. The natural recoil of the tissues will bring the spine back to neutral.

Tips: Least useful in cases where astride sitting can be a problem. **Extra considerations**: Try staggering the thumbs on either side of the spine to introduce a rotation element to the movement.

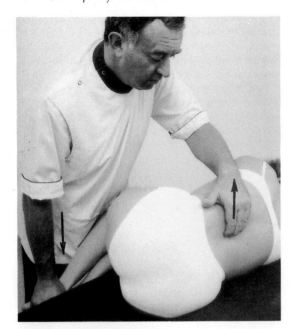

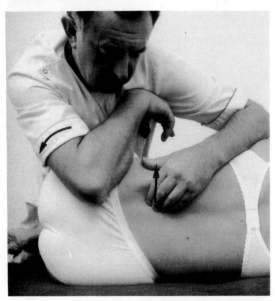

13.24 ◄ **Articulation into sidebending sidelying** Push down with one hand on the legs while pulling up on the spinous processes to induce sidebending. Increase the angle of hip flexion to direct the force to higher segments as desired.

Tips: Least useful in patients who have any hip disorder as this position may be a problem. Where the table has a hard edge the pressure may be uncomfortable for the thigh on the table. **Extra considerations**: Try introducing an element of extension to the technique to change the effect of the pure sidebending if necessary.

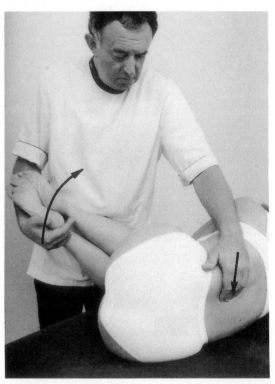

13.25 ▲ **Articulation into flexion/sidebending sidelying** Pull up with one hand on the spinous processes while the patient's pelvis is sandwiched between your body and arm and lean away from the spinal hand to produce sidebending. Varied degrees of flexion are applied by rocking against the patient's knees.

Tips: Most useful where very localized articulation is desired.

13.26 ▲ **Articulation into sidebending sidelying** Lift the patient's feet until tension is felt to accumulate under the other hand which pushes toward the table to produce sidebending.

Tips: Most useful where a strong generalized force is required. Least useful in the presence of any hip joint dysfunction. **Extra considerations**: Try varied degrees of hip flexion.

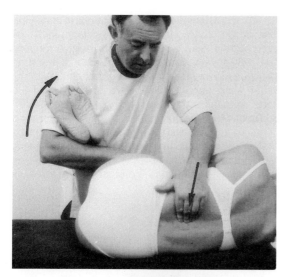

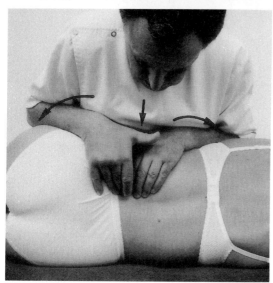

13.27 ◀ Articulation into sidebending sidelying
Take the patient's feet in the crook of your arm and fix against the upper thigh with your wrist. Your other hand pushes against the spinous processes toward the table. Varied degrees of flexion of the hips are applied to focus the forces to the segment desired.

Tips: Least useful in the presence of any hip disorder. Most useful where a very strong stretch is desired.

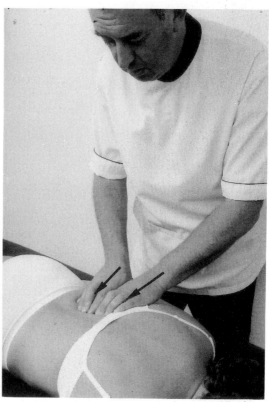

13.28 ▲ Articulation into sidebending sidelying
The patient is sidelying in a neutral position of slight hip flexion and you can push on the rib cage toward her head, on the pelvis toward her feet and on her spine toward yourself. The articulation movement is either a fixation with one hand and a pulling with the other or a movement of both. Varied degrees of rotation or flexion can be introduced as part of the overall leverage.

Tips: Most useful where any hip disorder prevents use of the hip as a lever and where strong localized forces are required. **Extra considerations**: A high compressive force toward the table helps to focus the technique.

13.29 ▲ Articulation into sidebending prone
Apply the fingers to the side of the spinous processes and push away from yourself to produce a sidebending and rotation force. This is most applicable in the upper lumbar area.

Tips: Least useful where the patient may find the prone position a problem. **Extra considerations**: Try placing the patient in some sidebending before the initiation of the technique.

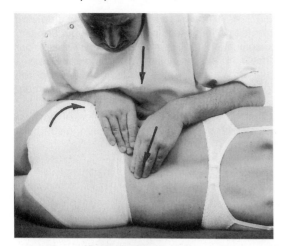

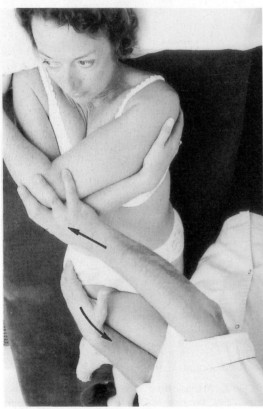

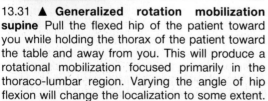

13.31 ▲ Generalized rotation mobilization supine Pull the flexed hip of the patient toward you while holding the thorax of the patient toward the table and away from you. This will produce a rotational mobilization focused primarily in the thoraco-lumbar region. Varying the angle of hip flexion will change the localization to some extent.

Tips: Least useful where specific localization is required.

13.30 ◄ Articulation into sidebending sidelying The patient is lying in a neutral position with hips only slightly flexed. Apply a compressive force to the pelvis with your body and caudal hand to produce sidebending away from the table. With the other hand apply a downward force toward the table to localize the sidebending.

Tips: Most useful where a localized force is required and it is necessary to avoid using the hips in the leverage. **Extra considerations**: Try using varied amounts of compression through either arm and rotation to enhance the sidebending force.

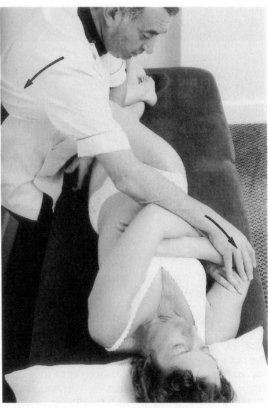

13.32 ▲ Generalized articulation into rotation supine Apply a force with your lower hand through the patient's hip using your wrist as a fulcrum. Use the other hand to hold the patient's folded arms away from you.

Tips: Least useful where specific localization is required. **Extra considerations**: Try placing the patient in some sidebending before the onset of the technique to enhance the effect.

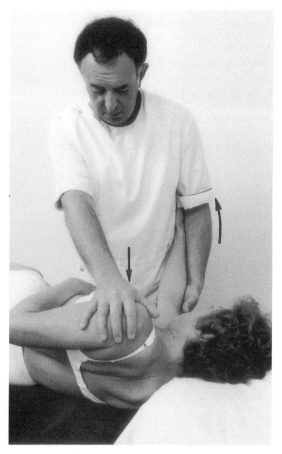

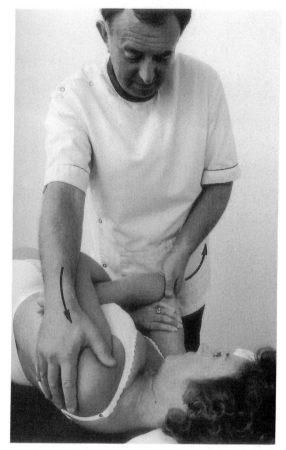

13.33, 13.34 and 13.35 Thrust sidelying, building of upper lever component. There are many ways of introducing the upper component to the lumbar roll position for applying a thrust. Each has its advantages and disadvantages. Individuals will have to experiment to find their own preferred method. Photograph 13.33 shows the operator clasping the patient's forearm under his arm. While pushing the other shoulder toward the table he is pulling the lower scapula out of the way. The pull can be either into pure rotation or sidebending either way according to the direction he takes the arm. In photograph 13.34 the patient's arms are folded and the operator is lifting on the lower elbow while holding down on the upper shoulder. It is less easy to introduce a sidebending component with this hold. In photograph 13.35 the operator is sliding the lower scapula forward while holding down on the upper shoulder. This hold allows sidebending to either side to be introduced if necessary and does not involve any strain on the patient's shoulder.

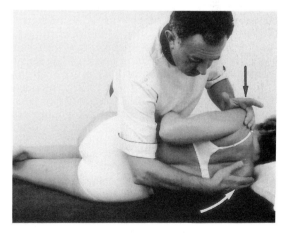

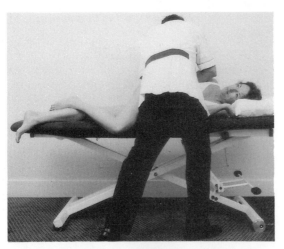

13.36 ◄ **Thrust using lumbar roll sidelying rear view** The operator is applying a classical combined lever and thrust technique. This rear view shows operator posture and how both feet are pointing to the head of the table with the rear heel just off the floor. Note that the weight is applied to the patient's pelvis with the thrusting hand. The other arm is only lightly fixing on the lateral aspect of the thorax and NOT the anterior aspect of the shoulder. The patient's body is rolled toward the operator who is, therefore, only slightly flexed and is able to apply the rotary force of the technique simply by a flexing of his knees.

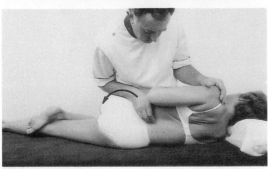

13.37 ▲ **Thrust using minimal leverage sidelying** The patient is positioned in a balanced sidelying position and a very small element of rotation has been introduced from above. Apply the hand to the patient's shoulder to produce a compressive force toward the table and your other arm is then flexed to 90° and held close to your side. Gather some skin from your forearm and the patient's buttock by gripping the buttock with the forearm and pulling it into you before applying the downward compression force. The force is applied as a combination of (a) compression to the table, (b) localized compression over the segment, (c) rotation of the pelvis by you flexing your knees and (d) a sidebending of the pelvis away from the shoulder. In minimal leverage thrust the amplitude is very short and the velocity is high.

Tips: Most useful where it is desired to produce facet separation with minimal distortion of the spinal area or torsion through the rib cage. **Extra considerations**: The final vectors of force direction will be slightly different in each subject. Although the directions given will apply in most cases, it must be remembered that an increase of one force direction will automatically reduce the quantity necessary for others. The order in which they are applied may also be changed to suit the circumstances. Considerable experimentation will be necessary to find the optimum for each operator's particular skill, the patient's morphology and the facet orientation. This depends to a large extent on palpatory awareness.

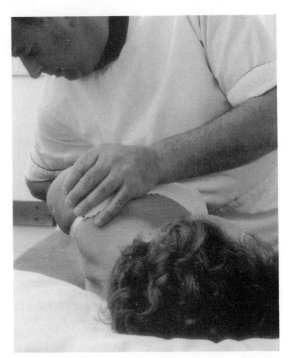

13.38 ▲ **Thrust, upper hand hold, combined leverage and thrust, sidelying** The operator has placed the patient in position for the thrust, and this photograph shows the rotation of the upper lever. Note that the patient's upper shoulder is behind the lower one, but only by a small amount. The operator's head is vertically over the lumbar spine although the abducted arm is going to apply the thrust. A compression force is applied to the shoulder with only enough backward pressure to act as an equal and opposite force to the thrusting hand. It does NOT enter into the thrust other than as a stabilizer.

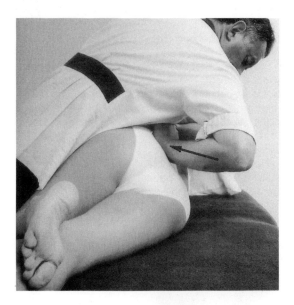

13.39 ◄ **Thrust, lower hand hold, combined leverage and thrust, sidelying** Roll the patient's body toward you and apply the heel of your hand to the ilium so that it is possible to produce a rotation and extension force as necessary. Your pelvis and side must be applied to the patient's thigh, and you must fix the patient's thigh to the table with your thigh.

Tips: Most useful for larger operators, and where an extension force is needed. This hold can also be used for a direct sacral thrust. **Extra considerations**: Some of the thrust force comes from a downward movement of the operator's body along with the hand force.

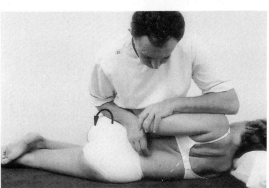

13.40 ▲ **Thrust using minimal leverage, alternative shoulder hold** Apply a downward pressure through the pelvis, after gathering some tissue under the applied forearm to induce compression and some rotation. Place your hand in direct contact with the vertebra at the apex of the force. Your other arm compresses the patient's thorax through the shoulder toward the table. The final thrust direction is a combination of compression, rotation and some sidebending as necessary.

Tips: More useful in larger patients where it may be too far to reach up to the axilla with the stabilizing hand. Less useful for operators with long arms, who may find it difficult to apply the hand to the spine at the same time as the usually applied part of the forearm to the ilium. This action will cause hyperflexion of the elbow and if repeated many times will make the risk of injury to it extremely high!

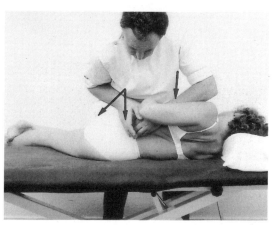

13.41 ▲ **Thrust into flexion using combined lever and thrust sidelying** The initial patient positioning involves using some flexion and afterwards you apply a compressive, rotary and flexion force to the pelvis. Note that the patient's lower leg is off the edge of the table and that you must be square to the table rather than in the usual position of facing toward the opposite top corner. The combined effect of this is to produce a flexion gapping force that may be very useful in hyperextended patients.

Tips: The final flexion is the gapping force and sufficient free play must be left to allow this to operate.

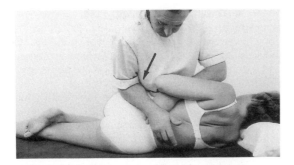

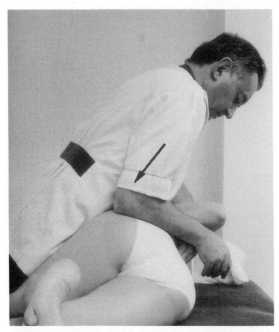

13.43 ▲ Thrust into rotation combined lever and thrust sidelying This view shows the lower arm hold used in photograph 13.42. The medial aspect of the elbow is applied to the small plateau on the lateral aspect of the ilium between gluteus maximus and gluteus medius. The soft tissues have been gathered first and the forearm muscles have been rolled to form a cushion between your ulna and the patient's pelvis.

Tips: It is worth spending some time experimenting to find the most comfortable way of applying the lower hand hold. It is often useful to apply the arm, and then, keeping contact with the patient, adduct it so that your forearm muscles are rolled between your ulna and the patient. Avoid using the back of the ulna or the point of the elbow. The forearm will be at approximately 60° to the long axis of the table. If it is at 90° this is likely to be very uncomfortable for the patient.

13.42 ◄ Thrust into rotation combined lever and thrust sidelying The hold used here is specific for the lumbo-sacral and L4/5 levels. The difference in this hold is that your lower hand is not in contact with the patient. The upper hand is threaded through and is palpating the relevant spinal level. The upper hand is used to apply a compression force at the target segment. If the lower hand were to be in contact with the spine the thrusting elbow would become excessively flexed and liable to injury.

Tips: The optimum plane for the thrust will be easier to find if the patient, as a whole, is rolled gently back and forth on the table within the thrust position. This does not mean that the levers alter at all, but that a momentum force is being used in rolling while keeping the levers the same. It is also easier to apply the thrust from a dynamic rather than a static position.

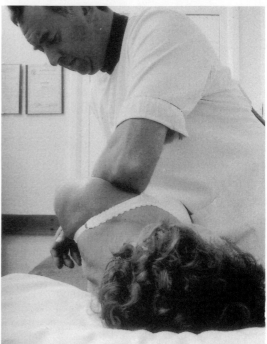

13.44 ▲ Thrust into rotation combined lever and thrust sidelying This view shows the upper arm hold used in photograph 13.42. Notice that the operator is standing fairly upright and that his arm pressure is not on the shoulder but rather the antero-lateral aspect of the thorax. He is using ulnar deviation of the wrist to bring the ulnar border of the hand against the lower ribs. To avoid the force dissipating when the thrust is applied, ensure your shoulders are pulled down by active contraction of your latissimus dorsi muscles on both sides. A useful rule is that if you can see your shoulders, except out of the corner of your eyes, they are too high.

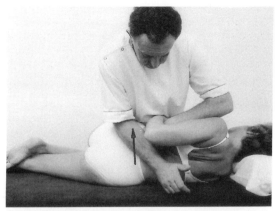

13.45 ▲ Thrust into rotation combined lever and thrust sidelying The hold shown here is for a pure rotary thrust where the operator is focusing the forces and then will simply flex his knees to introduce the rotation. This direction of force is most useful in patients who have very sagittal lower lumbar facet planes.

Tips: The optimum plane and timing for the thrust will be found if the patient's body is kept slowly rolling back and forth.

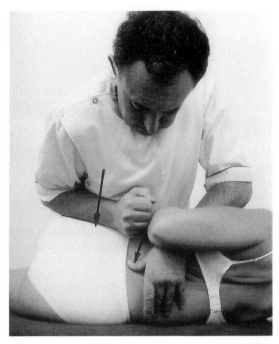

13.47 ▲ Thrust into rotation combined lever and thrust sidelying Hold directly on the spinous process of L4 or L5 to help make the force specific. Apply the thrusting arm to produce a direct compression and rotation force through a very small amplitude.

Tips: The stabilizing hand is not applied to the anterior of the thorax in this case but more to the lateral side of the ribs as the force should not reach much above the segment concerned. Most useful where excessive rotation of the thoracic spine is best avoided.

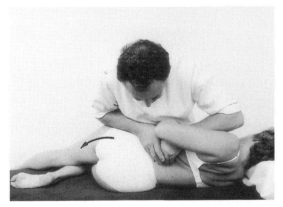

13.46 ▲ Thrust into sidebending combined lever and thrust The normal position of the patient's legs for HVT (high velocity thrust) techniques is reversed in that the upper leg is straight. This will introduce a sidebending toward the table and you can apply forces to emphasize this fact. The final thrust uses rotation and flexion or extension as necessary but will be primarily into rotation.

Tips: Most useful in cases where the sidebending force is desired to open an inter-vertebral foramen and possibly decompress a nerve root.

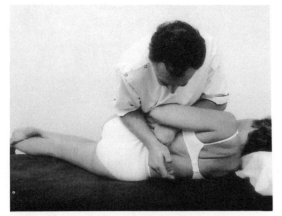

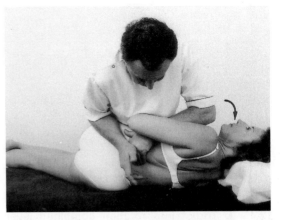

13.48 ▲ Thrust into extension combined lever and thrust sidelying Pull the lumbar spine into extension with your stabilizing hand and then while maintaining this vector perform the thrust into rotation and compression, avoiding flexion. If it is desired to gap the facet nearer the table, this is possible with the following vectors. Extension is maintained and a sidebending force is applied away from the table and then a compression thrust is used.

Tips: Most useful in patients who have very tight fascia, as their superficial posterior tissues will come on tension too early in flexion and prevent the technique reaching the facet joints. Paradoxically this is also effective in some very flexible patients where extension will produce an easier localization than flexion. This is because they automatically fall into extension and, rather than trying to fight this, the extension can be used as one of the components of the technique. The ability to gap the lower facet is very useful where there is nerve root impingement, as rotation, with the patient lying with the painful side uppermost, may be impossible.

13.49 ▲ Thrust using combined lever and thrust with patient assistance Focus forces in the usual way to the lumbo-sacral facet and then ask the patient to turn her head to look over her shoulder. This will often cause the barrier sense in the joint to be enhanced which may aid the thrust.

Tips: Most useful in patients who are very flexible where it is difficult to produce an accurate focus. It is also a useful distraction for patients who find it very difficult to relax. **Extra considerations:** Try asking the patient to look toward the table – this will have the effect of slackening the levers.

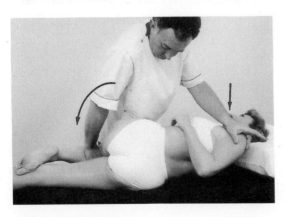

13.50 ◀ Thrust combined lever and thrust sidelying Fix behind the patient's knee and against the upper shoulder and apply a rotary force to the lumbar spine. The patient's body is rocked back and forth until a sense of focusing of forces is produced. The thrust is applied with a short amplitude, high velocity force toward the floor with the knee hand. Although this hold can be a very generalized manipulation, some operators find it is possible to be very specific to a particular segment. The tendency, however, may be for any relatively hypermobile segments to gap leaving the restricted ones unaffected.

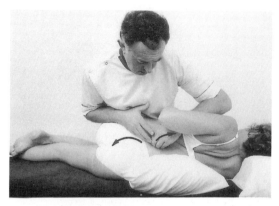

13.51 ▲ Thrust into sidebending combined lever and thrust sidelying Place a pillow under the patient's side which will produce sidebending toward the table. Accumulate the forces at the target segment and apply the final thrust directly into sidebending by pulling up on the spinous process with the fixing hand and thrusting toward the feet with the other.

Tips: Most useful where there may be nerve root pressure or foraminal encroachment and it is desired to open the foramen during the technique. Some treatment tables have moveable sections capable of producing the initial positioning rather than needing to use a pillow.

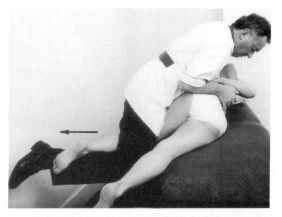

13.53 ▲ Thrust using sciatic stretch sidelying This hold uses similar principles to photograph 13.52 except that you hook your leg around the patient's foot. At the time of thrust you can straighten your leg to increase the traction component through the patient's leg. This clearly has disadvantages, as you are standing on one leg, but is sometimes a useful technique. It is often possible to produce a force specific to the sacro-iliac with this hold.

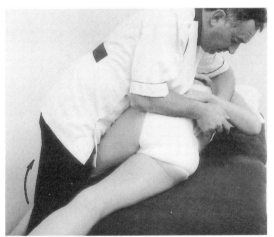

13.52 ▲ Thrust using sciatic stretch sidelying Sandwich the patient's leg between your thighs and after accumulating tension at the facet joint flex the thigh until sciatic stretch begins. Apply the thrust into rotation while maintaining the sciatic stretch. This can be useful in cases of long-term sciatica where it may be possible to break some adhesions around the nerve root. Great care must be taken not to over-stretch the nerve and traumatize it. Some adhesions will be stronger than the normal tissues, and if this is the case, damage can occur if excess force is used.

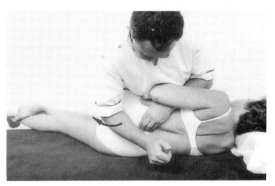

13.54 ▲ Thrust into flexion using minimal lever and thrust sidelying Compress the lateral wall of the thorax into the table with the stabilizing hand. Apply a compressive force directly over the sacrum with the other and then the thrust is performed as a short, sharp flick into flexion of the sacrum to specifically gap the lumbo-sacral facets.

Tips: Most useful in cases of acute spasm where any torsion is best avoided. **Extra considerations**: This is an extremely difficult technique to perform effectively. However, it is well worth the effort of practising it, as it is then possible to manipulate cases where most other techniques would be too painful due to the leverages necessary.

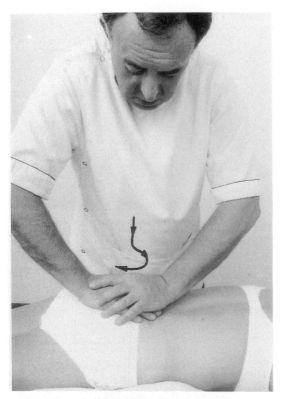

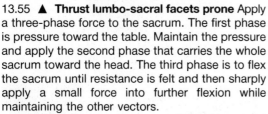

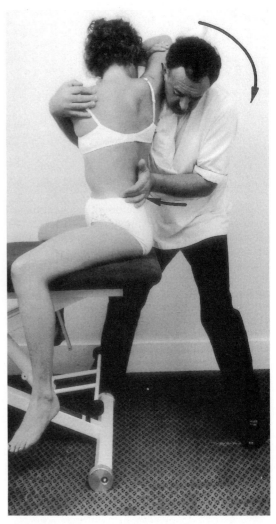

13.55 ▲ Thrust lumbo-sacral facets prone Apply a three-phase force to the sacrum. The first phase is pressure toward the table. Maintain the pressure and apply the second phase that carries the whole sacrum toward the head. The third phase is to flex the sacrum until resistance is felt and then sharply apply a small force into further flexion while maintaining the other vectors.

Tips: Most useful where specific lumbo-sacral gapping is required without spinal torsion. Least useful in patients where prone lying is a problem for any reason. Try adding a sidebending or rotation vector to direct the forces more specifically to one side or the other.

13.56 ► Thrust lumbo-sacral supine Hold the pelvis firmly down onto your hand, cupping the sacrum, and apply a traction force to the sacrum until some sense of resistance is achieved. Flex the distal interphalangeal joints of your sacral hand to pull effectively toward the feet with the fingers. Then use a short, sharp tug on the sacrum to specifically gap the lumbo-sacral facets.

Tips: Most useful in heavy or pregnant patients where torsional manipulation would be a problem.
Extra considerations: Try varying the hip flexion and initial sidebending position of the patient as well as the phase of respiration.

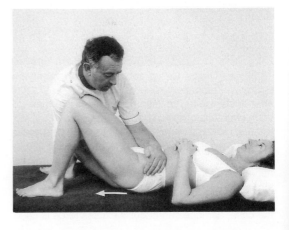

13.57 ◄ (see facing page, top right) **Thrust into rotation combined lever and thrust sitting** The patient sits astride the table to help stabilize the pelvis and places her folded arms over the operator's padded shoulder. Keep the patient's head vertically over her pelvis throughout. Introduce sidebending of the spine away from you and then, while maintaining this, rotate the spine until tension accumulates under your hand applied to the spinous processes. You and the patient turn as a unit and the thrust is performed during this turn by the spinal hand accelerating slightly into rotation.

Tips: Most useful in large heavy patients where their weight in compression on the spine assists the technique. Least useful where the sitting astride position may be a problem. **Extra considerations**: Try varying the compressive force forward toward you to minimize the rotation element. Do not lose the sidebending when applying the rotation or the focus of tension will be lost, and strain can occur at the sacro-iliac joints.

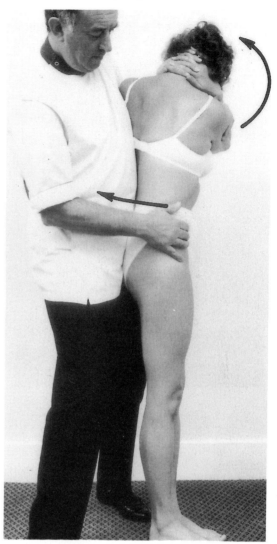

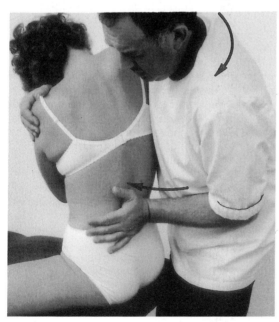

13.58 ▲ **Thrust into rotation combined lever and thrust sitting** This shows an alternative hold for the same technique as photograph 13.57. It may be more useful in large subjects where you may prefer to avoid taking the weight through your shoulder. This technique may be useful where no treatment table is available as it can be performed on a chair with the patient sitting astride the chair.

Tips: Keep the patient's head vertically over the sacrum throughout the technique.

13.59 ▲ **Thrust into rotation combined lever and thrust standing** Fix the sacrum with your hip on the forward leg and rotate the patient to that side with your hand interlaced between the patient's clasped hands. Your other hand holds back on the ilium and then you sidebend the patient toward your fixing hand. When tension accumulates, sharply increase the pull with both hands.

Tips: Most useful in flexible subjects where the slight pull of psoas in this position will help limit spinal movement and aid focusing the forces. This technique may be useful where no treatment table is available.

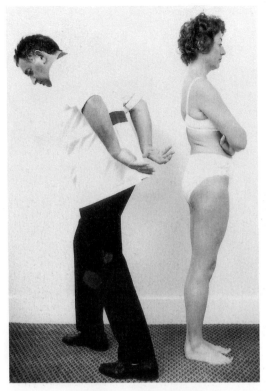

13.60 ◄ Vertical adjustment position standing
This shows the most common hold used where the operator is cupping his hands to clasp the patient's folded arms by the elbows. Note that one foot of the operator is in front of the other and that although he is flexed from the hips his spine is relatively straight.

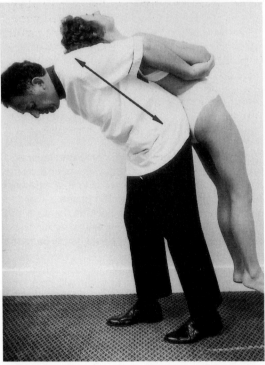

13.61 ◄ Vertical adjustment standing The hold shown in photograph 13.60 is applied and the patient is lifted so that your sacrum fits into her lumbar spine. Maintain firm compression of the patient's back against yours. You rise onto your toes and the adjustment is performed by dropping to your heels and firming your grip at the same moment. Your knees should never fully extend.

Tips: Ensure that the patient can extend her lumbar spine before performing this technique or it is likely to produce a lot of pain, as she will be in quite a considerable amount of extension at completion. Most useful where there is a vertical compressive component to any dysfunction such as disc herniation or overriding of facets. It is also useful in heavy patients where some element of traction can be very beneficial. This technique can often undo fixations that rotary techniques will leave partly unresolved and is usually best applied after rotary techniques. Least useful when the operator is shorter than the patient unless he stands on a suitable platform or step. **Extra considerations**: It is important that the operator pulls firmly through the elbows toward himself to add a compressive element. This helps to limit upper lumbar movement and increases friction so that the lifting force is less of a strain. The movement in the technique is synonymous with shaking the feathers down in a pillow. This technique would appear to be quite a strain on the operator but if performed properly the weight is taken mostly on his sacrum. There is not necessarily a big vertical compressive force on the operator's spine. With practice small amounts of sidebending and rotation can be used to focus the forces to particular locations within the lumbar spine.

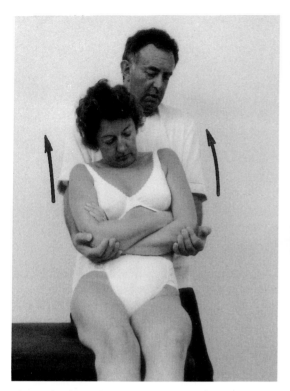

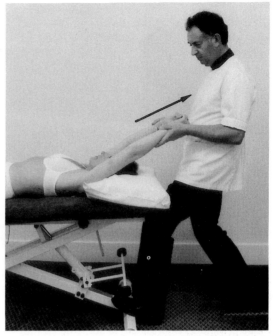

13.62 ▲ **Vertical adjustment sitting** Lift the torso of the patient through the folded arms, possibly using a pillow in the lumbar lordosis as a fulcrum. The adjustive force is a short sharp lift at the end of the accumulation of tension. There are several other hand holds for this procedure that may be tried. You could have the patient clasp the hands behind her neck. The patient could grip opposite shoulders, or she could be clasped around the lower thorax.

Tips: Most useful in small, light patients and where a narrow table is available so that the operator can bring the patient close to him. **Extra considerations**: Small elements of sidebending and rotation can be introduced by pulling differentially on the elbows or by the patient crossing the ankles or knees.

13.63 ▲ **Adjustive traction supine** Clasp above the patient's wrists and apply a steady pull until force is felt to accumulate at the lumbo-sacral joint. This is confirmed by watching the pelvis tilt. Keep the arms at approximately 30° from the horizontal. Apply a short, sharp tug through the patient's arms without releasing any of the tension produced.

Tips: Most useful in very tall subjects where a standing adjustment may be difficult. Least useful in the presence of any shoulder dysfunction that may be irritated by the traction force. It is essential to pre-load with the initial traction or the force will be dissipated before it reaches the lumbo-sacral.

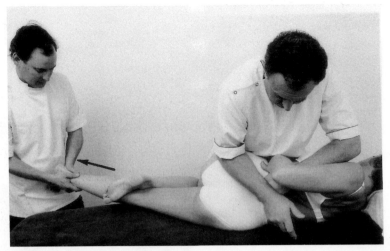

13.64 ▲ Thrust sidelying using second operator Apply forces in the normal way to focus to a particular joint. The second operator applies a slowly increasing traction force through the ankle until you tell him to stop. You will be able to do this as you should feel an enhancement of localization during this traction component. The thrust can then be performed while the traction is maintained.

Tips: Most useful in very flexible subjects where it is difficult to accumulate tension unaided. This is also a useful method where there is some nerve root impingement as the traction may allow a rotary force to reach the facet while the foramen is being opened slightly. **Extra considerations:** The second operator, with a minimum of practice, will also be able to feel tension accumulating as the levers are applied.

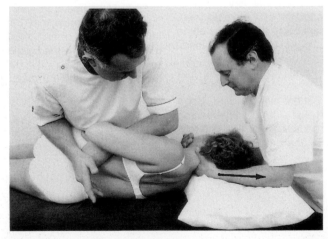

13.65 ▲ Thrust sidelying using second operator This technique uses exactly the same principles as those in photograph 13.64, except the second operator is applying traction to the neck until the required tension is felt by the first operator.

Tips: With a third operator this technique can be combined with the previous technique in photograph 13.64 if even more traction is required.

13.66 ▶ **Thrust sidelying two operator technique**
The patient is in a semi-Simms position and the first operator has lifted the patient's flexed knees while pushing toward the floor with the heel of his hand applied to the spinous processes. The second operator rests his thorax on the patient's scapula and while applying traction through the patient's wrist, is fixing under the spinous processes with his other hand. The forces are accumulated by the contra-rotation of the upper part of the patient's body toward the table and the lower part away. The thrust is performed by the second operator fixing while the first operator presses down on the spinous processes and sharply lifts the patient's knees toward the ceiling. Varied angles of hip flexion in the patient will direct the force higher or lower in the lumbar spine. It is critical to keep the patient's hips flexed throughout or the tension is very easily lost.

Tips: See photograph 13.67 for clarification of hand positions. Most useful where conventional rotary techniques are ineffective as this technique works on the principle of backward rotation of the lower component that will sometimes break fixation in a way not previously achieved. Least useful in very heavy patients where the strain on the operator lifting the legs may be too great. **Extra considerations**: This technique needs some practice to achieve appropriate coordination between operators.

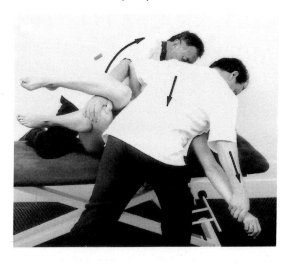

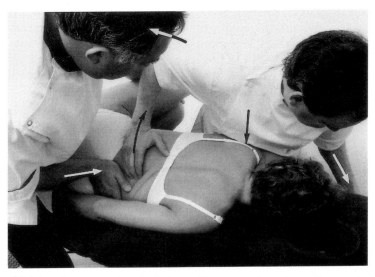

13.67 ▲ **Thrust sidelying two operator technique** The rear view shown here of photograph 13.66 clarifies the hand hold and patient position.

There are probably more differences of opinion amongst osteopaths as to how to deal with dysfunction of the sacro-iliac articulations than for any other area of the body. There are multiple theories of movement directions and type of lesioning. I have attempted to simplify the issue into the two main types of lesioning positions of anterior and posterior rotation. This is not to say that other types of dysfunction do not occur, but to say that they seem to be fairly rare. Treating the sacro-iliac joint as a rotary articulation will deal with the vast proportion of joint problems of a mechanical nature without excessive complication and therefore uncertainty. It is possible for the sacrum itself to become distorted, as in life it is a somewhat flexible structure. It can produce apparent sacro-iliac dysfunction which is, in fact, due to sacral torsion. Some techniques for addressing this problem are included in this section. Others are more appropriate when considered with the lumbar spine, as the sacrum can sometimes be classed as a vertebral, midline structure. The principles of treatment, therefore, are those of spinal joints.

The sacro-iliac, or to be more accurate the ilio-sacral articulations have a very limited range of mobility. However, that mobility is often very easily induced, and therefore it is extremely easy to 'overlock' when trying to produce a specific force. Then, as no movement can be felt, even more force is used and pain, trauma and ineffective technique is the result. The sacro-iliac articulations respond far better to delicate, careful applications of force in very specific directions.

Special precautions include the elimination of pathological states in the bones themselves, and the possibility of inflammatory disorders. If the sacro-iliac dysfunction is recurrent the possibility of it being part of a postural compensation must be considered. Excessive recurrence and a sense of precariousness should alert the practitioner to the possibility of hypermobility. This, nevertheless, may manifest as recurrent locking.

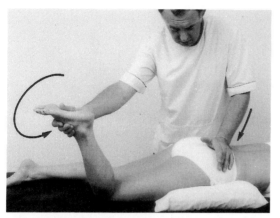

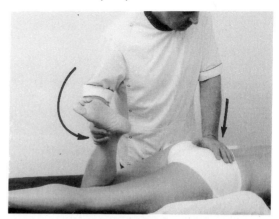

14.1 ▲ Articulation of sacro-iliac further side prone Find the approximate angle of the joint plane using your cephalic hand, and apply gentle pressure. The other hand takes the leg through a circumduction movement until a sense of potential for mobility is perceived through the applied hand. At this point of stressing the joint, a pressure along the line of joint movement is applied. The arc of movement in the circumducting leg when a sense of resistance from the sacro-iliac is reached will vary slightly from person to person. It is sometimes difficult to isolate the sacro-iliac movement from hip movement in this hold.

Tips: Most useful in patients who are not too acute and can lie prone. Least useful in acute cases, or in the presence of any lumbar disc syndrome where the position may be a problem. May be difficult in very large patients to reach across this far for small operators. **Extra considerations**: It is very easy to apply too much pressure with the cephalic hand, feel nothing, and therefore, press even harder. If a sense of movement cannot be felt, change angle or reduce pressure; do not increase force. Use of a pillow under the abdomen can aid comfort and finding the best angle for the joint.

14.2 ▲ Sacro-iliac articulation nearer side prone Operator applies gentle pressure along perceived plane of joint with cephalic hand and then performs a circumduction movement with other hand controlling leg. As sense of tension accumulates in sacro-iliac joint, firmer pressure is applied to ilium along joint plane to mobilize joint. The arc of movement within the circumduction where the joint play will be felt varies slightly with different patients.

Tips: Most useful in larger patients where reaching across may be a problem when working on the other side. Least useful if the table is not adjustable, and it is not possible to get the angle of the articulating arm vertical. Not comfortable in acute patients where lying prone is a problem, or in the presence of lumbar disc lesions where extension may be painful. **Extra considerations**: Use of a pillow under the abdomen will often make the correct joint plane accessible.

14.3 ◄ Sacro-iliac articulation anteriorly side-lying The patient is put into some rotation of the spine, and the upper leg flexed to a comfortable position. The operator firmly grasps the ilium between his own forearm, abdomen and other hand. A rocking back and forward along the plane of the joint can be applied. Sufficient rotation must be applied to obliterate most of the lumbar movement, as otherwise the rocking action will simply produce flexion and extension of the lumbar area.

Tips: Most useful in patients who cannot lie prone such as pregnant women, and acute lumbar pain syndromes. Least useful in very flexible subject where the lumbar movement tends to absorb the forces. **Extra considerations**: Harmonic technique can be performed in this position if the upper part of the body is made to oscillate, and if the ilium is held very firmly, an anterior gapping can be applied if the operator flexes his own knees and holds the pelvis in the same plane. This hold can also be used for lumbar sidebending and several other directions of articulation with a little thought.

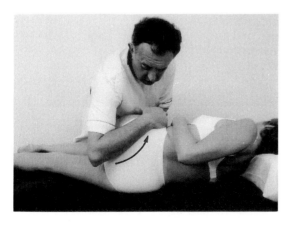

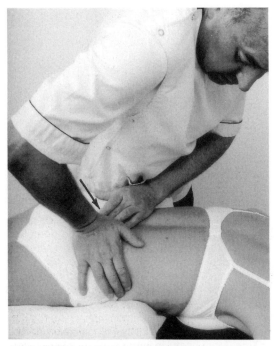

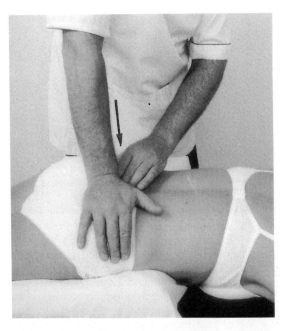

14.4 ▲ Sacro-iliac springing prone This is as much a testing hold as it is a treatment technique. The operator is palpating in the sulcus of the sacro-iliac joint on the opposite side, and the other hand is applying a force vertically towards the table. If movement is felt in the sacro-iliac it must be hypermobile, as the plane of the joint is far more medial to lateral than vertical. Rotary movement of the lumbar spine is sensed with this pressure also, and if excessive gives a clue as to possible cause of dysfunction states.

Tips: The pressure must be applied carefully over the posterior superior iliac spine as otherwise only soft tissue mobility will be sensed. Least useful in acute subjects where lying prone is a problem. **Extra considerations**: This hold develops into the next one illustrated as a means of sensing from where movement is being induced.

14.6 ► Harmonic technique pelvis supine Operator cups anterior superior iliac spines in the palms of both hands and initiates an oscillatory movement into rotation of the pelvis. This can be diagnostic as well as therapeutic, as differences in rotary capability of the pelvis on the lumbar spine can be sensed.

Tips: A pillow behind the knee may change the angle of the pelvis and make movement easier. Least useful in cases of sacro-iliac hypermobility as this pressure may induce pain in the joint concerned. This is in itself diagnostic.

14.5 ▲ Sacro-iliac articulation and springing prone This illustration directly follows on from the previous one. The springing hand has gradually changed direction until the plane of the joint has been sensed, and the combined sense of proprioceptive awareness with the springing hand and tactile sensing with the other hand allows the optimum direction of movement to be used. If the best direction for joint play cannot be sensed, use less force not more as the applied weight of the hands may have obliterated the free play, and more pressure will only rotate the lumbar spine and not have any more effect on the sacro-iliac joint.

Tips: Gradually moving the shoulder of the springing hand through a circle will allow the optimum direction of force to be assessed. A pillow under the abdomen may help to reduce the lumbar lordosis, and make the sacro-iliac joint more accessible. Least useful in acute lumbar pain syndromes where lying prone may be a problem.

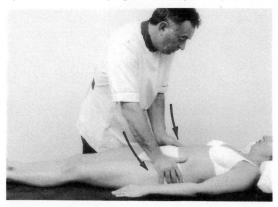

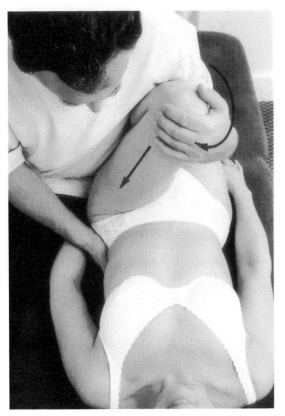

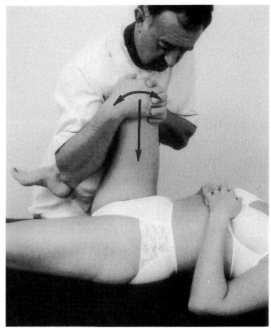

14.7 ▲ **Sacro-iliac articulation supine** The fingers of the palpating hand are placed so that the tips are in the sulcus of the joint and while gentle downward pressure is applied toward the table the knee is taken through a circular movement to mobilize the joint.

Tips: Excessive pressure toward the table should be avoided as this will obliterate joint movement. Within the arc of circumduction of the knee, a point of resistance will be felt and this can be emphasized with increased downward pressure at that time to optimize the mobilizing force. Most useful where patient cannot lie prone for any reason. Least useful in the presence of osteoarthrosis in the hip or knee.

14.8 ▲ **Sacro-iliac thrust into anterior direction supine** The optimum direction of the joint is found and then a downward pressure is applied with some internal rotation of the hip to put the hip capsule on some tension. The knee will be approximately over the midline of the body in most cases. Small adjustments of flexion and extension of the hip will be necessary to find the optimum, and then a short sharp downward force is applied to direct the ilium into an anterior rotation direction. At first this may seem to be doing the opposite of what is intended, but it should be remembered that the sacro-iliac joint is superior to the hip, and therefore when a pressure is applied towards the table, the ilium will be rotated forward, not backward. If, however, the hip is taken further into flexion, the ilium will be rotated backward.

Tips: Very accurate joint plane sense is required for this technique, and it may be necessary to feel this with fingers in the sulcus of the joint first, and then remove the hand and apply it to the knee. Most useful in simple uncomplicated sacro-iliac dysfunction in fairly stiff subjects where the force will not be dissipated into the lumbar spine. Least useful in cases where there is osteo-arthrosis of the hip and this pressure will be uncomfortable or impossible.
Extra considerations: May be repeated several times as a springing rather than a specific thrust if correct barrier sense cannot be found.

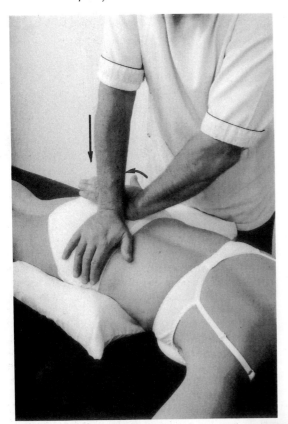

14.9 ◄ Sacro-iliac thrust and articulation anteriorly prone The plane of the joint has been found with the caudal hand and while maintaining this direction of force, the operator applies the other hand to the sacrum near to the other sacro-iliac joint. The sacral hand becomes a fixing hand, and the sacro-iliac can be mobilized with springing into an anterior direction. If a crisp barrier is sensed, a thrust can be applied, but, owing to the small range of movement of the joint, this will be a very short amplitude.

Tips: The sacral hand can be placed in such a way to tip the sacrum into flexion, rotation or sidebending to optimize the tension at the sacro-iliac joint. Different phases of breathing can be used as felt appropriate. If the thrust is applied when the patient is holding a full breath in, the pelvis will become firmer, and the thrust may be easier. In a very tight subject, exhalation may be more useful. Most useful in uncomplicated sub-acute or chronic cases. Least useful in acute cases or where the patient may find lying prone a problem.

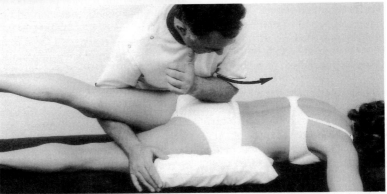

14.10 ▲ Thrust sacro-iliac anteriorly prone The medial aspect of the elbow is applied over the posterior superior iliac spine and along the crest of the ilium. The other hand levers against the table and the other thigh, to produce an anterior rotation movement of the ilium. Adjustments will be necessary of the adduction and extension of the thigh to produce the optimum tension in the joint. At the point of accumulation of forces, the thrust is applied along the crest of the ilium.

Tips: Most useful in small patients, and where there is no problem lying prone. Least useful in acute cases where the prone position may be a problem. **Extra considerations:** Care must be taken not to hyperextend the lumbar spine and thus cause pain. In this respect keeping the anterior of the pelvis on the table is a help. If the correct tension sense does not accumulate, reduce tension rather than increase it, as it is very easy to over-lock. Different phases of respiration may help to produce the best barrier.

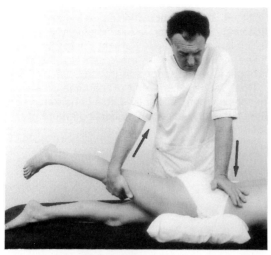

14.11 ▲ **Thrust sacro-iliac anteriorly prone** Pressure is applied to the posterior superior iliac spine of the opposite ilium in the direction of the joint. The other hand lifts the thigh into extension and some adduction of the hip until tension accumulates at the sacro-iliac. Varied rotation of the hip will aid the build-up of tension. The thrust is applied with the hand on the ilium, not the lifting hand.

Tips: Most useful in chronic cases where fixation is liable to be more crisp and, therefore, more easy to release. Least useful in acute cases where lying prone may be a problem or where the patient is very heavy, making lifting of the leg a problem. **Extra considerations**: Keep the pelvis firmly applied to the table as otherwise hyperextension of the lumbar spine can occur. A pillow under the abdomen may assist patient comfort. Different phases of breathing will often assist in accumulation of optimum tension.

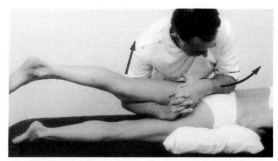

14.12 ▲ **Thrust sacro-iliac anteriorly prone** The thrusting hand is applied behind the posterior superior iliac spine, and the fingers of the other hand interlock with the thrusting hand so that the leg can be lifted until tension is felt to accumulate. Adduction of the leg will help the build-up of tension.

Tips: Most useful in patients who are fairly tight as tension will accumulate more easily. Least useful where there is any hip dysfunction or where extension of the lumbar spine is going to be a problem. **Extra considerations**: If the operator is small, the position may be difficult, as the leg-lifting hand is drawing the operator toward the feet of the patient, and thus reducing the force available at the sacro-iliac. Use of a pillow under the abdomen can be useful to avoid hyperextension of the lumbar spine.

14.13 ◄ **Thrust/articulation sacro-iliac anteriorly supine** The patient has firmly clasped the other thigh into flexion to lock the lumbar spine. The operator has fixed the patient's leg between his thighs and is assisting the patient in holding the other leg in flexion. He applies a downward force to the knee so that the sacro-iliac is torsioned forward on the sacrum. If tension is sufficient, a thrust can be applied toward the table.

Tips: Most useful in young and fairly fit patients as the position can be rather extreme. The position of extreme flexion of the other hip puts the lumbar spine in a flexed position which can help to obliterate movement which may be useful. Least useful if there is any hip disorder. **Extra considerations**: A useful fulcrum can be made if the patient is capable of lying with the sacrum on the edge of the table. This position is also a differential test of lumbar and sacro-iliac dysfunction. If pain is reproduced in this position, as the lumbar spine is not involved in the movement, it can be reasonably assumed that the sacro-iliac is the source of the symptoms. If pain gets much worse as the patient releases the other knee, there is a good chance that it is movement of the lumbar spine which is implicated in the pain syndrome.

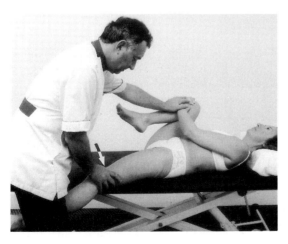

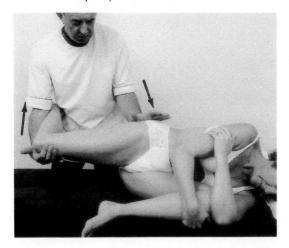

14.15 ▶ Thrust using leg tug sacro-iliac anteriorly supine The hand hold is shown before being applied to the foot. Note that one hand is supinated and the other pronated. The thumb of the pronated hand is interposed between the third and fourth fingers of the other hand. This has the advantage that as the operator leans back, without actively gripping, the hold becomes tighter automatically.

Tips: Experimentation will reveal which is the most comfortable way to interlock the hands.

14.16 ▶ Thrust anteriorly sacro-iliac using leg tug supine The hold shown in photograph 14.15 is applied and the lower extremity is taken into some flexion to clear the other leg as adduction is applied. Apply adduction and internal rotation of the hip until the fascia lata and hip capsule, respectively, are on tension. A preliminary traction force is used until tension is felt to accumulate in the sacro-iliac and then without releasing the tension a sharp longitudinal tug completes the thrust.

Tips: Least useful where there is any knee or hip dysfunction or in very lax subjects where the force will be dissipated. **Extra considerations**: Greater efficiency is sometimes achieved if the patient is asked to hold their breath or to cough coincident with the thrust. Try bracing the patient's other leg on the table against the operator's thigh.

14.14 ◀ Thrust/articulation sacro-iliac anteriorly sidelying This position is fundamentally the same as photograph 14.13 except that the leg has been flexed at the knee. The movement is now much stronger as the quadriceps is put on tension earlier.

Tips: Varying the flexion of the knee can focus the tension more efficiently. **Extra considerations**: The same implications of the testing nature of this position apply as for photograph 13.15.

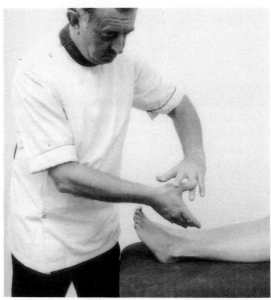

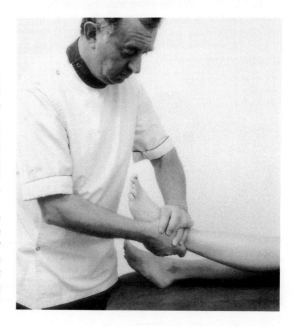

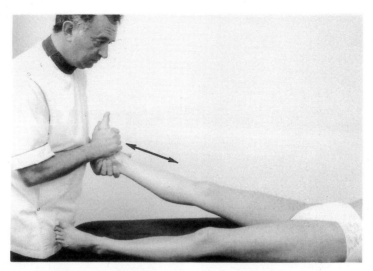

14.17 ▲ Harmonic technique for sacro-iliac This technique shows longitudinal harmonic technique to the pelvis and particularly the sacro-iliac.

Tips: Refer to earlier section relating to harmonic technique.

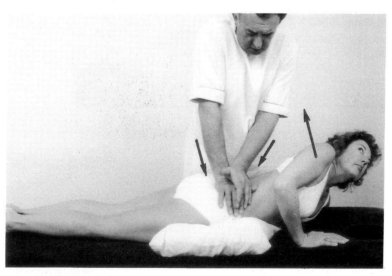

14.18 ▲ Thrust sacro-iliac anteriorly prone Operator focuses forces applied to posterior superior iliac spine along the plane of the joint and fixes pelvis to the table. Patient performs a one-handed push up and as tension accumulates at the joint, operator applies a very short amplitude thrust.

Tips: Most useful in very mobile subjects where the use of active muscle contraction in the patient helps reduce spinal mobility. **Extra considerations**: Try adjusting initial sidebending to find the optimum tension.

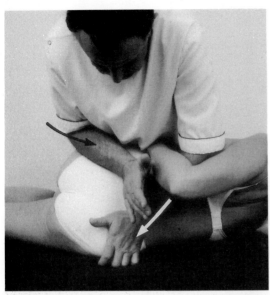

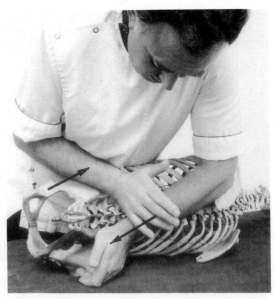

14.19 ▲ Thrust to sacro-iliac anteriorly sidelying
This is a modified lumbar roll position. The cephalic hand of the operator is pushing towards himself on the posterior superior iliac spine of the ilium on the table. The other hand is applying a rotary force on the pelvis so that the lower sacro-iliac is gapped. Firm compression with both hands is necessary to focus the forces at the target joint. Excessive rotation of the spine must be avoided.

Tips: Most useful where there is a disc syndrome making rotation to the other side difficult. Least useful in very large subjects where it may not be possible to achieve sufficient compressive force.
Extra considerations: With compression maintained, roll the pelvis forward and backward to find the optimum barrier sense.

14.20 ▲ Thrust to sacro-iliac anteriorly sidelying shown on skeleton This photograph may clarify the hand position of photograph 14.19.

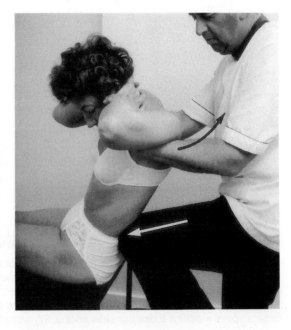

14.21 ▶ Thrust to sacro-iliac anteriorly sitting
The operator's knee pushes firmly forwards against the posterior superior iliac spine. The patient is flexed slightly and rotated down until tension accumulates at the operator's knee. The thrust is a combination of a slight increase of rotation of the patient's body and a forward movement of the knee against the ilium.

Tips: This is a very long lever technique and rarely used; however, there may be some cases where it can be a method of choice, particularly those where it is desired to have the spine vertical, thereby slightly driving the sacrum down between the ilia.

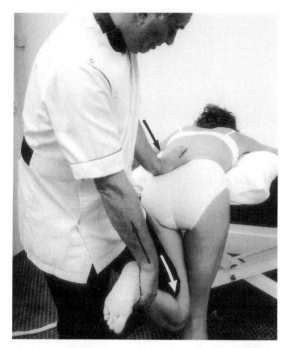

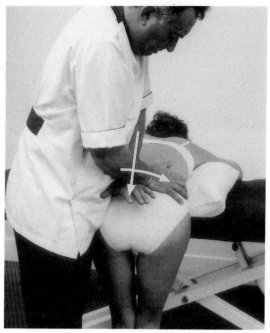

14.22 ▲ **Thrust to sacro-iliac anteriorly part standing** Patient lies across the table keeping the other foot on the floor. The operator applies the heel of his thrusting hand to the posterior superior iliac spine and his knee in the popliteal space of the flexed knee. He pushes down with his knee while pulling up with the hand holding the ankle until tension accumulates at the sacro-iliac. The thrust is mostly a force with his hand but the knee and other hand assist slightly.

Tips: This will be a rarely used manoeuvre but was taught by Andrew Taylor Still. Most useful where lumbar torsion is to be avoided. Least useful where there is any knee dysfunction. **Extra considerations**: The barrier sense will accumulate more easily, in most cases, if the patient holds the breath for the thrust.

14.23 ▲ **Thrust sacro-iliac anteriorly part standing** The patient lies across the table which has been lifted to the height of the patient's pelvis. She flexes her knees slightly so that the anterior superior iliac spines support her weight. Pressure is applied along the plane of the joint with one hand and the other stabilizes the sacrum. The thrust is applied forwards on the posterior superior iliac spine to break fixation of the sacro-iliac furthest from the operator.

Tips: Most useful where it is necessary to avoid torsion of the lumbar spine. Least useful where the patient is elderly and the position may be difficult to attain. **Extra considerations**: The sacrum-stabilizing hand can hold the bone in a variety of directions. It will be necessary to experiment to find the optimum direction which focuses the forces at the sacro-iliac. It will usually be easier to accumulate tension if the patient holds the breath for the thrust.

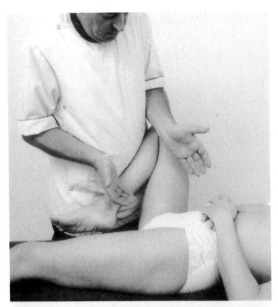

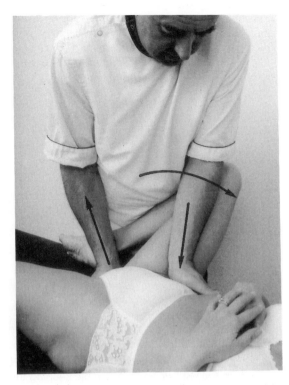

14.24 ▲ Thrust sacro-iliac posteriorly supine
This photograph shows the hand hold and patient positioning for this technique. The palm of the cephalic hand will be applied with the anterior superior iliac spine. The other hand will be placed under the ischial tuberosity and the flexed knee and hip are positioned across the operator's abdomen.

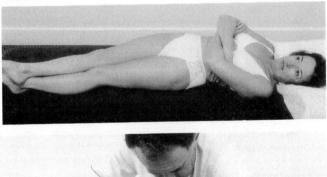

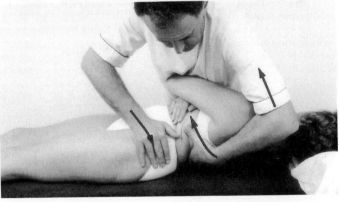

14.25 ◄ (see facing page, top right) **Thrust/ articulation sacro-iliac posteriorly supine** The hold shown in the previous photograph is applied and the operator is pushing the thigh into abduction with his elbow. The thrust is performed as a combination of pushing back with one hand, pulling up with the other and a bending of the knees to further abduct and flex the hip. This will drive the ilium back on the sacrum.

Tips: Most useful in patients with a fairly rigid lumbar spine where the force will focus more easily in the sacro-iliac. Least useful in the presence of any hip dysfunction. **Extra considerations**: Barrier sense may accumulate more easily if the patient holds the breath at the time of the thrust.

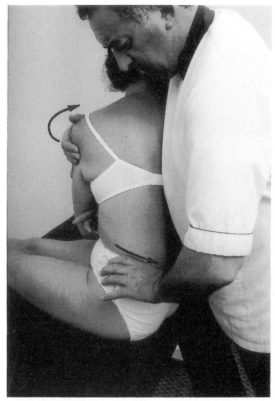

14.26 ◄ (see facing page) **Thrust position sacro-iliac posteriorly supine** The patient is positioned into sufficient initial sidebending so that when the operator applies the other components, the sidebending may reduce, but will not be completely lost.

14.27 ◄ (see facing page) **Thrust sacro-iliac posteriorly supine** The so-called 'Chicago' technique has been applied with the operator's cephalic hand maintaining sidebending and producing a rotation of the patient's torso towards him. His other hand holds the ilium against the table, and as tension accumulates in the sacro-iliac a short amplitude thrust is applied to the anterior superior iliac spine.

Tips: Initial positioning of the patient is critical with this technique. The sidebending must not be lost or the force will dissipate higher in the spine. The direction of force applied to the ilium will govern whether the technique focuses at the sacro-iliac or the lumbo-sacral. If the thrust is applied with the cephalic hand, it will tend to focus forces on the thoraco-lumbar junction. It may be necessary to experiment to find the optimum. Most operators find that tension accumulates best if the patient's leg on the operator's side is crossed over the other one, but sometimes the opposite is true.

Tips: Least useful for small operators working on large patients where it may be impossible to reach sufficiently well to accumulate the correct tension.

14.28 ▲ **Thrust sacro-iliac posteriorly sitting** The patient has folded her arms and the operator has rotated her whole torso down to the sacrum. He holds back on the ilium with index finger and thumb. He applies a rotary force away from the ilium with the other hand and as tension accumulates he thrusts backwards on the ilium. Side-bending toward the thrust side is maintained at all times to help focus the forces as otherwise they will dissipate through the lumbar spine.

Tips: Most useful in tight subjects who have no major spinal dysfunction. Least useful in very tall subjects where it will be difficult to control the levers. **Extra considerations**: It may sometimes aid the technique if the patient sits astride the table.

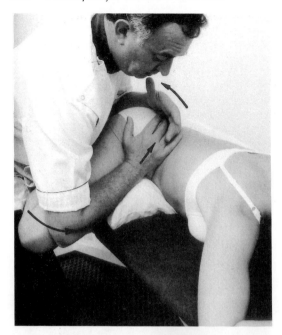

14.29 ◄ Thrust/articulation sacro-iliac posteriorly prone The operator has abducted and flexed the patient's hip and knee and the tibia is resting on his own flexed thighs. He fixes the whole lower extremity between his forearm and abdomen and cups the anterior superior iliac spine in the palm of his thrusting hand. The wrist of his other hand has applied pressure behind the ischial tuberosity and the two hands together pull the ilium backwards. The thrust is applied with a combination of operator's hands and body.

Tips: Least useful where the patient may find prone lying a problem. **Extra considerations**: It is important to hold the ilium and pelvis against the table as abduction is applied to the hip, as otherwise rotation occurs into the lumbar spine and the force will not accumulate at the sacro-iliac.

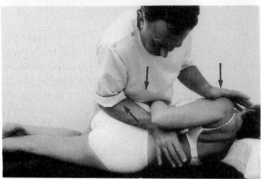

14.30 ▲ Thrust sacro-iliac posteriorly sidelying This is a modified lumbar roll position. The operator has applied only a small amount of rotation to the thorax and lumbar spine but has substituted compression toward the table, through the shoulder. The thrusting forearm is placed behind the ilium and the elbow pushes the ischial tuberosity towards himself to rotate the ilium backwards. The thrust is applied with a compression force from the operator's body at the same time as an adduction and external rotation of his arm applied to the ilium.

Tips: Excessive rotation of the lumbar spine will dissipate the force up to the thoraco-lumbar junction; hence the use of compression. A gentle oscillatory rolling of the whole patient will enhance the ability to find the optimum thrust plane. Least useful in very flexible subjects where the thrust will merely produce lumbar flexion.

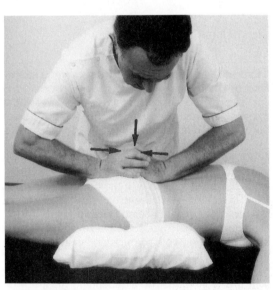

14.31 ▲ Thrust to sacrum prone This shows a recoil technique where the operator has applied a slight compressive force to the sacrum toward the table and then squeezes the sacrum between both hands to slightly buckle it. The technique is performed with the release of tension allowing the natural recoil of the bone to act as the mobilizing force. This may need to be repeated two or three times.

Tips: Most useful where despite ilio-sacral gapping, some dysfunction remains which may be due to intra-sacral distortion. **Extra considerations**: It may be found that compressing the sacrum more on one side than the other will produce a more specific result.

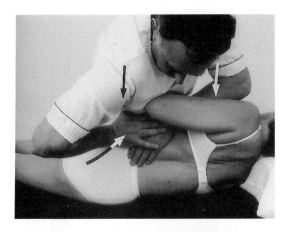

14.32 ◄ Thrust to sacrum sidelying This is a modified lumbar roll position. The operator has applied compression to the pelvis and the thorax to reduce the range of rotation necessary to reach the sacrum. The thrust is a combination of an increased compressive force on the ilium with the operator's chest at the same time as the heel of his hand drives the sacrum forwards.

Tips: Most useful where torsion of the sacrum rather than the ilium is the prime element in the dysfunction. Least useful in very flexible or very large subjects. **Extra considerations**: The direction of the sacral thrust can vary according to the optimum sense of barrier accumulation.

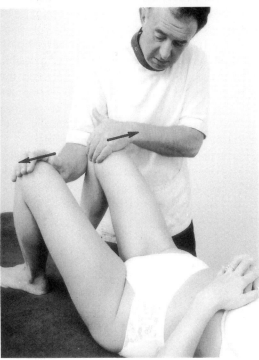

14.33 ▲ Thrust to symphysis pubis supine This is a combined technique where the operator holds the patient's knees apart as she attempts to draw them together. The patient does not use full power but allows him to gradually work the knees further apart until tension accumulates at the joint. He applies a short amplitude thrust into abduction of the thighs while the patient maintains muscle tone.

Tips: Vary the range of hip flexion and knee flexion to find the optimum. Ensure the amplitude of the thrust is very short. Least useful when the patient is very strong and the operator is small.

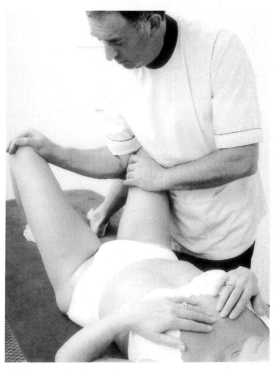

14.34 ▲ Muscle energy technique symphysis pubis supine See earlier section on principles of muscle energy technique.

Tips: Vary the angle of hip flexion and knee flexion to achieve the optimum. This hold only allows an isometric muscle energy technique as the patient presses against the operator's flexed hand and elbow between the knees.

As the glutei are such strong muscles and are in close proximity to the sciatic nerve they may play an important role in production and maintenance of sciatic pain syndromes. Hypertonic glutei can affect posture and prevent normal mechanical relationship of the hips to the rest of the body. There may be a tendency for the hips to rotate outwards and thus upset locomotion, sitting and standing postures. Lumbar origin pain syndromes will often present as tense painful areas in the glutei, piriformis and gamelli, and work on these can be helpful in treatment of such cases.

Particular caution is rarely necessary in working on the glutei except that a Ewing's tumour in the bone or the ilium itself can present as gluteal pain. Due to the sensitive nature of the area, particular care needs to be taken with the treatment here so that no accusations of improper handling can occur. Informing the patient of the purpose or a particular procedure should eliminate this problem.

The coccyx is commonly a site of pain although many cases are due to referred pain from the lumbar spine. It is, however, possible to have a dysfunctional junction between the sacrum and the coccyx. There are techniques that approach the joint through the rectum, but external techniques are generally preferred by patients and operators alike!

Particular precautions include the possibility of fracture if there has been direct trauma, and rare cases of referred pain from the rectum in the presence of a space-occupying lesion.

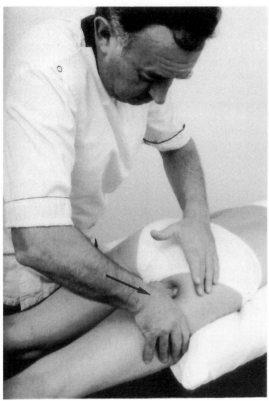

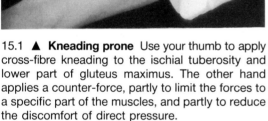

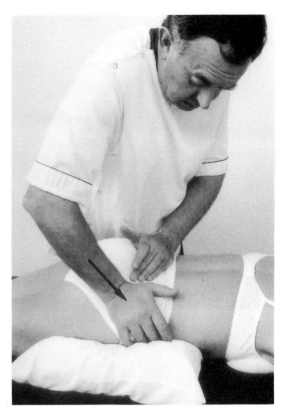

15.1 ▲ **Kneading prone** Use your thumb to apply cross-fibre kneading to the ischial tuberosity and lower part of gluteus maximus. The other hand applies a counter-force, partly to limit the forces to a specific part of the muscles, and partly to reduce the discomfort of direct pressure.

Tips: Most useful in cases of ischial tuberosity bursitis, muscle strains and residual sciatica. Least useful where prone lying might be a problem. **Extra considerations**: The pillow under the abdomen is for patient comfort. Try using varied degrees of abduction in the thigh, or a pillow under the tibia to flex the knee and reduce stretch on the posterior thigh muscles.

15.2 ▲ **Kneading prone** Apply a kneading force to the glutei, gamelli and piriformis on the opposite side of the patient. The other hand monitors the stretch produced, and spreads the effect of the hold to reduce any discomfort.

Tips: Least useful where prone lying may be a problem. Exquisite tender areas will often be found in the glutei in lumbar dysfunction syndromes, and although these are often due to referred pain, they can be maintaining factors. Recovery can be enhanced if these muscles are relaxed to allow freer pelvic movement. **Extra considerations**: The pillow under the abdomen will usually aid patient comfort. Try abducting the leg by varied amounts to find the optimum.

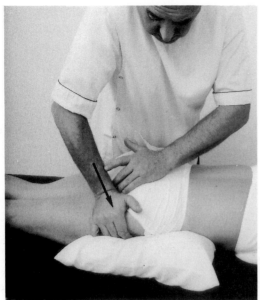

15.3 ◄ Kneading prone Work on the lower part of the glutei and the piriformis while holding back on the belly of the muscle with the other hand, to localize the force. The lateral muscles of the thigh can also be addressed in this position.

Tips: Most useful in cases of residual sciatica where there is a muscular component as a maintaining factor. Least useful where prone lying may be a problem. **Extra considerations**: The pillow under the abdomen will usually aid patient comfort. Try varying the abduction of the thigh to find the optimum for the technique.

15.4 ▼ Inhibition prone Apply a direct pressure over the piriformis with your thumb. Maintain a steady pressure and internally rotate the hip until tension is felt. Inhibition implies a steady pressure, usually while a lever is applied, and a finite time must elapse until a sense of release is attained.

Tips: Most useful in cases of persistent piriformis tension as in some sciaticas. Least useful where prone lying is a problem. **Extra considerations**: Try varying the hip abduction in the initial set-up for the technique. This may be a very uncomfortable procedure, but within about 10–15 seconds the muscle will be felt to relax, often accompanied by an immediate relief of symptoms.

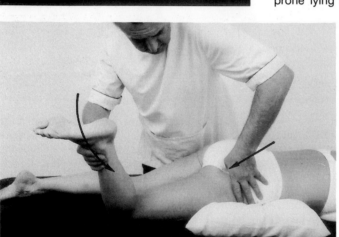

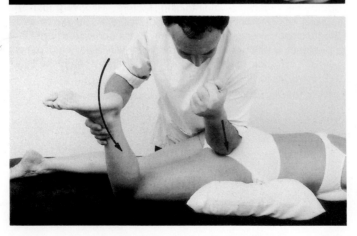

15.5 ◄ Inhibition prone Carefully apply the tip of your elbow to the piriformis while maintaining the internal rotation of the hip with the other hand applied to the ankle.

Tips: Most useful in cases of severe, long-term spasm of piriformis. It is also the method of choice when the operator's thumbs are not strong enough. Least useful where prone lying may be a problem. **Extra considerations**: The pillow under the abdomen is to increase patient comfort. This is clearly a powerful technique, and needs sympathetic care in handling to avoid excessive pain; however, it can be extremely useful.

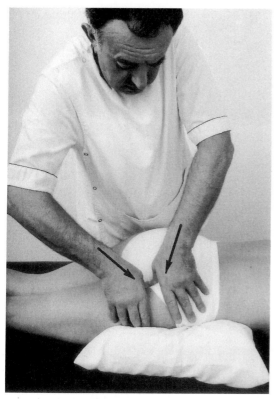

15.6 ▲ Inhibition prone Apply a double thumb pressure to the piriformis with the pads of the thumbs overlaid. This has the advantage over the elbow hold of being a little more gentle, yet very specific.

Tips: Most useful in cases of sciatic nerve irritation where the piriformis is involved, and inhibition alone is required, without stretch. The previous holds for working on piriformis use some longitudinal stretch. Least useful where prone lying is a problem.

15.8 ▶ Articulation of sacro-coccygeal joint prone Internally rotate the hip with varied degrees of knee flexion as suitable for the case. Hold back on the coccyx with the other thumb. The technique is performed with either a pressure on the coccyx, a circumduction of the leg, or both simultaneously.

Tips: Least useful where prone lying is a problem. This hold is more suitable than the one in photograph 15.7 if a gentler procedure is required as it avoids stressing the hip.

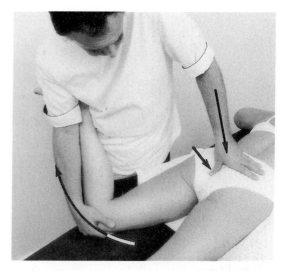

15.7 ▲ Articulation of sacro-coccygeal joint prone Abduct and internally rotate the hip carefully, as this is potentially a very strong hold. Hold back on the coccyx with your thumb. The technique can be performed as a force with either hand, or both simultaneously.

Tips: Least useful where prone lying is a problem. **Extra considerations**: Try asking the patient to temporarily hold the breath to assist in firming up the pelvic floor.

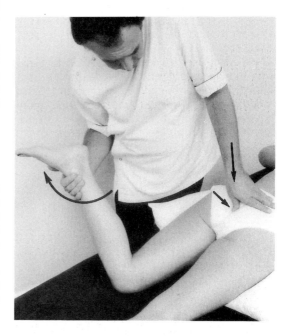

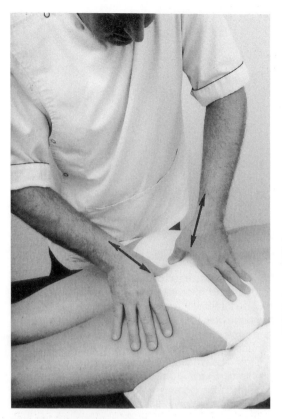

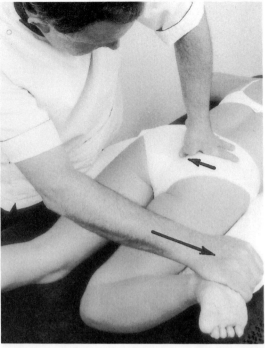

15.9 ▲ Articulation of sacro-coccygeal joint prone
Spring alternately on the sacrum and the coccyx.
Different lateral pressures can be introduced if
required to find the optimum barrier for the
articulation.

Tips: Most useful where it is desired to avoid
using the hip as a lever. Least useful where the
prone lying position may be a problem. **Extra
considerations**: To make the technique more
effective try using patient breath-holding to drive
the pelvic floor down and firm up the area.

**15.10 ▲ Articulation of sacro-coccygeal joint
prone** Hold the coccyx toward yourself while
internally rotating the opposite leg.

Tips: Most useful where one hip has a dysfunction
making it unusable as a lever, so the contralateral
side is used. Least useful where prone lying may be a
problem or where the reach may be too great for a
small operator. **Extra considerations**: Try using
varied degrees of hip abduction to amplify the
technique.

TECHNIQUES FOR THE THORACO-LUMBAR JUNCTION AREA

16

When referring to the thoraco-lumbar region we are encompassing the area from about the tenth thoracic to the second lumbar vertebrae, not just the twelfth thoracic to first lumbar articulations. The term refers to an area rather than a specific segment.

Like all the junctional areas of the spine, there are differences from adjacent areas. As the curves are changing and the stability of one area meets the relative mobility of the other, difficulties occur. From a technique and treatment viewpoint the presence of the autonomic outflow to the coeliac plexus, and the diaphragmatic attachments, further complicate this area. Osteochondrosis is extremely common and often causes the characteristic flexion deformity, premature arthrosis, and stiffening which make the application and choice of technique difficult. As the prostate and uterus drain through their veins into this area, the possibility of secondary meta-static deposits from these sites must always be considered in history, examination and diagnosis.

Excessive torsion of this area in treatment can produce nausea. Poor application of technique and excessive leverage into rotation can lead to sacro-iliac joint strain. Careful consideration of appropriate modifying factors, and greater use of compression rather than rotation can help to avoid this problem.

Techniques for the area can be difficult in extremely mobile young subjects, as it is not easy to isolate the area, but high force should not be used instead of skill.

The area can be considered as part of the lumbar spine, the thoracic spine, or an area in its own right. It should be possible to employ techniques that reach the area without excessive force, but owing to the length of the levers necessary, suitable protection of adjacent areas is important.

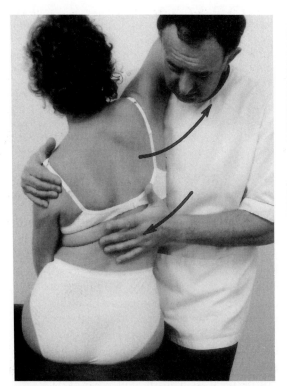

16.1 ▲ Articulation into sidebending sitting The patient sits across the table at one end with one arm over the operator's shoulder. Apply a side-bending force by pulling with one hand while giving a counter-force with the other. Rock from your front to your back foot to produce the desired movement.

Tips: Control of the compression through the fixing hand on the patient's shoulder is critical in this hold. Note that the patient's head remains over her pelvis. The spine is being buckled specifically at the thoraco-lumbar area.

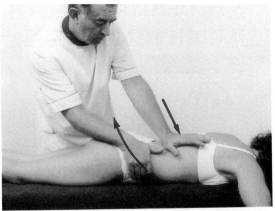

16.2 ▲ Articulation prone Stand below the patient's pelvis and pull up against the anterior superior iliac spine. Fix with the other hand over the transverse processes at the thoraco-lumbar area. If a suitable barrier accumulates, this can be made into a rotation and extension thrust although to avoid pain the amplitude must be kept very small.

Tips: Try placing the patient in some sidebending first which will have the effect of making the technique reach the deeper or more superficial tissues according to the direction of the sidebending. Try asking the patient to turn her head to one side or the other. Try having her arms by her sides, under her shoulders, under her forehead or over the sides of the table. Each change will make a difference to the technique. Try applying the technique at varied phases of breathing.

16.3 ▶ Articulation prone Lift the thigh just above the knee of the prone patient. Fix with the other hand over the transverse processes of the thoraco-lumbar area. Adduct the thigh and extend it. Force will be transmitted through to the upper lumbar area. The pull on psoas is very powerful and in most subjects it will direct forces to the area without excessively stressing the lumbar area.

Tips: Least useful in very heavy subjects where lifting the leg would be a problem. Most useful where strong articulation is necessary.

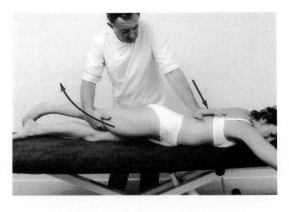

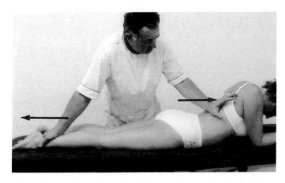

16.4 ◄ **Thrust prone** The patient lies prone in a 'sphinx' position. Clasp her ankles between thumb and index finger and index and middle finger of the pronated hand. Apply the other hand over the spinal level desired and initiate a rocking motion of the patient from end to end of the table. As you are rocking, increase the traction force with both hands until tension is felt to accumulate under the spinal hand. Apply a small thrust against the spinous process into extension, or against a transverse process into rotation.

Tips: Try asking the patient to stagger her elbows slightly which will introduce a preliminary sidebending or rotation to the area. It may be necessary to have the patient drop her feet over the end of the table if they are uncomfortable. Try using varied phases of respiration to find the optimum barrier.

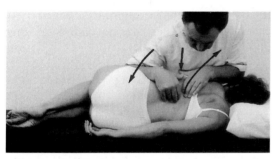

16.5 ▲ **Thrust sidelying** The patient is placed sidelying with her lower arm behind the thorax. Push backwards against the anterior aspect of the pelvis to stabilize it. Push the spine backwards from below to introduce rotation. Pull forward against the transverse processes of the vertebrae above with the other hand and use the forearm to stabilize the scapula. Rock the whole patient into a small amplitude of rotation to find the optimum point of tension and then apply the thrust with the upper hand while maintaining the lever position with the lower.

Tips: This technique requires quite firm compression with both hands into the table as well as into rotation. It is critical not to release the fixation produced by the lower hand at the moment of the thrust as the focus is liable to be lost. Try varied phases of breathing.

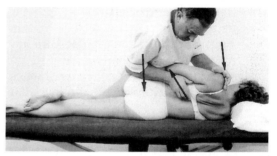

16.6 ▲ **Thrust sidelying** The patient is sidelying in a classical lumbar roll position. Apply the levers in the usual way for the thrust with some small variations. Use a substantial element of compression through the pelvis toward the table. Use a compressive force through the shoulder toward the table and slightly toward the patient's head. The thrusting hand is pushing into compression against the lamina of the vertebral segment desired. As the forces accumulate, the thrust is applied with the lower hand pulling the vertebra and the pelvis toward you as a unit. This ensures that the force is not dissipated in rotation of the lumbar spine. This is primarily a compression thrust with a small local rotary force at the contact point at the moment of full compression.

TECHNIQUES FOR THE THORACIC SPINE

17

The term 'thoracic' will be used in preference to the term dorsal, which has now been largely superseded. If the reader is accustomed to 'dorsal', he will need to make a mental translation at each reference. The thoracic spinal area is more accessible than the lumbar in that the embryological curve is maintained. The facet joints are liable to be involved in mechanical dysfunction syndromes as they are in apposition during normal posture, not just in flexion of the spine. Despite the torsional nature of movement in the thoracic area, disc lesions are much less common than in the other areas. However, when they do occur, they produce equally serious problems. The flexible nature of the thoracic area in rotation means that it is often necessary to use a large element of 'contra-rotation' to produce locking in manipulative technique. This in itself, if excessive or poorly controlled, will be painful and result in over-locking. There can be a tendency to apply more leverage when suitable resistance is difficult to feel, which leads to even more discomfort.

Special precautions for the area must include the possibility of bony weakness such as osteoporosis and secondary deposits. There is potential for damage in cases of advanced osteoarthrosis with ligamentous stiffening, particularly if excessive force is used.

The autonomic chain is very close to the thoracic spine and this means that applying any physical therapy can produce undesired or unexpected autonomic changes in the body. These may include sweating, sense of coldness, fatigue, yawning and breathing and digestive changes. While adverse reactions of this sort are usually temporary, and not too alarming, it is best to be aware of this possibility so that the practitioner can advise the patient accordingly.

Prognostic factors for a poor result include the patient with very 'stringy' muscle tissue in the area. This awareness can allow the practitioner to be more accurate in prognosis early on in a treatment series. 'Stringy' muscle has undergone some partial fibrotic changes, which are by their very nature only partly reversible. This is not uncommon in the thoracic area and it should direct treatment to the cause of the dysfunction, rather than just the painful area.

It is often useful to consider phases of breathing when performing technique in the thoracic area. Most thrust technique is easier if performed as the patient exhales. There are times when this is not the case. If it is necessary to stabilize a very mobile subject, asking them to hold the breath may be of more help. Experimentation is necessary to find the best method for each patient.

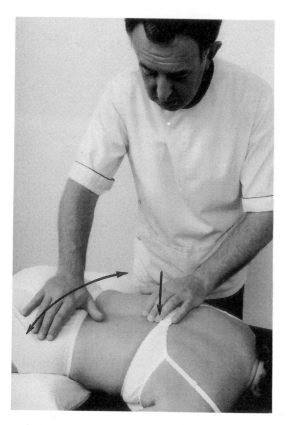

17.1 ◀ **Harmonic technique prone** Use your upper hand to fix or focus the harmonic rocking of the pelvis induced by your lower hand. The amplitude of the harmonic movement will increase depending how far up the thoracic spine you fix as the lever lengthens. See earlier section relating to harmonic technique.

Tips: Although this is a therapeutic procedure, it performs a useful diagnostic test that will rapidly find areas of diminished flexibility.

17.3 ▼ **Articulation in sidebending and extension sitting** The patient rests her folded arms on the operator's shoulder and upper arm and he is reaching around to clasp the paravertebral regions on each side. Rock into sidebending and, therefore, induce sidebending in the patient. Pull your hands toward yourself against the fulcrum of the shoulder and induce extension into the patient's spine.

Tips: Try adding rotation to either side before or after the other movements to help focus them.
Extra considerations: Fix the patient's knees, padded if necessary, against you.

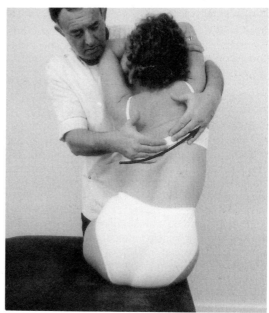

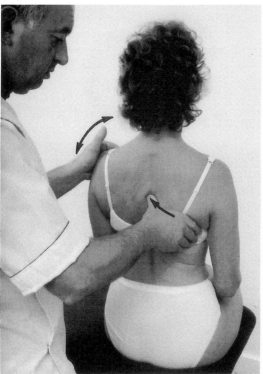

17.2 ◀ **Articulation into rotation sitting** Fix against the spinous process at a chosen level and rotate the rest of the body back against this level by pulling the shoulder backwards. The natural recoil of the body will take it forward again so that you can move up or down to the next segment and repeat the exercise.

Tips: This can be a diagnostic exercise or a mild therapeutic technique.

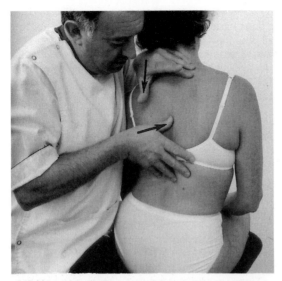

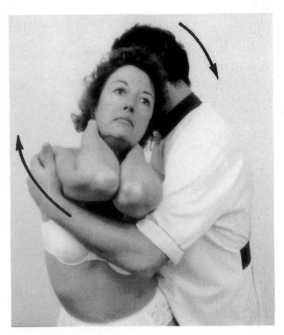

17.4 ▲ Articulation into sidebending sitting Sit or stand close to the patient's side and hook your abducted arm over her shoulder. Apply your thumb or thenar eminence against the spinous process and buckle the body into sidebending while using your thumb as a fulcrum.

Tips: Most useful in fairly stiff subjects where only small movement is required. **Extra considerations**: Try using circumduction movement of the upper body around the thumb to induce other ranges of movement.

17.5 ▲ (top right) Articulation into sidebending sitting The patient sits with hands clasped behind the neck. Clasp the far shoulder of the patient. Hold her near shoulder firmly against your chest and keeping her head directly above her pelvis, buckle the spine over your thumb or thenar eminence applied to a spinous process. Firm compression of the patient against the operator is necessary and the movement comes from a slight flexing of the knees.

Tips: Try adding other ranges of movement to the sidebending to help focus it. Try circumduction.

17.6 ▶ Articulation into sidebending sitting The patient sits with folded arms. Lift the further elbow while pressing down on the near shoulder with your axilla. Buckle the spine around your thumb or thenar eminence applied to the near side of a spinous process. It is necessary to have firm compression of the patient into the operator and the sidebending movement occurs as you flex your knees.

Tips: Most useful where it would be difficult for the patient to clasp hands behind the neck.

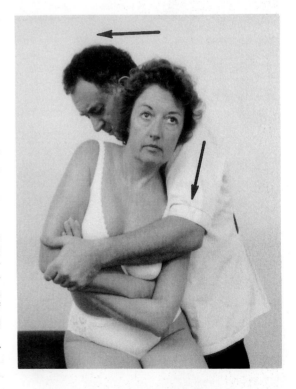

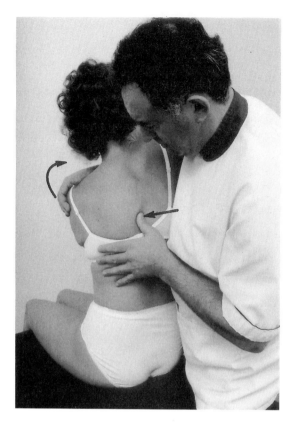

17.7 ◄ **Articulation into rotation sitting** The patient folds her arms and the operator reaches either across the folded arms, or through them, to clasp the further shoulder. Compress the patient into your chest and apply a thumb or thenar eminence to one or more spinous processes. Induce a small amount of sidebending away from yourself and rotate the patient's and your body together to focus the force at the contact point.

Tips: Try circumduction instead of simple rotation to address different parts of the dysfunction.

17.8 ▼ (bottom left) **Articulation into rotation sitting** The patient clasps her hands behind the neck. Reach around to clasp her far shoulder and apply your thumb or thenar eminence to one or more spinous processes. Compress the patient into yourself and induce rotation down to your applied thumb by twisting your body and the patient's as a unit.

Tips: The thumb applied to the spinous process can be on the nearside to push further rotation or on the far side to block rotation below that point. **Extra considerations**: If the patient is very flexible, an astride sitting position may be more efficient as it limits thoraco-lumbar mobility with the legs abducted in this way.

17.9 ▼ **Articulation into extension upper thoracic area sitting** The patient folds her arms and rests them on the operator's upper chest. Thread your forearms through her folded arms and using your hands as a fulcrum lever the spine into extension.

Tips: Try making this into a circumduction movement. Brace the operator's thighs against the patient's knees – padded, if necessary.

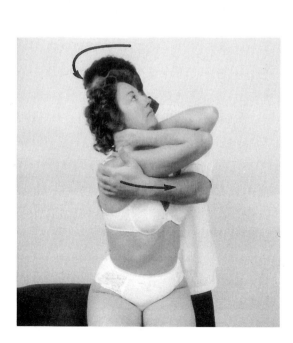

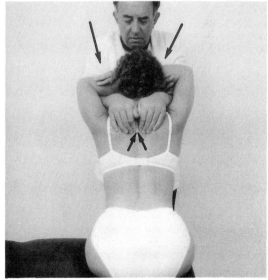

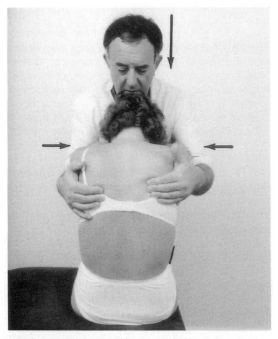

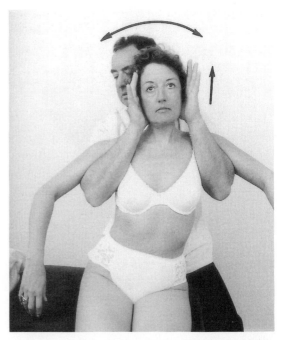

17.10 ▲ Articulation into flexion sitting The patient folds her arms and drops her head forward onto the operator's chest. Fix the top of her head with your chin and apply a lateral compression force, to the thorax, through your wrists and forearms. Pull up under the angles of a chosen pair of ribs while bending your knees to induce a localized flexion.

   Tips: Try inducing some sidebending movement or circumduction. Fix the patient's knees against the operator's thighs, if necessary.

17.11 ▲ Traction and sidebending articulation sitting The operator threads his arms under the patient's arms. Lift under the patient's mastoid processes with the heels of your hands. The lift also takes place through the axillae. Lean the patient against your chest and while maintaining the lift, introduce circumduction to reach the mid thoracic area.

   Tips: Most useful in smaller patients and children as the lift can prove hard work if applied to larger adults.

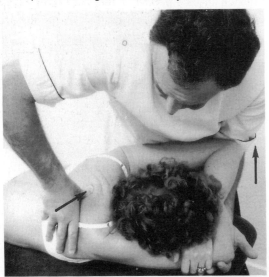

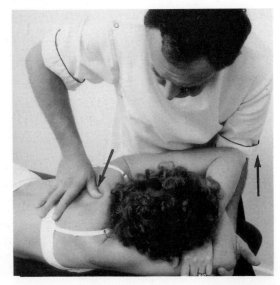

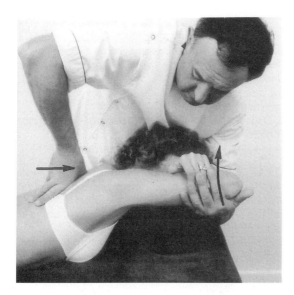

17.14 ◄ **Articulation into extension prone** The patient lies prone with her arms folded under the forehead. Lift the folded arms, head and thoracic spine into extension while counter-fixing with your other hand.

Tips: Least useful where the patient is very large as considerable effort would be required to perform this technique. **Extra considerations**: Try introducing sidebending or rotation to help focus the forces.

17.12 ◄ (see facing page, bottom left) **Articulation into rotation prone** The patient lies prone with her arms folded under the forehead. Fix a thoracic spinous process toward yourself and with your other hand under the patient's folded arms introduce rotation down to the fixing hand. Note that the patient is not being lifted as the operator's upper hand acts as a fulcrum and rests on the table.

Tips: Most useful where it is desired to limit rotation down to a specific segment as the thumb will act as a block to movement below this point. **Extra considerations**: Try adding different combined forces of sidebending or extension to the rotation.

17.13 ◄ (see facing page, bottom right) **Articulation into extension prone** The patient lies prone with her arms folded under the forehead. Lift the folded arms, head and thoracic spine into extension while counter-fixing with your other hand.

Tips: Least useful where the patient is very large as considerable effort would be required to perform this technique. **Extra considerations**: Try introducing sidebending or rotation to help focus the forces.

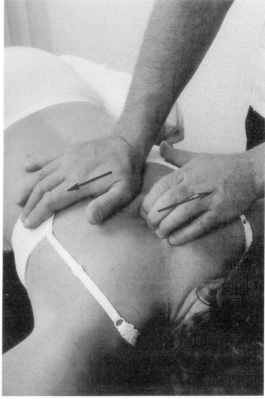

17.15 ▲ **Springing prone** Apply a classical 'push and pull' technique by bracing several spinous processes with the heel of one hand to rotate them away from yourself. Brace several adjacent ones above to produce a rotation force between the hands. Naturally, the technique can be used with the hands reversed.

Tips: Try fixing with one hand and mobilizing with the other and vary the patient's head rotation to find the optimum.

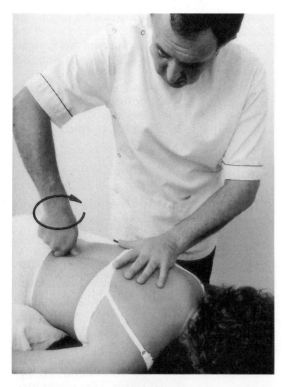

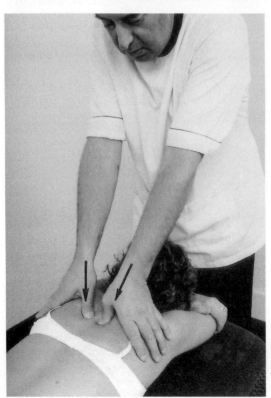

17.16 ◄ Articulation into rotation prone The operator is working specifically on one segment, taking hold of it as if it were a wing nut. Push toward the table to absorb the spring. Apply the thumb and index finger on opposite sides of adjacent spinous processes. They introduce the rotary force as you pronate your forearm.

Tips: Least useful where the spine is very tender. The force needed to make this technique effective would be too great in cases of severe restriction.

17.17 ▼ (bottom left) **Springing postero-anterior prone** The patient is lying prone, in this case with her hands folded under her head. Stand at the head of the table and use the pads of your thumbs to spring the chosen level directly anteriorly. Press with the thumbs over the laminae of the vertebrae, not the spinous processes as they can tend to be sensitive.

Tips: Most useful where specific segmental dysfunction is present. **Extra considerations**: Try springing on one side only, or staggering the thumbs to work on adjacent segments. Try having the patient's arms by her side or over the edge of the table.

17.18 ▼ Thrust starting position supine The patient grasps opposite shoulders without crossing her forearms. The operator has rolled the patient toward himself and is sliding his hand under the spine. He is using a flat hand, but can apply a variety of possible holds to the target segment. Note that the patient's head is left on the pillow and that she is only rolled far enough to allow the hand to be slipped underneath. This has become known as the **dog** technique after Fryette saw this being done badly and commented, 'I wouldn't do that to a dog!' If he had seen it done well, he would not have made that comment, but the name has stuck since then!

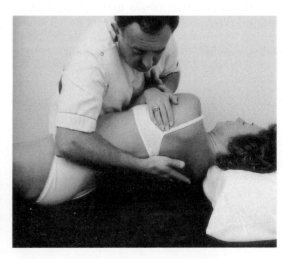

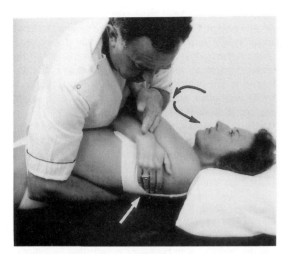

17.19 ▲ Thrust to mid thoracic spine supine
The hold shown in photograph 17.18 is adopted and the patient is rolled over onto the hand. Test for free play in the primary lever direction of traction. Focus all other components of flexion, rotation away from yourself, sidebending toward yourself and slight compression and sideshifting away. If this seems excessively complex, you should simply concentrate on bringing your elbows in toward your sides; this will automatically produce the correct components. The underneath hand performs a small pronation and traction toward the pelvis to help tighten up the levers. At the point of barrier accumulation, emphasize the pronation of the lower hand and apply the thrust through your upper hand and chest into traction pushing her elbows toward her shoulders. It is usually possible to reach from about the third to the tenth thoracic vertebra with this hold.

Tips: This is not a flexion thrust. It is not a compression thrust. The use of all the secondary levers is designed purely to help minimize the amplitude of the primary lever of traction. **Extra considerations**: Many varieties of hand hold underneath are possible. A flat hand pronated slightly is most comfortable for the patient. The hand can be applied with the fingers loosely clasped. It can be applied using a fist so that the spinous processes fit into the space between flexed fingers and thenar eminence. The underneath hand is as much a part of the technique as the upper hand. If the hold causes pain to the operator in the lower hand, try pushing the hand firmly into the thoracic spine, rather than simply resting it on the table. Leave a small space between the back of the hand and the table so that the wrist is as much part of the fulcrum as the hand. Try using varied quantities of patient head rotation to help focus the technique. Generally rotation away from the operator will tighten the levers.

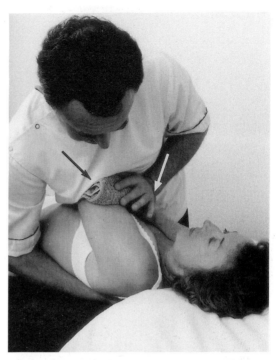

17.20 ▲ Thrust to mid thoracic spine supine The patient is only crossing one arm over her chest. The operator is using a pad between his chest and the patient's elbow. His upper hand is applied to the pad to direct the force more accurately. It is usually possible to reach from about the third to the tenth thoracic level with this hold.

Tips: Most useful for the patient with a shoulder dysfunction as the painful shoulder can be left out of the hold. All other factors are as the details in photograph 17.19.

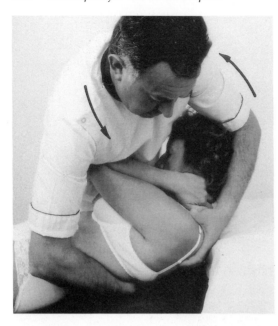

17.21 ◄ Thrust mid thoracic area supine The patient clasps her hands behind her neck. Lift her upper body with your upper hand and slip your lower hand under the patient to apply it to the target vertebra. Flex the patient down to the segment and while holding her steady, apply a thrust with your thorax to the patient's elbows. In this variation of the basic technique it is difficult to reach much above the fifth thoracic level in most subjects.

Tips: This is a mobile technique and it is not usually possible to stay in the thrust position for more than a few moments. It is much more difficult to use varied secondary levers with this hold and it tends to become a flexion and compression thrust. As the secondary levers are not used to any great extent, this can become a rather forceful variation. It is more difficult to be specific with this technique and, therefore, it can become a technique for gapping several facets at once. This means that a restricted segment in the midst of a mobile area may not be mobilized effectively.

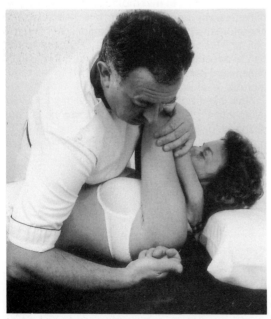
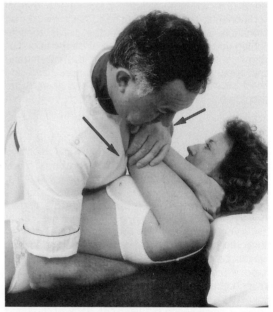

17.22 and 17.23 ▲ Thrust upper thoracic area supine The patient clasps her hands behind her neck. The operator makes a loose fist and slips it under the patient to fit the spinous processes into the palm. Flex the patient's elbows and apply all the usual components. The thrust is performed into traction and some compression when the levers have focused.

Tips: Most useful for upper thoracic area from second to fifth levels.

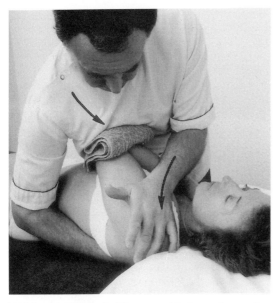

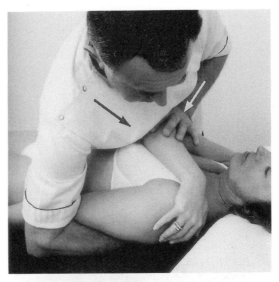

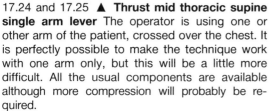

17.24 and 17.25 ▲ Thrust mid thoracic supine single arm lever The operator is using one or other arm of the patient, crossed over the chest. It is perfectly possible to make the technique work with one arm only, but this will be a little more difficult. All the usual components are available although more compression will probably be required.

Tips: Most useful in cases where any problem with one shoulder or the other makes the normal hold impossible.

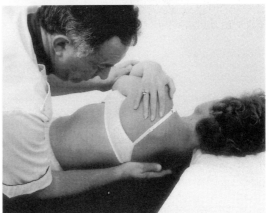

17.26 and 17.27 ▶ Thrust mid thoracic area from same side The patient crosses her chest with her arms in the usual way avoiding crossing the forearms. Roll the patient away from you to slide your hand under the spine from the nearside. Roll the patient onto your hand and apply your forearm to her folded arms. (Note that the completed hold is shown from the other side for clarity.) Test for free play in the primary lever direction of traction while adding the secondary components to bring the target joint to the optimum thrust focus.

Tips: Most useful in very large subjects where it may be impossible to reach all the way around. This hold can also be used for costo-vertebral and costo-transverse joints. It is also a useful method when an operator, for any reason, finds use of one particular hand a problem, as it means that the same hand can be used from both sides, whereas with the conventional hold he would need to change hands to reach the other side.

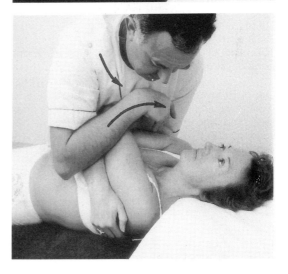

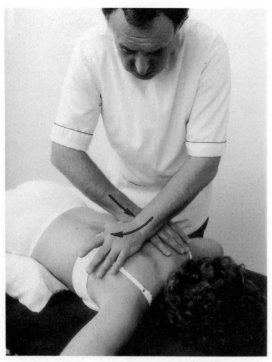

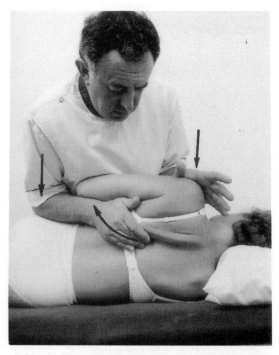

17.28 ▲ **Thrust using crossed hands mid thoracic area prone** The patient lies prone with her arms over the sides of the table to spread the scapulae. Apply your crossed hands to opposite sides of the spine. The far hand is slightly supinated to bring the pisiform into contact with a transverse process. The near hand is pronated to bring the hypothenar eminence into contact with a transverse process of the same or adjacent vertebra. The thrust is applied after the slack has been taken out of the tissues with a downward pressure and a small element of sidebending.

Tips: Most useful in fairly flexible subjects. **Extra considerations**: Try changing the hands to make the far hand push toward the head and the near one push toward the feet. It may be necessary to change the applicator to use the thenar eminences for some operators. The thrust is usually co-incident with exhalation to avoid rib damage. Try varying the patient's head rotation to find the optimum.

17.29 ▲ **Thrust mid thoracic area sidelying** The operator is using his lower arm to stabilize the pelvis in this modified lumbar roll position. The upper, or fixing, hand is maintaining a downward pressure to produce a compression force. The actual thrust is applied with a direct compression force into the table and against the transverse process of the level desired.

Tips: Most useful in cases where compressive forces on the chest might be undesirable for any reason. **Extra considerations**: Although this position might seem difficult, or even impossible for the purpose intended, it needs remarkably little practice to be made into an efficient technique. The control of the two very long levers is critical. Careful study of the photograph will reveal the compressive and torsional forces being applied. Try varying the phase of breathing to find the optimum tension.

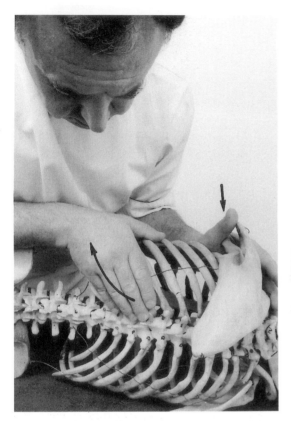

17.30 ▲ Thrust mid thoracic area sidelying, shown on skeleton The hold shown in photograph 17.29 is applied here to the skeleton for clarity. Note that the lower hand is applied to the transverse processes and the ribs. The lower elbow is applied to the lateral aspect of the pelvis. The upper hand is pushing the shoulder back slightly, but mostly down into the table.

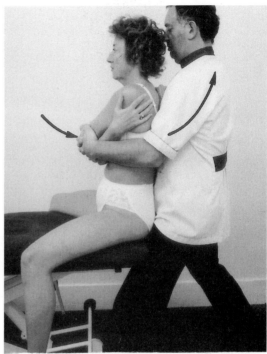

17.31 ▲ Thrust mid thoracic area sitting The patient clasps round her chest gripping opposite shoulders. She has not crossed her forearms. Pull in toward yourself on her elbows using a pad, if necessary, as a fulcrum between your chest and the desired level of the patient's spine. You need to pull in on the elbows to produce a compression while engaging the barrier in a traction, flexion, sidebending and opposite rotation direction. The thrust is an accentuation of the primary lever of traction. **Extra considerations**: Lateral compression is available simply by the operator bringing his elbows toward his sides. If the elbows are staggered slightly one above the other, an automatic sideshift will be introduced. Note that the patient is sitting astride the table in this illustration. This is not an essential part of the technique but may help fix the pelvis in a very mobile subject. Try varying the phase of breathing to find the optimum.

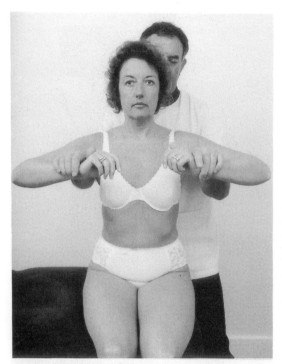

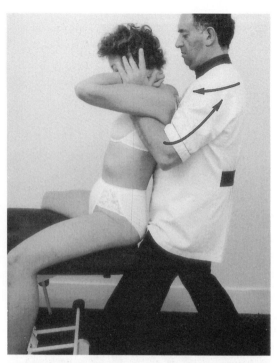

17.32 ▲ **Thrust mid thoracic area sitting (taking up the hand hold)** The operator is clasping the patient's wrists. Ask her to interlace her hands behind her neck. Taking up the hold in this way avoids having to thread your hands through her elbows, and makes the grip much easier to access.

17.33 ▲ **Thrust mid thoracic area sitting** The operator has taken up the hold in the way shown in photograph 17.32. Place a pad if necessary between your chest and the patient's spine. Pull her into flexion down to the segment desired, compress toward your chest and induce some sidebending and opposite rotation. The thrust is applied with a combination of a lift of your body from the knees, and an increase of compression of the patient against your chest. The forces are produced by pulling in on her arms at the same time as the lift.

Tips: Least useful where a shoulder problem might make the hold painful or difficult. Try a lateral compression of the chest in mobile subjects to absorb the free play in the thorax. Try making the thrust after a circumduction of the patient's body so that the technique becomes a movable procedure rather than just a lifting exercise. **Extra considerations**: Note that the patient is astride the table in this illustration. This is not essential to the technique. Nevertheless, in mobile subjects the astride position will help to absorb excessive free play in the lumbar spine. Note that the patient's elbows remain pointing forward; if they are allowed to splay to the side the patient's shoulders may be strained. Try varying the phase of breathing to find the optimum tension for the thrust.

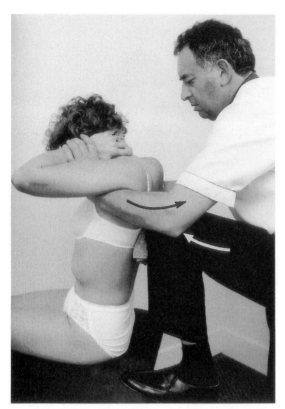

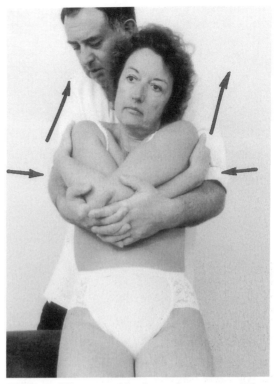

17.34 ▲ Thrust mid thoracic area sitting, knee fulcrum The patient is sitting with hands clasped behind her neck. Thread your hands through the arms and grip the patient's wrists to pull her into flexion down to the level desired. Apply your padded knee to the spinous or transverse process. The thrust is performed with a small lifting force through the patient's arms, against a very small increase of pressure with your knee.

Tips: Note that the patient's elbows remain pointing to the front; they are not allowed to splay out as this can strain the shoulders. This is a very powerful technique, and if performed with excessive force could very easily become traumatic. Try varying the phase of breathing to find the optimum tension for the thrust.

17.35 ▲ Thrust mid thoracic area sitting patient's arms across chest The patient clasps opposite shoulders without crossing her forearms. Grip her elbows and pull her into your chest over a suitable pad, if necessary, applied to the desired spinal level. Apply a lateral compressive force to absorb the free play in the thorax. Stagger your arms slightly to produce a small component of sideshift as you squeeze the thorax. The patient leans back against you and you flex her spine until the barrier accumulates. The thrust is performed with a small increase of the compression coinciding with a lift directly into traction. Small vectors of sidebending and rotation can be introduced as necessary.

Tips: Try varying the phase of breathing to find the optimum barrier. Note that in this photograph the patient is sitting across the table. If the table is very wide, this will mean that she is too far from the operator to make the technique efficient. Either a narrower table would be necessary or she could sit astride the table. Another alternative might be to use a stool.

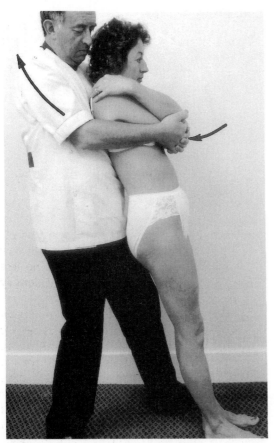

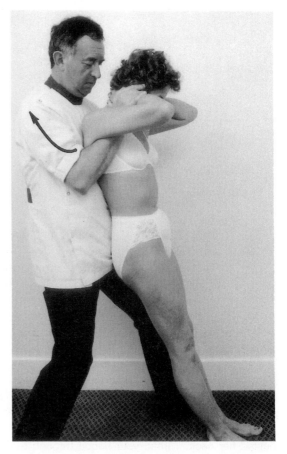

17.36 ▲ Thrust mid thoracic area standing The patient clasps opposite shoulders without crossing her arms. Pull her into your chest with a suitable pad interposed if necessary. Grip her elbows and pull her into compression, some sidebending and opposite rotation. Flex down to the segment desired and then lean her back against you as you drop your weight onto your back leg. The patient has been told what to expect. At the optimum tension, apply a small increase of compression at the same time as a small lift by shrugging your shoulders.

Tips: At all times the patient remains in some flexion. This is not so much a lifting force as a resistance to dropping of the segments above the fulcrum. The primary lever is a traction force.

17.37 ▲ Thrust mid thoracic area standing, hands clasped behind neck The patient clasps her hands behind her neck. Pull her against your chest with a suitable pad interposed if necessary. Warn her that she is to be pulled off balance. Apply a compression, sidebending and opposite rotation force while pulling her into flexion down to the segment desired. At the point of optimum tension, perform the thrust with a small shrug of your shoulders.

Tips: Note that the patient's elbows remain pointing to the front. If they are allowed to splay, there is a possibility of straining her shoulders.

The ribs and thorax present certain of their own particular problems from the point of view of efficient performance of technique. These problems mainly relate to the variations in shape of the thoracic curve in different individuals and the need to modify approaches accordingly. There are several pathological conditions that need particular care. Although this is not the place to be detailing all these, the reader is encouraged to think in particular about osteochondrosis, osteoporosis, scoliosis, and myeloma. All these are examples of the type of conditions where special consideration as to type of approach is needed as there will be deficiency of bone strength.

The rib articulations are rarely dysfunctional by themselves, and it has been stated that in a given case, the thoracic spine should receive attention first and subsequently the ribs. If rib articulations are addressed first, they may be disturbed again when any thoracic spinal technique is performed thereby rendering the rib work ineffective.

Although there are usually twelve pairs of ribs, they vary progressively from above down, in shape and movement possibility; technique will inevitably vary according to the area being worked. The techniques, therefore, are divided broadly into those applicable on the lower, middle and upper ribs. Naturally these demarcations are artificial, and there will be some overlap.

Technique classifications have often referred to the nature of movement of ribs. They demarcate the 'bucket-handle' type of movement from the 'pump-handle' type. This classification is not used here as rib dysfunction is considered simply in respect of good function or lack of it. The choice of technique is by the quality and quantity of the dysfunction found rather than by any pre-conceived notion of specific functional movement possibilities. Although this does not accord with traditional thinking when working on ribs, it is no less effective in actual practice, and considerably simpler to apply.

Due to the springy nature of the ribs in normal subjects, it is usually necessary to absorb some of that spring in performing techniques. This is done by using several vectors of force of compression in more than one direction. This can be either along or across a particular rib so that the amplitude of a force applied need not be too great. Torsion with this method of approach is less necessary, and discomfort is reduced with these carefully applied compressions.

The control of rhythm is clearly necessary, particularly in rhythmic techniques that have to be repeated several times. Phases of breathing also need to be taken into consideration. Many techniques require either exhalation to induce relaxation or, alternatively, inhalation to create a firming up of the part and improving the access to the optimum motion barrier.

The choice of position to perform the technique, such as supine, sidelying, etc., is going to be governed by the most comfortable position for the patient at the time, and the position most effective for the requirements of the treatment and technique being given. As a rule, sidelying is more comfortable than supine, and supine is more comfortable than

prone. Sitting is better where larger movements are necessary, but this requires more
cooperation from the patient and control by
the operator. It is preferable to avoid the
necessity of changing the patient's position
excessively during treatment and the relative
size of operator and patient may also deter-
mine the optimum position in which most
techniques can be performed.

Because of the deep nature of the intercostal
muscles, direct soft tissue work is less effective
here than in some regions, and stretching
and articulation will be more useful. Thrust
techniques have a particular use when there
has been a traumatic onset to a particular
syndrome. They play a smaller part in more
chronic conditions, except at the outset, to
break fixation and pave the way for more
rhythmic approaches later. Care should
always be taken of the aesthetic nature of the
procedure being used. This is particularly
true when working on female patients so as
not to put pressure on breast tissue which
could be embarrassing and possibly painful.

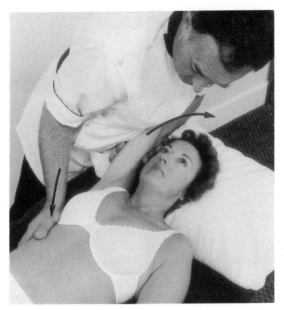

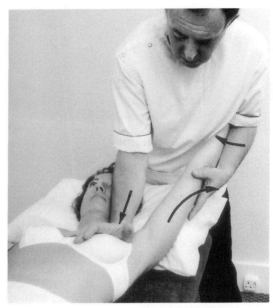

18.1 ▲ Articulation of mid ribs supine Hold the patient's arm in extension, and use internal rotation to put the shoulder capsule on tension. Apply the applicator thumb and thenar eminence to the costal interspaces. Rock from one foot to the other and apply a careful pressure to the lower of a pair of ribs so it is possible to increase their spacing and mobility. This hold can be used from twelfth to third rib.

Tips: Most useful in kyphotic patients where the ribs will be in close apposition. Least useful in large-breasted women where it may be impossible to get to the ribs without intruding on the breasts. **Extra considerations**: It may be useful to use different phases of respiration.

18.2 ▲ Articulation of upper ribs Stand at the head of the table with the patient's arm extended and internally rotated. Apply a force through the shoulder and ribs by rotating your body. Keep the patient's arm held firmly into your side so that the rotation movement causes rib articulation forces to develop.

Tips: Most useful where the first three or four ribs are involved in a dysfunction syndrome. Least useful where there is any shoulder problem making the arm movement difficult in this plane. **Extra considerations**: With tension maintained try using a harmonic oscillation in this position.

18.3 ▶ Articulation of lower ribs Apply a slight compressive force to the thoracic cage and use the thumbs to carefully hold the ribs being worked towards the pelvis while you rhythmically lean back. The patient here is holding a towel between her hands as the stretch round the operator to clasp her hands may be too great.

Tips: Least useful in patients where shoulder movement of this amplitude may be a problem. **Extra considerations**: Try using a harmonic oscillation in this position.

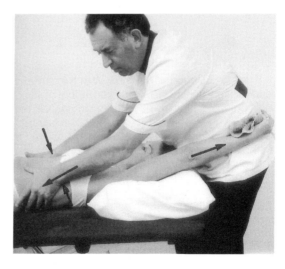

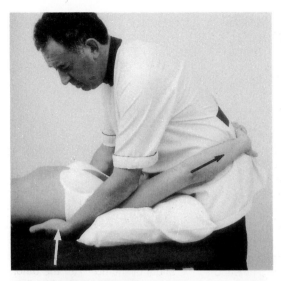

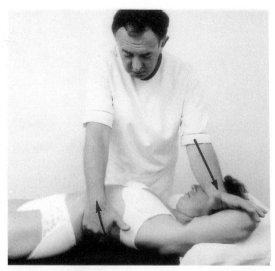

18.4 ▲ Articulation of mid ribs Apply a slight lateral compression force to the upper thorax to limit movement there, then, with the back of the hands resting on the table, apply an anterior force to the shafts of the ribs. At the same time apply a traction by leaning back and, thereby, produce a stretch from the patient's linked hands.

   Tips: Most useful in kyphotic patients where rib 'spreading' is an important element of treatment. Least useful where the shoulders cannot adopt the position. **Extra considerations**: Try using different phases of respiration.

18.5 ▲ Articulation of lower ribs The patient links her hands behind her head and then you apply a resistive force to her elbow. You can lift the lower ribs by twisting your own body with relatively fixed arms.

   Tips: Most useful where there is a need to elevate and spread the lower ribs strongly. Least useful where the shoulder cannot be used in this range of movement. **Extra considerations**: Try using varied phases of respiration.

18.6 ► Articulation of mid ribs With the patient's hands linked behind her neck you apply a lifting and spreading movement to the mid ribs on the opposite side. This is particularly effective in patients who have a very flexed thoracic spine, for example from age, osteoporosis or osteochondrosis. It will only be effective as far as the sixth or seventh rib, as the scapula intervenes.

   Tips: Least useful in large subjects where the reach may be too great for smaller operators. **Extra considerations**: Try using varied phases of respiration and varied amounts of preliminary sidebending of the patient's body.

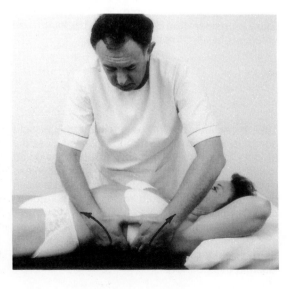

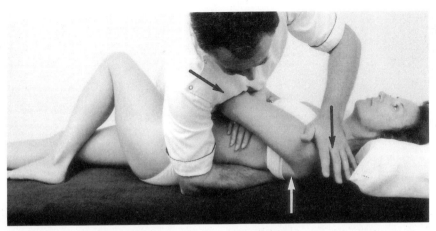

18.7 ▲ Articulation of mid and upper ribs This hold uses initial patient positioning as the opposite leg is flexed at the hip and adducted to produce some rotation of the pelvis toward the operator. The arm is placed under the side of the patient. Apply the thenar eminence to the angle of the rib. With the other hand, hold down the shoulder and pronate the applicator forearm to apply the mobilizing force. Stabilize the patient's folded arms with a traction force applied with your own chest if required.

Tips: Most useful in very tight subjects where the springing force developed in this way will help mobilize the individual joints effectively. Least useful if the rib heads are very tender to pressure. **Extra considerations**: Try using varied phases of respiration and head rotation to optimize the tension.

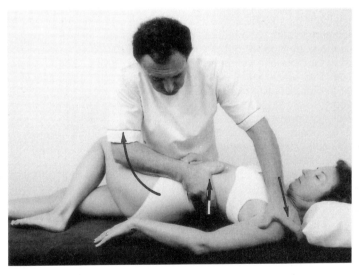

18.8 ▲ Articulation of mid to lower ribs The applicator here is the border of index finger and second metacarpal. They apply an extension and separating force, while the patient's shoulder is held down with the other hand and the elbow of your applicator hand rotates the patient's pelvis towards you.

Tips: Most useful where a strong mobilizing force is required. Least useful where rotation in the thorax may be a problem. **Extra considerations**: Try using different phases of respiration and varying the patient's initial position to help localize the force.

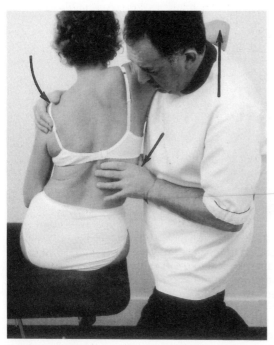

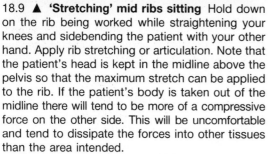

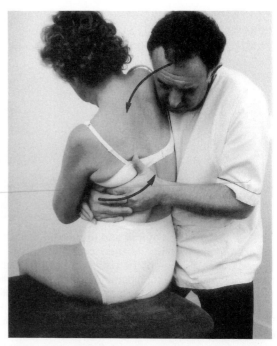

18.9 ▲ 'Stretching' mid ribs sitting Hold down on the rib being worked while straightening your knees and sidebending the patient with your other hand. Apply rib stretching or articulation. Note that the patient's head is kept in the midline above the pelvis so that the maximum stretch can be applied to the rib. If the patient's body is taken out of the midline there will tend to be more of a compressive force on the other side. This will be uncomfortable and tend to dissipate the forces into other tissues than the area intended.

Tips: Least useful in very flexible subjects where it would be difficult to localize the force. **Extra considerations**: Try using different phases of respiration and try circumducting the patient's body around the fixed applicator hand as an alternative approach.

18.10 ▲ Articulation of mid to lower ribs sitting This hold can be used where there is a scoliosis, as the ribs can be worked on the convexity. It requires a firm compression between the bodies of the operator and the patient, and whilst the hands are held relatively fixed the oscillation of body movement will perform the articulation. **Extra considerations**: Try using varied phases of respiration and different amounts of active flexion and extension in the patient.

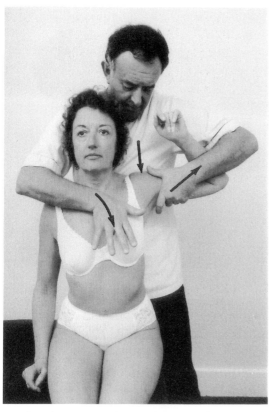

18.11 ◄ Articulation of upper ribs sitting Apply the hand to the costo-chondral junction and keep it relatively fixed while you abduct and externally rotate the shoulder to a comfortable limit. Then, hold the shoulder and perform the articulatory force by pressing forwards against the scapula to induce a force localized to the rib. Sometimes a slight increase of traction through the arm assists the technique. **Extra considerations**: Try using varied phases of respiration.

18.12 ▼ (bottom left) **Articulation of costo-chondral joints** Hold back on the sternum and apply a traction, external rotation and abduction force to the shoulder. Then lean forward against the patient's scapula to produce a gapping force. Lower down the rib cage, more initial rotation needs to be induced in the patient's body to establish localization.

   Tips: Least useful in cases where shoulder dysfunction would cause pain in this position. **Extra considerations**: Try using different phases of respiration.

18.13 ▼ Articulation of mid to lower ribs Side-bend the patient over your padded knee and compress her firmly against your side. The mid ribs will require more extension of the patient's body than the lower.

   Tips: Least useful if the patient is very large and the operator very small. **Extra considerations**: Try using varied phases of respiration.

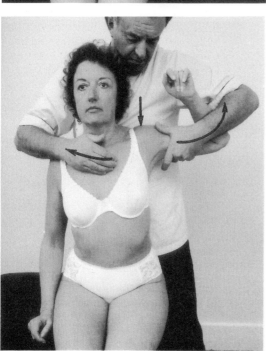

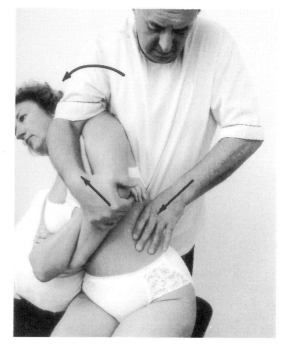

18.14 ▶ Articulation of mid ribs sidelying Use your upper hand to apply a posterior to anterior force while your elbow maintains the patient's shoulder in extension, abduction and external rotation. This transmits the force to just below your fingertips where the other hand applies a slight compressive force and holds down on the rib towards the pelvis. It is possible to reach up to about the fourth or fifth rib except in very mobile subjects, where the scapula gets in the way.

Extra considerations: Try using varied phases of respiration.

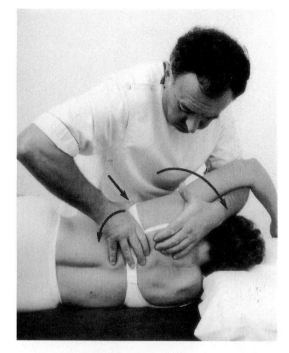

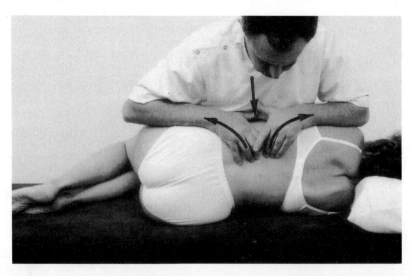

18.15 ▲ Articulation of mid to lower ribs sidelying Apply a downward force through both forearms on the lateral border of the scapula and the pelvis. Use a small component of postero-anterior force and then, while maintaining these, separate your hands slightly to produce the required direction of force.

Extra considerations: This position can be used for harmonic technique where the focus is made with the hands and then the whole patient's body rocked around them. Try using varied phases of respiration.

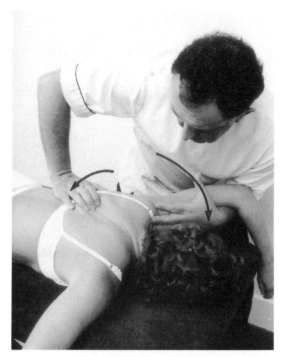

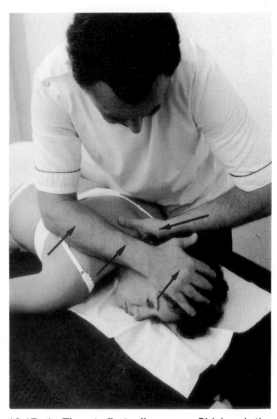

18.16 ▲ **Articulation of mid ribs prone** Extend and abduct the shoulder and then, while the rib is held toward the pelvis with the fingertips and thumb, further abduct the shoulder to reach the fixation point so that articulation can be performed.

Tips: Least useful in patients where prone lying is a problem and where there is shoulder dysfunction.
Extra considerations: Try using varied phases of respiration.

18.17 ▲ **Thrust first rib prone** Sidebend the neck toward the rib and rotate it away. Produce a component of sideshifting with the stabilizing hand. Form an apex by pressure of your metacarpophalangeal joint as close to the head of the rib as possible. When you have taken up the slack, the direction of force will be approximately toward the opposite axilla. The hand holding the head is a stabilizer in this technique and does not enter into the thrust. As the technique is mostly used on ribs that have been fixated relatively superiorly by the pull of the scaleni, it is normally performed as the patient exhales.

Tips: Most useful where a treatment table head-piece can drop below horizontal to take the whole neck into some flexion. Least useful where the patient is over the age of 40, where neck extension and rotation may be limited. **Extra considerations**: Avoid this technique where there is a brachial nerve compression syndrome on the same side, as it may aggravate nerve root pressure.

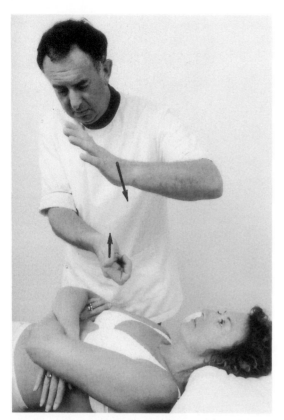

18.18 ▲ **Thrust hand position first, second and third rib**

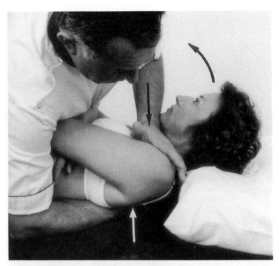

18.19 ▲ **Thrust first, second or third rib supine**
Use the hand hold shown in the photograph. Apply your hand to the head of the rib, keeping it in some pronation so that the thenar eminence is applied to the angle of the rib. Apply the other hand just lateral to the costo-chondral junction, and use your thorax to push downwards on the folded arms and toward the head, to produce traction and some compression. As the patient lifts her head from the pillow, barrier sense will accumulate on the thenar eminence. It is then necessary to make a small increase of pressure toward the table with the upper hand, and a further sharp pronation with the table hand to complete the thrust.

Tips: Most useful in very tight subjects where neck levers are best avoided. **Extra considerations**: If excessive pressure is applied to the rib head too early, the patient will be unable to lift the head. Try using varied phases of respiration.

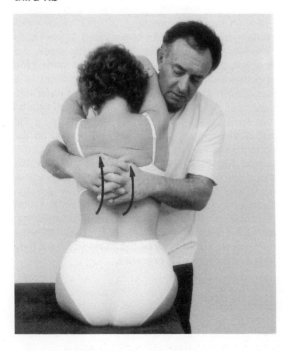

18.20 ◄ **Thrust mid ribs sitting** Pull the patient's body into extension and apply a localized force using your thumb directed to the angle of a rib. Sidebend the spine over that thumb and then rotate it away to produce locking of the spinal column. Then apply a short amplitude thrust in an upward and forward direction which will break fixation in the costo-vertebral or costo-transverse articulations, depending on the amount of preliminary rotation. More rotation directs the force laterally to the costo-transverse articulation.

Tips: Least useful in very flexible subjects where it is difficult to produce localization. This technique may be impossible in large patients as the reach for the operator may be too great. **Extra considerations**: The patient may be more comfortable with a pillow between her arms and the operator's shoulder. Try using different phases of respiration.

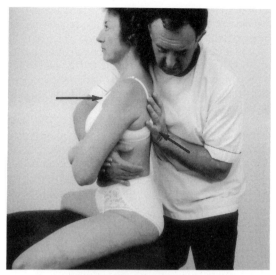

18.21 ▲ Thrust starting position for mid ribs sitting Apply the hypothenar eminence to the angle of the rib and stretch the other arm across the thorax to compress the ribs slightly from front to back. This compression of the chest makes the thrust point more accessible. Then rotate your and the patient's body, pushing the rib forward. At the last moment introduce a sidebending toward the rib with enough extension to focus the forces. The extension is produced partly by pressure on the rib angle, and partly by asking the patient to extend her head and neck. Most techniques do not require a specific order of components. However, in this hold it is far too easy to over-lock if the balance between the components is wrong. If the order described is used there is a greater probability of balance between comfort and effectiveness.

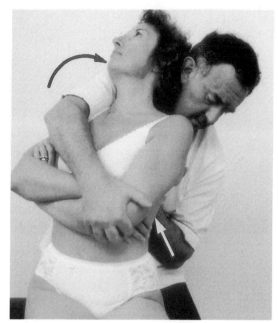

18.23 ▲ Thrust for middle ribs sitting This shows essentially the same technique as photograph 18.22 but an alternative hand hold across the thorax has been taken and the patient is sitting across the table rather than astride.

Tips: This hand hold may be better as it avoids the breast area in female patients.

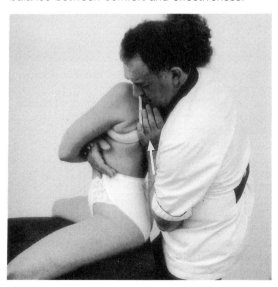

18.22 ◄ Thrust for mid ribs The operator has applied the rotation away from the rib and the side bending down to it until the forces accumulate as in photograph 18.21. The patient then extends her head. Apply a compressive force between the two hands and perform the thrust with the pisiform vertically on the angle of the rib. If the thrust force is more anterior than vertical, pain will be induced and the technique will be less effective.

Tips: Least useful where the operator is smaller than the patient and where the reach around may be a problem. **Extra considerations**: This is one of the few thrust techniques where generally it is better not to apply very much in the way of soft tissue procedures first. It is often difficult to accumulate useful tension if the structures have been previously relaxed. Try using varied phases of respiration. (The sitting astride position shown here is not an essential part of the technique.)

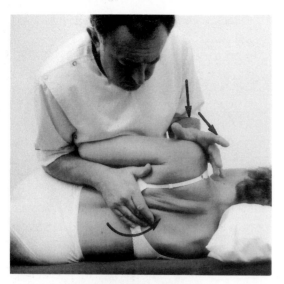

18.24 ◄ **Thrust for mid ribs sidelying** This is a modified lumbar roll position with hand applied directly over the costo-transverse articulation on the side of the thorax closest to the table. Use the other hand to compress the pectoral girdle directly toward the table and prevent forward rotation of the body. Apply the force with the whole of the thrusting arm and hand and use a direct compressive force anteriorly and slightly superiorly to produce gapping of the joint.

Tips: Most useful in tight subjects as their stiffness helps to produce a localization more easily. Least useful where the operator is small and it may be difficult to apply sufficient compressive force for localization. **Extra considerations**: Try different phases of respiration.

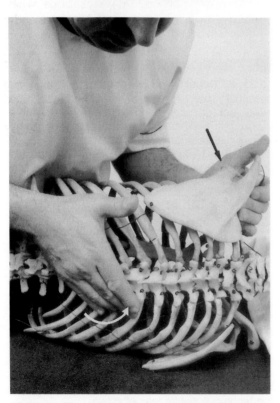

18.25 ▲ **Thrust to mid ribs sidelying shown on skeleton** The exact positions of the fingers of the thrusting hand in the previous illustration are seen more clearly here. Although this may seem a rather unusual way of reaching the mid ribs, it is particularly useful where excess torsion would be a problem. The controlled compressive force allows the target rib to be reached. If a pure rotation force were to be used instead of the compression, the whole lumbar spine would be at risk of strain.

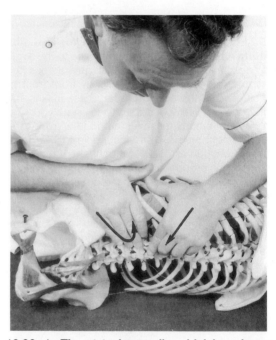

18.26 ▲ **Thrust to lower ribs sidelying shown on skeleton** A modified lumbar roll position has been applied and the finger tips of the thrusting hand have been directed toward the table. This will reduce spinal movement. A force is applied then toward the operator to gap the rib articulations while the other hand holds back on the spinous processes. The critical element in this technique is the control of compressive force to focus the forces accurately.

Tips: Most useful where torsion of the whole thorax is best avoided as compression substitutes for rotation. Least useful in the presence of lumbar or sacro-iliac dysfunction as some stress inevitably occurs at these regions.

The soft tissue articulation of the scapulo-thoracic junction is frequently involved in tension states and postural control of the pectoral girdle. Fibrotic muscle bands are frequently found under the scapula, and these can limit mobility and be a source of symptoms in themselves. Restricted mobility of the scapula can put undue strain on the shoulder joint itself. In cases of shoulder dysfunction this can make the difference between comfort, reasonable usage, and mechanical problems.

From a practical viewpoint the difficulties lie mostly in finding ways to access the area underneath the scapula. Techniques must be used which allow the scapula to be partly separated from the thoracic wall to allow the operator's fingers or hand access to the muscles. Very tight fascial states will make this difficult, but these patients are the subjects most likely to benefit from such approaches.

There are few special precautions when working on this area except to be aware of the forces being put through the shoulder joint. It is necessary to avoid excessive stress on the gleno-humeral joint in the process of reaching the scapulo-thoracic junction. Deep emotional tension often manifests here, and release of the muscles can produce emotional release, so the thinking practitioner should be prepared for this possibility.

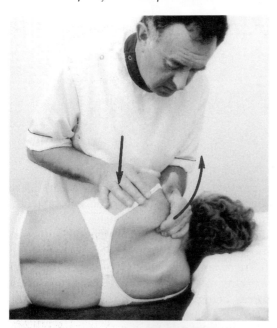

19.1 ◄ Kneading of soft tissues on superior and medial part of scapulo-thoracic junction side-lying Fix the scapula slightly down toward the table with the stabilizing hand while the other applies kneading to the horizontal fibres of trapezius, and the rhomboids. As these muscles are involved in respiration, it may be best to use the exhalation phase of breathing to enhance the relaxation response.

Extra considerations: Try holding the muscles on tension and moving the whole body against the tension in very tight subjects rather than moving the muscles against the body.

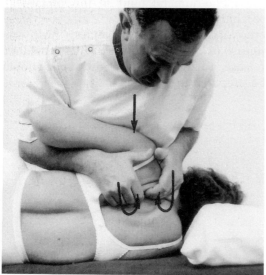

19.2 ▲ Kneading and stretching rhomboids and subscapularis sidelying Push the patient's shoulder and upper arm toward the table with your thorax and arm to wing the scapula. Then push the finger tips up into the space formed so that they can work directly on the muscles. Kneading can be performed directly or the whole scapula can be lifted while being held against your chest to perform stretching. If you sidebend your body it is possible to work the upper or lower parts of the area.

Extra considerations: Can be used as an inhibition technique with sustained pressure.

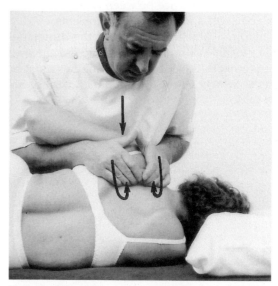

19.3 ▲ Articulation of scapulo-thoracic junction sidelying Fix the scapula and shoulder between your thorax and finger tips and rhythmically roll the patient's upper body into rotation. This will have the effect of mobilizing the scapula on the thorax.

Extra considerations: Try taking the whole scapula superiorly and inferiorly.

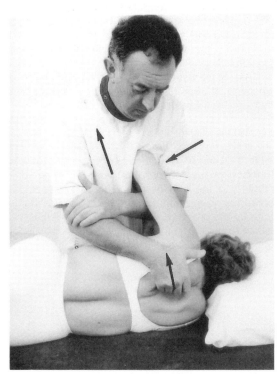

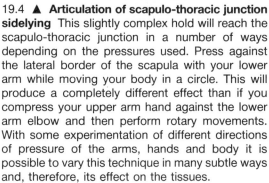

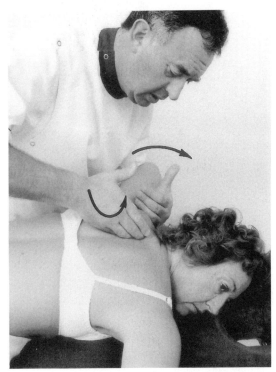

19.4 ▲ Articulation of scapulo-thoracic junction sidelying This slightly complex hold will reach the scapulo-thoracic junction in a number of ways depending on the pressures used. Press against the lateral border of the scapula with your lower arm while moving your body in a circle. This will produce a completely different effect than if you compress your upper arm hand against the lower arm elbow and then perform rotary movements. With some experimentation of different directions of pressure of the arms, hands and body it is possible to vary this technique in many subtle ways and, therefore, its effect on the tissues.

Tips: Most useful where stretch rather than kneading is the preferred method. Least useful where there is shoulder dysfunction making this position difficult for the patient.

19.5 ▲ Kneading and articulation of scapulo-thoracic junction prone Abduct the patient's arm to an appropriate point and rotate it as necessary with your lateral hand. You can reach the deep interscapular muscles and pull the scapula into different degrees of rotary movement.

Tips: Least useful where prone lying is a problem for any reason. **Extra considerations**: Try changing the patient's head position to vary the tension on the scapular muscles.

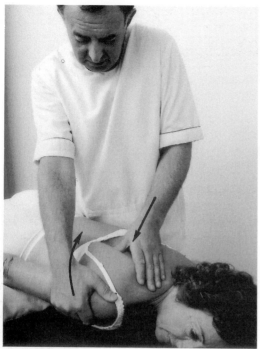

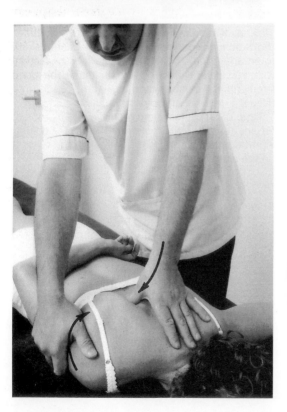

19.6 ◄ Kneading scapular muscles prone Pull the shoulder toward you and backwards to wing the scapula and apply the thumb of the other hand to work on the muscles that have been taken off tension.

Tips: Most useful in very tight subjects and where it is required to work on the posterior thoracic wall. Least useful where prone lying may be a problem and where operator thumb strength may be insufficient for the technique.

19.8 ▼ Kneading and friction of scapulo-thoracic junction prone Perform the work with fingertips applied to the soft tissues. This allows a wider spread of pressure that may be less uncomfortable than thumb pressure. Some operators will find this easier to perform if their thumbs are too mobile for the other holds.

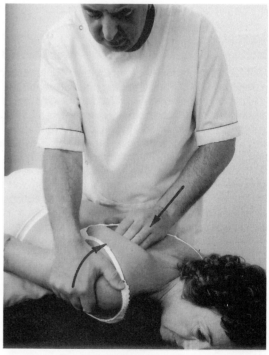

19.7 ◄ Kneading and articulation scapula prone Place the patient's arm in strong internal rotation and pull the shoulder toward you and backwards to make the subscapular muscles more accessible. The thumb is performing the kneading work.

Tips: As photograph 19.6.

The cervico-thoracic, or cervico-dorsal, region can be a source of more frustration in attempting to achieve successful technique results than almost any other area. There are many reasons for this. The area is junctional which means that there will be a change in orientation of anatomical curves. There is a mobile area of the neck meeting a less mobile area of the thoracic spine and ribs. There are emotional factors which manifest in the area relating to stress and tension. The use of the arms puts mechanical strains on the area, requiring it to be stable, and this very stability means that the range of movement of the joints is somewhat limited. This can lead to a greater susceptibility to mechanical strain in these joints if they are taken out of their normal range in an uncontrolled fashion.

Particular care should be taken with regard to the possibility of pathological conditions in the area affecting bone strength, such as secondary deposits from primary carcinoma in the lung and thyroid. Severe brachial nerve entrapment syndromes require particular caution if the neck is going to be used as a lever. The presence of extreme hypertension can manifest as a very hypertonic state in the muscles of the cervico-thoracic area. Inability to get adequate relaxation in the area should alert the practitioner to this possibility. As a precursor to incipient cardiac infarction there can also be a characteristic feel to this area, presumably due to aberrant viscero-somatic reflex patterns. This manifests as an increasing state of tension with a 'sheet like' nature in that there is no specific point of tension. There is, rather, a generalized state that partly resolves with manual treatment only to recur very rapidly. This is difficult to describe, but once it has been felt, will never be forgotten. This muscular state disappears almost immediately after a myocardial infarction, presumably due to the changes in the reflex patterns. There may be other factors in operation here such as changes in life-style, the shock to the system, and many others, but it is, nevertheless, quite characteristic.

Some of the techniques are modified versions of cervical holds, some modified thoracic ones, and some are specific to the area itself. There is no inherent benefit in any one over another, except there may be times when it is necessary to avoid the neck or the thorax for some reason. It is, therefore, necessary to have a range of techniques available to affect the area by a variety of means.

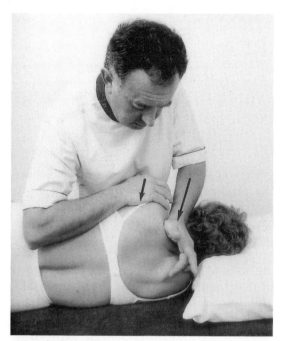

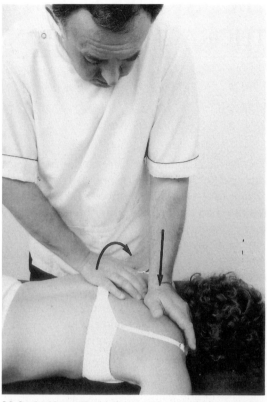

20.1 ▲ Kneading sidelying The patient is side-lying nearer you than the back of the table. Fix the upper scapula with your forearm and hand and apply the kneading to the trapezius and rhomboids towards the spine with the thenar eminence.

Tips: More useful for patients who might find prone lying a problem. Better for tight-muscled subjects where the action of pushing the muscles toward the spine may be easier than pulling away using the more traditional methods.

20.2 ▲ Kneading prone The patient is prone with her arms over the sides of the table and her face in a breathing hole in the table if available. Fix the nearer side of the spine with the lower hand into a slight rotation toward you. Use the thenar eminence of the kneading hand to push against the muscles on the opposite side toward the table and away from the spine.

Tips: Try using the expiration phase of breathing to give the best relaxation effect.

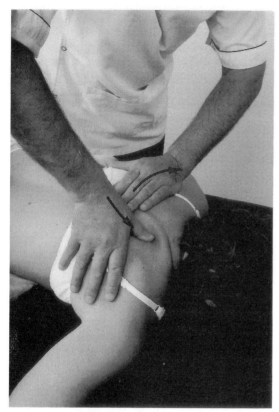

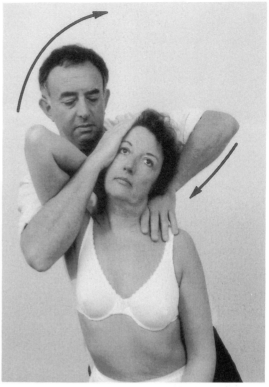

20.3 ▲ **Kneading prone** The patient is prone with her face in a breathing hole in the table if available. Her arms are over the sides of the table. Fix the spine with the upper hand to prevent too much rolling of the spine into rotation and apply the kneading with the other hand. Take up some skin slack and use the thumb or thenar eminence to perform the kneading to trapezius and rhomboids.

Tips: Least useful if the operator has any problem of thumb instability.

20.4 ▲ **Articulation sitting** Stand behind the seated patient and have her place one hand behind her neck. Fix with your thumb against a spinous process directed toward her other axilla so that the thumb forms a fulcrum for a sidebending movement. Reach under her flexed arm with your arm and fix against the side of her head. Keep the vertex in the midline and introduce the sidebending movement with both hands simultaneously.

Tips: Try circumducting the patient's body around the fixed vertebra to make a stronger and more variable force. Avoid continuing this movement for a long duration as there will be a tendency for ulnar nerve irritation from your arm pressure under her flexed arm.

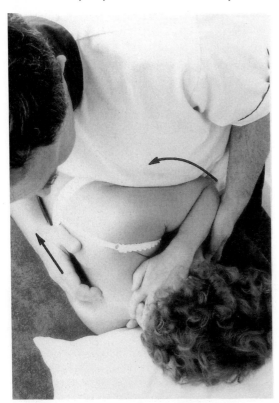

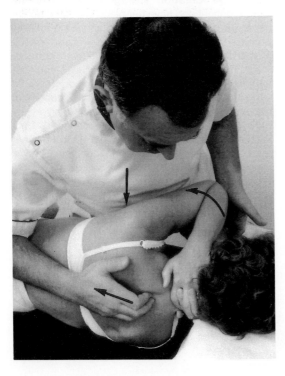

20.5 ◄ **Articulation sidelying** The patient clasps her hands behind her neck in the sidelying position. Fix on the spinous process of the target vertebra with the fingers of one hand. Clamp the patient's flexed arms between the side of your thigh, hand and forearm. Introduce flexion and extension with small amounts of any other movements by making a small rotation movement of your body.

Tips: Least useful where there is any shoulder condition which may make this position difficult for the patient. Try using only one arm flexed and gripping the neck rather than both.

20.7 ▼ **Articulation sidelying** Fix the patient's flexed arms between your body and abducted upper arm. Grip around her hands with your upper hand so that the movements of flexion, extension and small amounts of rotation and sidebending can be introduced. Fix the spinous process of the target vertebra with the other hand to act as a counter-force to the movement induced.

Tips: Least useful in nervous patients as this position is somewhat claustrophobic. Not very useful if there is any shoulder condition which may make the position difficult to attain. Try using only one flexed arm instead of two. Most useful where it is desired to block out cervical movement.

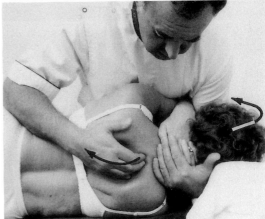

20.6 ◄ **Articulation sidelying** Fix the under-surface of the patient's flexed upper arms against your side and hold her elbows. Use a firm grip on the spinous process of the target vertebra with the other hand. Introduce flexion and extension by rocking your body into rotation, thereby carrying her arms back and forth.

Tips: Least useful where the patient has any condition of her shoulders making the flexed position difficult. Try using one flexed arm only. Most useful where it is desired to eliminate neck movement from the equation as her hands will help do this.

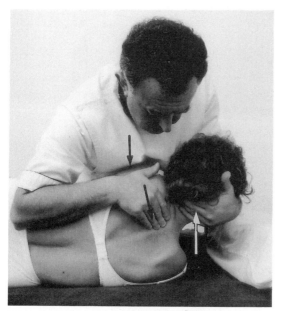

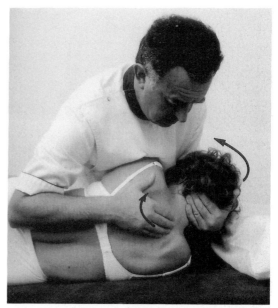

20.8 ▲ **Articulation sidelying** Flex both of the patient's arms to pull the scapulae apart. Support her head and mid neck with your upper hand. Use the fingertips of the other hand to push against the spinous processes of the area to introduce a sidebending articulation with some possible rotation. Lift the head using the tips of the fingers under the neck to limit the movement to the lower cervical and upper thoracic area.

Tips: The lower down the neck you fix with the upper hand, the more localized the force becomes, and the more the upper neck is protected from strain. Avoid having your upper arm biceps against the patient's eyes; rather, fix against the forehead. Use some downward compression through the upper scapula to stabilize the body. Least useful where there may be any neck instability, as however much protection is introduced, there will be some strain induced.

20.9 ▲ **Articulation sidelying** Flex the patient's neck and grip as far down as possible with the upper hand to avoid neck strain. Use the fingers of the other hand to pull the spinous processes against the movement of the upper hand. Most movement directions are possible with this hold.

Tips: The fixing hand protects the neck and allows reasonable localization of the articulation. Avoid crowding the patient's face with your upper arm or chest.

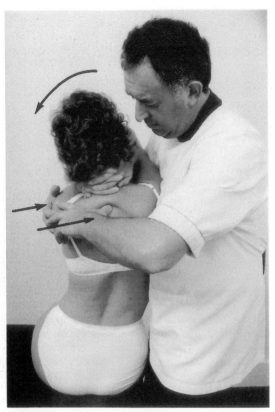
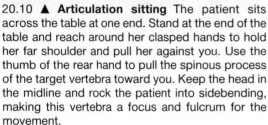
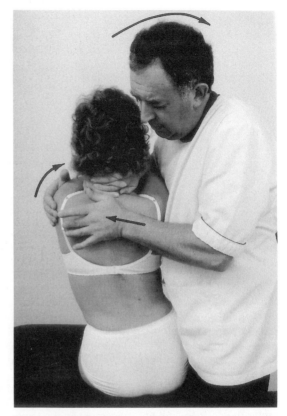

20.10 ▲ Articulation sitting The patient sits across the table at one end. Stand at the end of the table and reach around her clasped hands to hold her far shoulder and pull her against you. Use the thumb of the rear hand to pull the spinous process of the target vertebra toward you. Keep the head in the midline and rock the patient into sidebending, making this vertebra a focus and fulcrum for the movement.

Tips: Firm compression toward you will allow induction of movement to be produced by a rocking back of your body. Try introducing circumduction movements as well as simple sidebending. Least useful if the operator has an unstable thumb. In this case try substituting a thenar hold.

20.11 ▲ Articulation sitting The patient sits across the table at one end. Stand at the end of the table and reach around her clasped hands to hold her far shoulder and pull her against you. Use the heel of the rear hand to push the spinous process of the target vertebra toward you. Keep the head in the midline and rock the patient into sidebending making the vertebra a focus and fulcrum for the movement.

Tips: Firm compression toward you will allow the induction of movement by a rocking back of your body. Try introducing circumduction movements as well as simple sidebending. Least useful if the movement needs to be very specific to only one segment as this pushing movement will inevitably involve several vertebrae.

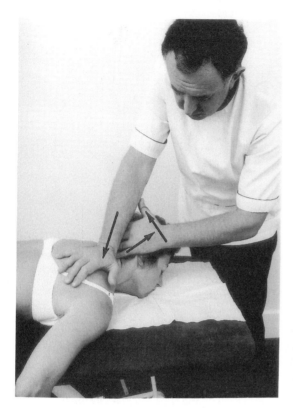

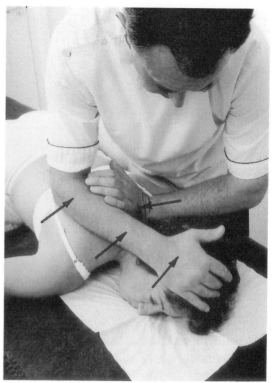

20.12 ▲ Thrust prone Sidebend the neck and head of the prone patient at the same time as you induce a slight rotation to the other side. Fix as low down on the neck as possible with the head hand to avoid excessive neck strain. Apply a compression force against the transverse process of the target vertebra toward the table and axilla with the thrusting hand. Gently rock the head on the chin to find the optimum barrier accumulation under the thrusting hand. At the point of optimum barrier, apply a very short amplitude thrust to the transverse process to gap the joint on the same side.

Tips: Least useful for patients who find the prone position a problem. Least useful for most patients over 45 years of age, as normal degenerative changes in the neck will make the lever uncomfortable. If a table with a dropping head leaf is available, it is possible to perform this technique on a wider range of patients as the slightly flexed position will remove some of the strain. Avoid pulling the head harder when the thrust is performed as this is often painful. Try varied balance between rotation and sidebending to find the best mix of effectiveness and comfort. Try moving the thrusting hand laterally to the angle of the rib to make this into a rib gapping technique.

20.13 ▲ Thrust prone Stand at the side of the table with the prone patient's head in rotation away from you. Fix the scapula with your lower hand and gently fix the head into rotation and a small amount of sidebending. Apply the heel of the thrusting hand against the side of the spinous process of the target vertebra toward the patient's axilla. Balance the forces so that the head hand does not move when the thrust is applied with the spinal hand to gap the facet on the far side of the patient's spine.

Tips: The direction of thrust governs which side will be gapped. If the force is toward the axilla, the other side will gap as the facets on the nearside are in apposition. If the force is predominantly into the table, there will be a tendency for the same side to gap. Avoid this position in patients over about 45 years of age as the strain on the neck may be unacceptable. Avoid the tendency to introduce excessive extension as this can be traumatic and, moreover, renders the technique less effective. Move the thrusting hand more laterally onto the angle of the rib to make this into a rib gapping technique.

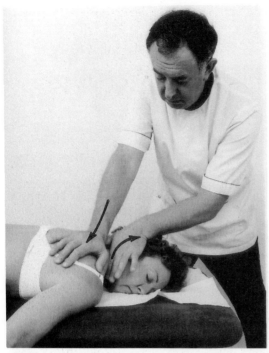

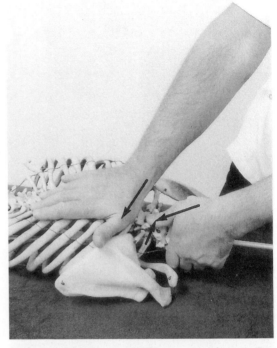

20.14 ▲ Thrust prone Stand at the head and slightly to one corner of the table with the patient's head turned away from you. Carefully fix the neck as low down as you can reach with the upper hand. Fix the spinous process of C7 with the thumb of this hand to limit movement to the upper thoracic area. Apply the thenar eminence of the thrusting hand to the transverse process of the target vertebra, pushing it toward the axilla. Stabilize the rotation with the head hand, and increase the pressure with the thrusting hand until a suitable barrier accumulates. Apply the thrust with the lower hand only to gap the facet on the thrusting side.

Tips: Apply the thrust to the angle of the rib to make this into a rib gapping technique. Avoid this position in patients over about 45 years of age as the neck extension may be uncomfortable. It is possible to perform this at a more advanced age if a drop leaf table is available.

20.15 ▲ Thrust prone (shown on skeleton) The technique shown in photograph 20.14 is demonstrated here on the skeleton to show the position of the hands more accurately.

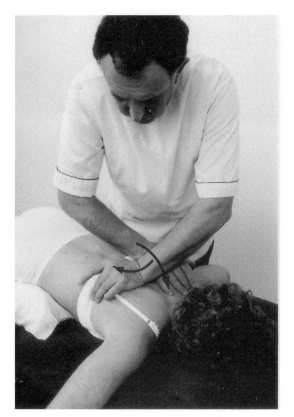

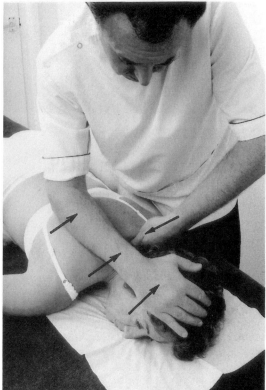

20.16 ▲ Thrust prone Stand at the side of the prone patient and apply the hypothenar eminences of both hands to opposite sides of the spine at adjacent segmental levels. Apply some pressure onto the transverse processes to induce some compression and sidebending. Rotate your body to emphasize this movement and vary the pressure with the hands to introduce some rotation to the movement until a suitable barrier is found. The thrust can be applied with one hand, the other hand, or both.

Tips: Try reversing the hand position to find the optimum for each case. As each vertebra has multiple joints, every change in angle or pressure will vary which will be the target joint. A sidebending thrust rather than a compression thrust will be more comfortable, and less potentially traumatic in cases of possible rib fragility.

20.17 ▲ Thrust prone Fix the scapula with the forearm and the head into rotation away from you with the lower hand. Introduce a very small element of extension and sidebending with the head hand. Push against the spinous process of the target vertebra with the thumb of the thrusting hand into sidebending and slight compression into sideshifting. The thrust is applied into sidebending with the thrusting hand while maintaining the head position with the other hand. This will gap the facet on the far side. If the force is directed more toward the table with the thrusting thumb, it will tend to gap the facet on the nearside.

Tips: Least useful where the operator has problems with thumb stability. The fixation of the scapula and head gives some protection to the neck providing they are held steady during the thrust.

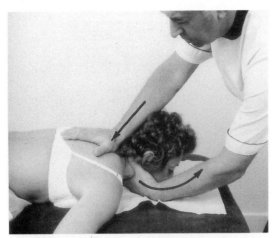

20.18 ▲ Thrust prone Rest the patient's head on her chin and gently support it with one hand avoiding throat pressure. Cup one spinous process with the area between the thenar and hypothenar eminences of the other hand and apply a pressure toward the sternum. Carefully oscillate between the hands until a suitable barrier accumulates under the thrusting hand. The thrust is a very short amplitude force while maintaining the head steady. Avoid excessive neck extension that can become traumatic.

Tips: This is a technique that is potentially dangerous, and must only be used with great care in suitable subjects.

20.19 ▶ Thrust sitting Stand behind and slightly to one side of the seated patient. Apply the thumb against the side of a spinous process of the target vertebra to induce sidebending and rotation. Support the patient by pulling her against your abdomen with the hand, and introduce slight rotation by pulling back against the clavicle. Flex your other arm and apply the inside of the forearm against the side of the head and face to produce a direct sideshifting force. Form a fulcrum of the vertebra and thumb while performing slight circumduction to the body to accumulate the best thrust barrier. When the tension is optimum, apply the thrust with the thumb toward the opposite axilla while the neck is fixed by the other hand.

Tips: Least useful for operators who might have instability in the thumb. Try using the thenar or hypothenar eminence instead. Vary the flexion and extension of the head, and try antero-posterior shifting to aid the focus of forces. If the thrust is applied against the spinous process toward the opposite axilla, it will gap the facet on the opposite side. If the thrust is applied more in a forward direction it will tend to gap the facet on the same side. In this case there will need to be a vector of downward pressure introduced as well.

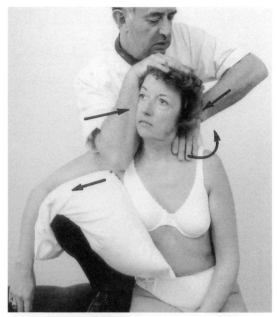

20.20 ▲ Thrust sitting This hold is substantially similar to photograph 20.19 except that the patient has placed her arm over a suitable pad on the operator's knee to act as a fulcrum. It is easier to induce sideshifting with this hold, and some patients feel more stable and secure. It is, however, more difficult for the operator to balance the forces as he is standing on one leg.

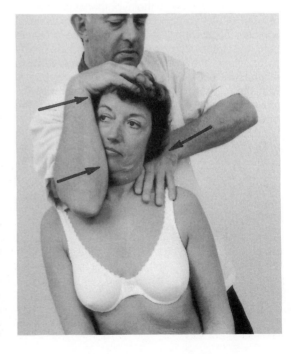

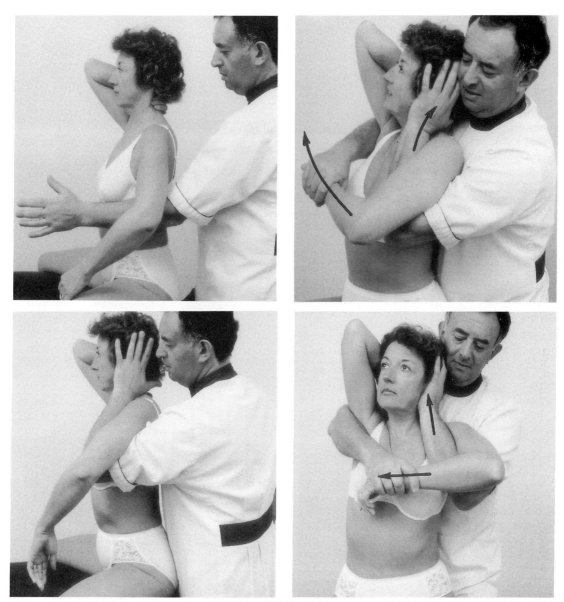

20.21, 20.22, 20.23 and 20.24 **Thrust sitting** This hold is very specific for the C7 to T1 joints. The sequence of photographs shows the order of application of the hold. Have the patient place one hand behind her neck and reach under the other arm with your thrusting hand. When you have reached as far as possible, flex your elbow to bring the heel of your hand against the fingertips of the patient that are flexed over the lower neck. Maintain some pressure there, and reach around her chest to grasp her wrist with your other hand. Apply some sidebending toward your thrusting hand, and rotate slightly away from this hand by pulling on the wrist. Pull the patient firmly against your chest to produce a direct antero-posterior compression. This will better help focus the other vectors of force. Apply the thrust vertically through the patient's fingers to gap the facet on the same side. (Note the astride position is shown for clarity only; it is not an essential part of the technique.)

   Tips: This is a complex technique, and several things can cause it to fail. The thrust must be vertical not anterior. The pull on the wrist must be quite firm to maintain the sidebending. Some extension is necessary, but too much will block the technique.

20.25, 20.26 and 20.27 **Thrust sidelying** Fix against the side of the spinous process with the thumb, heel of the hand or thenar eminence according to your preference. Lift the head into sidebending away from the table. Abduct the arm holding the head so that the patient's face is not obstructed and so it is possible to reach down to support the neck with the ulnar border of the hand. Introduce some sideshifting away from the table as well as a slight anterior shift of the neck. Fix against the upper scapula with your chest. Accumulate the barrier with a combination of sideshifting and sidebending away from the table, slight rotation toward the table, and compression against the shoulder. Apply the thrust with the chosen applicator to produce a rotation and sidebending of the target vertebra.

Tips: Note that the direction of the thrust can be varied to gap the lower or upper facet. Force directed toward the table will tend to gap the lower one, while force toward yourself will tend to gap the upper one. The lower down the neck you grip, the more the neck protection, and the less uncomfortable for the patient. The selection of applicator is dependent on operator thumb strength and ability to focus with the other parts of the hand.

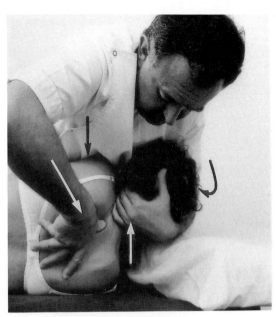

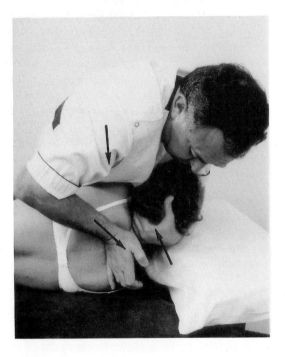

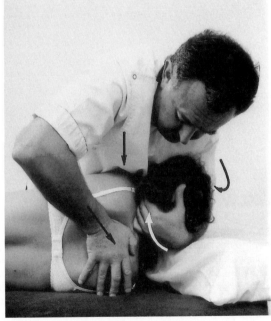

The cervical spine poses several problems for the manipulative practitioner. Patients are often nervous of having their neck handled. This is either through natural fear of damage to the area from its apparent fragility, or due to having had a previous bad experience. Some operators are also afraid of harming the patient with techniques in the neck and unconsciously transmit this to the patient. The patient then finds relaxation impossible, thus perpetuating the vicious circle.

There are clearly particular reasons for extreme caution in the neck, and it is wise to use as gentle technique as is possible consistent with a good result. Particular care should be taken in cases of hypertension, postural hypotension and vestibular origin dizziness. Each of these conditions can be irritated by excessive force or rapid movement. If a particular position irritates a brachial syndrome, it should also be stopped immediately. Nowhere is it more important to make technique slow, deliberate, and non-threatening than in the neck.

Discomfort and pain will often occur if not enough care is taken to keep the head substantially in the midline. Most of the thrust techniques require the vertex to remain almost central and the neck to be pushed or buckled into sidebending and sideshifting to achieve locking and localization. It may apparently be easier to produce an effective barrier if the head is taken out of the midline, but pain, distress and overstretch are the common undesirable results.

Some patients feel threatened if they cannot see the practitioner, and in these cases techniques should be performed from the side or front of the patient. Some patients intensely dislike chin hold techniques, and in these cases cradle hold methods are preferable. The use of rhythm is essential to produce a dynamic state of relaxation, and it is also easier to accelerate in thrust technique from a slightly moving pathway.

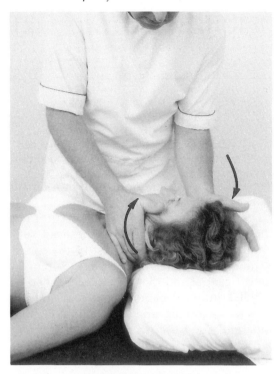

21.1 ▲ Kneading of soft tissues supine Stand at the side of the patient and stabilize the head with the upper hand. Pull up on the posterior and lateral tissues with the pads and fingertips of the active hand. Depending which fingers are used, the lower, mid or upper parts of the neck muscles are kneaded.

Tips: Try adding a sidebending movement with the head hand to emphasize the effect. Try not to slide over the skin excessively as this can be uncomfortable.

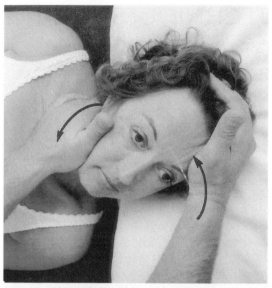

21.2 ▲ Kneading of soft tissues supine This operator viewpoint photograph shows the hold illustrated in photograph 21.1. Note that even though the head has been sidebent, the vertex remains in the midline. This avoids excessive facet compression on one side, and overstretch on the other.

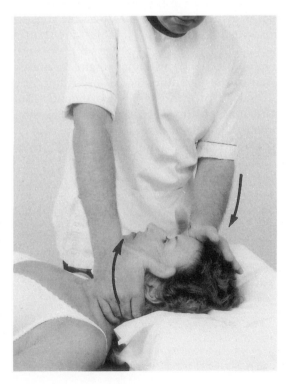

21.3 ► Kneading of soft tissues supine This photograph is of a similar procedure to that shown in photograph 21.1. However, it can be seen that by changing the hand hold slightly, you can pull into a combined extension and rotation at the same time as the kneading. This will have the effect of making the technique much stronger.

Tips: Try extending the neck with the kneading hand or fixing with this hand and extending with the other. Try using both hands together.

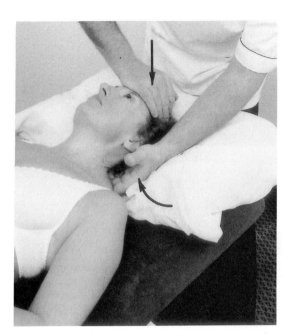

21.4 ◀ **Kneading of soft tissues supine** Fix the head into the pillow with one hand applied to the forehead. Apply the fingertips of the kneading hand parallel to the spinous processes. Push the fingers upwards into the neck and pull laterally while maintaining this upward push. The effect of this is to stretch the muscle tissue away from the spine while the neck remains static.

Tips: Use the back of the hand on the pillow as a fulcrum. **Extra considerations**: Try rolling the head slightly to enhance the effect of the kneading force.

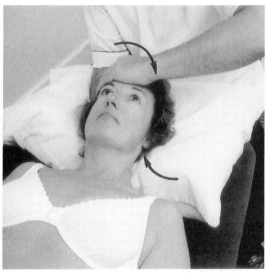

21.5 ▲ **Kneading of soft tissues supine** Fix the head into the pillow with the stabilizing hand. Use the fingers and thumb of the kneading hand to work on the posterior tissues of the neck on both sides at once.

Tips: With both fingers and thumb applied underneath it is easier to combine an articulation force at the same time rather than when just using the fingers. **Extra considerations**: Try adding a traction force.

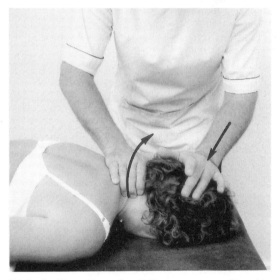

21.6 ▲ **Kneading of soft tissues prone** Stand to the side of the table and stabilize the head with the upper hand. Apply the kneading hand to the tissues on the other side of the neck and pull toward yourself.

Tips: This is not very comfortable for the patient unless a table with a breathing hole is used as excessive extension can result if insufficient care is taken.

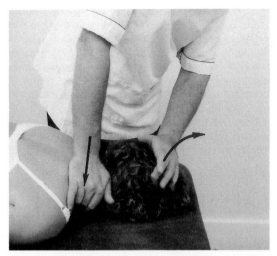

21.7 ▲ Kneading of lower soft tissues prone
Stand at the side of the table and stabilize the head with the upper hand. Use the heel of the kneading hand to push the trapezius and lower posterior cervical muscles toward the table.

Tips: This is not very comfortable for the patient unless a table with a breathing hole is used as excessive extension can result.

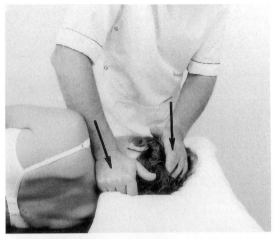

21.9 ▲ Kneading of soft tissues sidelying Stand in front of the patient and stabilize the head with the upper hand. Use the heel of the kneading hand to work on the lateral and posterior tissues uppermost to push them toward the spine.

Tips: Most useful in subjects with very tight fascial states as working toward the spine is often easier than working away. Try reaching round to the lower side and pulling up with the fingertips to work on the tissues nearer the table.

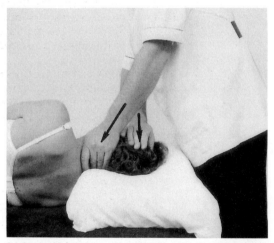

21.8 ▲ Kneading of lateral soft tissues sidelying Stand at the head of the table and stabilize the patient's head with the front hand. Use the thumb and thenar eminence of the kneading hand to work on the tissues on the side of the neck to produce the kneading force.

Tips: This hold allows the anterior tissues to be worked as well as the lateral ones. Try varying the rotation of the head with the stabilizing hand to direct the effect of the technique to different layers and parts of the muscles.

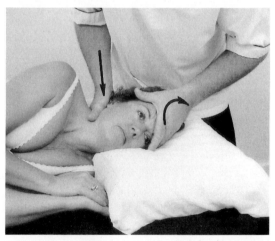

21.10 ▲ Kneading of soft tissues sidelying Stand at the corner of the table slightly behind the patient and stabilize the head with the upper hand. Use the thumb and thenar eminence of the lower hand to work on the soft tissues of the neck.

Tips: Try using a rotation force at the same time with the head hand to emphasize the effect of the force applied with the kneading hand.

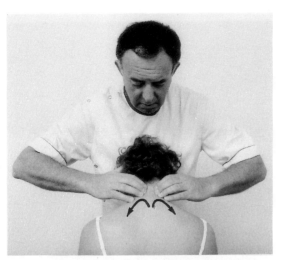

21.11 ◄ Kneading of soft tissues sitting The patient sits with her legs over the side of the table. Stand in front of her and stabilize her head on your chest; use a suitable pad if necessary. Reach round her neck and use the fingertips to pull the soft tissues away from the spine on both sides simultaneously.

Tips: Try adding a sidebending movement at the same time to aid the muscle stretch effect.

21.12 ▼ Kneading of soft tissues sitting The patient sits with her legs over the side of the table and her head is stabilized against your chest, suitably padded if necessary. Control her head with one hand and use the fingertips of the other to knead the soft tissues on the lateral and posterior parts of the neck.

Tips: This hold allows movements to be combined with the kneading as the head hand can control the directions more easily than if two hands are performing the kneading.

21.13 ▼ Kneading of anterior tissues supine Stand at the head of the table and fix the head into the pillow with one hand. Reach carefully round the anterior part of the neck to the scaleni muscle group and push toward the table with the thumb and thenar eminence. When the barrier has been engaged, keep the thumb still and roll the head away with the other hand to bow the muscles over the thumb.

Tips: If kneading is applied directly to the scaleni, it is extremely uncomfortable. Working on the muscles using this method allows quite strong stretch with far fewer problems.

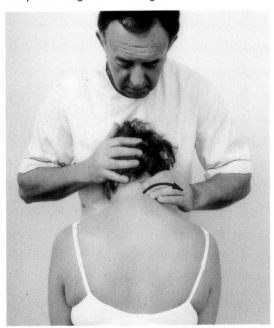

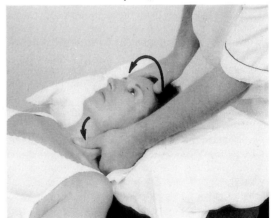

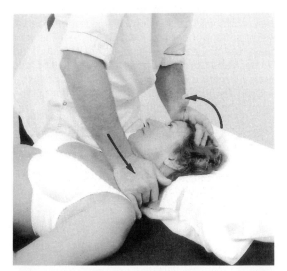

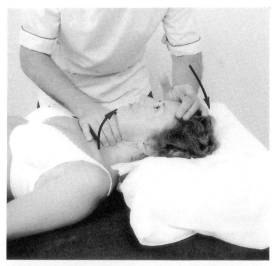

21.14 ▲ Kneading of anterior tissues supine
Stand to the side of the table and stabilize the head on the pillow with the upper hand. Use the heel of the lower hand to push carefully into the scaleni until resistance is felt. Hold the muscles on this slight tension and roll the head away to bow the muscles over the thenar eminence.

Tips: As the scaleni are so sensitive to pressure, this allows quite strong stretch and kneading effect by using a lever rather than pressure.

21.15 ▲ Kneading of anterior soft tissues supine Stand at the side of the patient and stabilize the head with the upper hand. Reach round the throat with the lower hand and pull the tissues toward the midline. When a small amount of tension has been achieved, push the head away to focus the forces in the throat and anterior tissues.

Tips: A direct stretch and kneading on these tissues can be very uncomfortable so this technique allows them to be worked with far less discomfort.

21.16 ▶ Stretching of lateral tissues supine
Stand to the side of the patient and cup the shoulder in the lower hand. Hook the upper hand around the occiput with the thenar eminence resting against the mandible. Stabilize the shoulder and rotate the head away from the shoulder until tension is felt to accumulate in the lateral tissues.

Tips: Try varied degrees of rotation to reach different depths of tissues. Try varied degrees of sidebending, either before or after the rotation to alter the tissue to be affected. Try reaching down the neck with the head hand to fix around the transverse process of a mid or even lower cervical segment. This will focus the force below the fingers to emphasize the stretch in the lower neck instead of the whole neck. Try varied directions of pressure on the shoulder, toward the table or toward the axilla for example. Try changing the order of application with each hand. Every minor change in order, amplitude or direction will vary the technique and only by experimenting in this way can you find the optimum for each case.

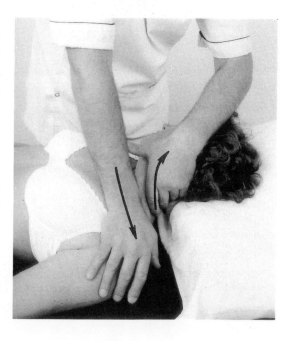

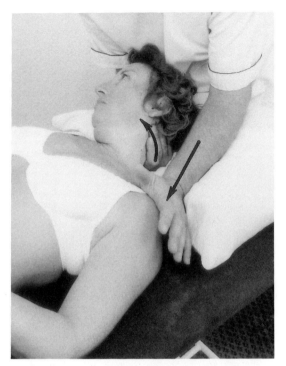
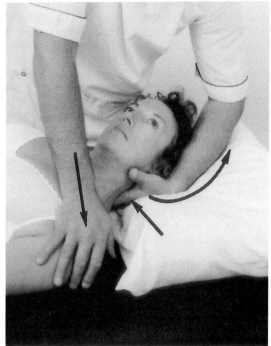
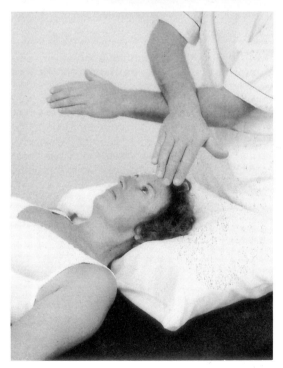
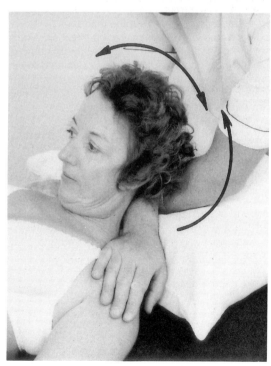

21.17 ◀ (see previous page, top left) **Stretching of lateral tissues supine** Stand at the head of the table and cup the occiput and upper neck in one hand. Fix on the distal part of the shoulder with the other hand. Apply a sidebending to the neck while rotating it away from the shoulder until a stretch is felt to accumulate in the tissues.

Tips: Try varied degrees of sideshift with the head hand to focus the forces at the area desired. See tips for photograph 21.16, as the same parameters apply.

21.18 ◀ (see previous page, top right) **Stretching of lateral posterior tissues supine** Stand slightly to the side of the head of the table and support the head in the palm of the upper hand. Fix the tip of the shoulder with the other hand. Apply the stretch with the head hand pulling into a combination of flexion, sidebending and rotation until the tension is felt to accumulate in the area desired. Note that the head hand has pushed up into the neck in this view to focus the force more specifically to the lower neck.

Tips: See tips for photograph 21.16 as the same variations apply in this hold.

21.19 ◀ (see previous page, bottom left) **Stretching of posterior tissues supine** (hand hold) Cross your forearms with the palms facing the floor. When they are placed under the head and the hands are against the shoulders it will be possible to lever downwards with the hands, and upward with the forearms to push the head into flexion. This will, therefore, stretch the posterior tissues.

21.20 ◀ (see previous page, bottom right) **Stretching of posterior tissues supine** The hand hold shown in photograph 21.19 is applied. Induce the flexion movement by shrugging your shoulders, or by slightly straightening your arms.

Tips: Try sidebending your body to produce a rotation of the patient's head which will tend to focus the force on one side more than the other. Try changing which arm is on top to see which reaches the target structure and tissue best in each case.

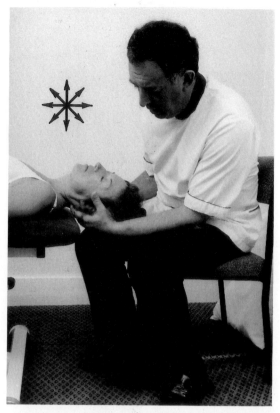

21.21 ▲ **Functional technique or strain and counter-strain hold supine** The patient lies with the head over the end of the table. Support the head in your palms with the fingertips of both hands contacting the articular pillars of the relevant segment. With this hold it is possible to introduce all possible movement parameters of the neck to find the optimum pathway of ease for the functional technique. See earlier section relating to functional techniques.

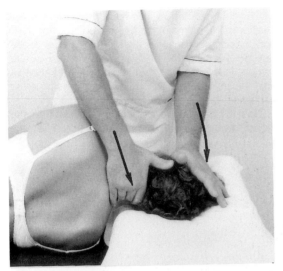

21.22 ◄ Articulation into sideshifting, sidelying Stand in front of the patient and stabilize the head into the pillow with the upper hand. Reach around the articular pillars with the lower hand and pull directly up toward the ceiling to induce a sideshifting movement. Focus the forces by emphasizing most of the lifting force with one finger while maintaining some pressure with the other fingers to reduce discomfort.

Tips: This hold allows an accurate test of individual segmental mobility as well as being a useful treatment technique. Restricted mobility will manifest as a distinct lack of sideshift capability.

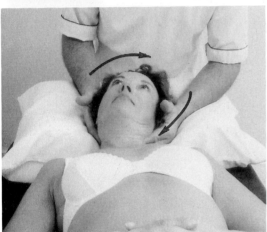

21.23 ◄ Articulation into sidebending supine The patient's head rests on the pillow. Push with the pads of the fingers of one hand over the transverse processes while pushing the head with the other hand in the same direction. Note that it is important to keep the vertex substantially in the central plane so that you do not induce excessive strain on the other side.

Tips: Least useful where the transverse processes are very tender for any reason. In this case, use the pads of the fingers and prise the head over them. This will be much less uncomfortable than pushing into the neck with the fingertips. **Extra considerations**: Paradoxically the operator performs rotation of his body to perform sidebending of the patient's neck.

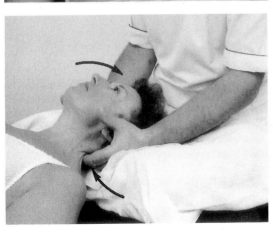

21.24 ◄ Articulation into extension supine Leave the head resting on the pillow and prise up toward the ceiling behind the articular pillars to induce extension. The backs of the hands remain on the pillow to act as a fulcrum for the movement.

Tips: Least useful in cases where extension movement may be a problem, such as postural hypotension or brachial neuritis syndromes.

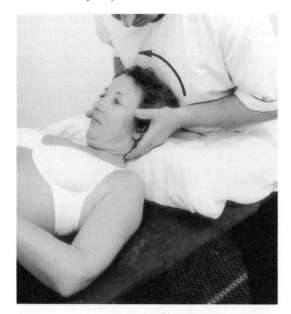

21.25 ◄ **Articulation into flexion supine** Lift the head with the palms of the hands and rest it on your upper abdomen or lower chest. Pull up against the desired level with the pads of the fingers to induce flexion. Use a small straightening of the knees to aid the movement which will also help avoid excessive fatigue in the hands.

Tips: Note that the elbows remain close to the sides throughout so that the movement is performed by the operator's body, not the arms.

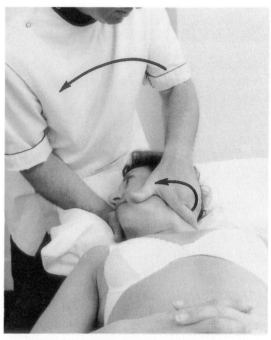

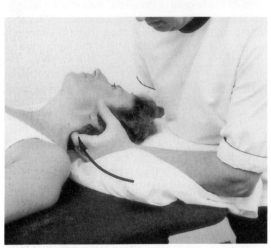

21.26 ▲ **Articulation into localized extension supine** Leave the head on the pillow and use the forearm as a fulcrum. Prise the target level up with the pads of the fingers into localized extension.

Tips: Avoid pressing too far laterally as the tips of the transverse processes are usually very tender.
Extra considerations: Try adding sidebending to the extension movement to localize it even more specifically.

21.27 ▲ **Articulation into rotation supine** Leave the head on the pillow and stand slightly to the side of the table. Rotate the head to the same side. Keep the vertex in the midline so that a pure rotation can be made. Support the head with one hand and allow it to slide under the head as the other hand pulls behind the transverse processes into rotation. Note that the index finger is applied at a target level to focus the force principally to one point.

Tips: Try standing in varied positions to find the best personal method, at the end of the table, to one side or the other. **Extra considerations**: Paradoxically the operator performs sidebending of his body to produce rotation in the patient's neck.

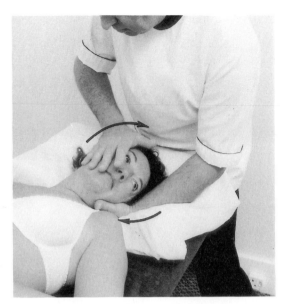

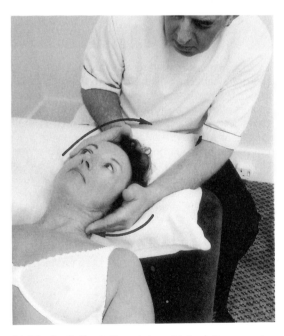

21.29 ▲ Articulation into sidebending supine For this alternative hold sit at the head of the table and use the fingertips of one hand to act as a fulcrum for the sidebending. Push with the other hand against the parietal area on the other side to induce the sidebending.

Tips: The sitting posture forms a useful variation for the operator who might find standing tiring, inconvenient or impossible.

21.28 ◄ Articulation into rotation supine Keep the head on the pillow and turn it to one side, allowing the underneath hand to slide under the head. Apply the other hand to the temporal and maxilla area of the upper side and pull into rotation.

Tips: It is easy to introduce different elements of sidebending along with rotation in this hold. Try rotating and then adding sidebending, or sidebending and later adding the rotation. The sum of the movement is similar, but the effect is completely different according to which tissue is put on tension first.

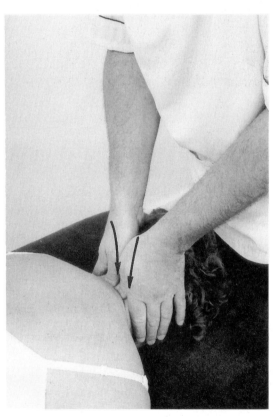

21.30 ▲ Springing into extension prone The patient lies prone, preferably with the face in a breathing hole in the table. Apply your pads of thumbs directly over the posterior aspect of the transverse processes of the target segment. Apply a direct posterior to anterior springing movement to produce localized extension.

Tips: Least useful where the patient may have a problem with prone lying. Least useful in cases where extension is best avoided due to any circulatory insufficiency causing potential obstruction of vertebral arteries.

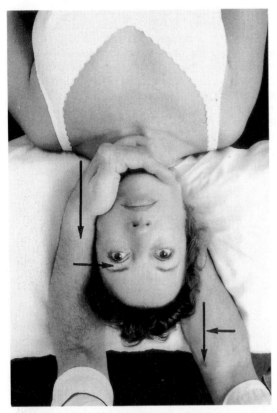

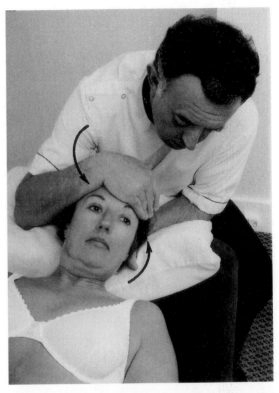

21.31 ▲ Traction supine This operator viewpoint photograph shows the hands applied to perform traction. The underneath hand has carefully gripped round the occiput with the head resting on the palm. The other hand is gripping around the chin and the heel of the hand is applied to the mandible. The wrist and forearm of the chin hand push slightly toward the opposite side to induce a slight sideshift. The occiput hand is introducing a variable quantity of sideshifting depending on the target segment. More sideshifting will drive the force lower in the neck. The wrist of the chin hand balances the pressure of the other hand. Once the sideshift is applied, the traction force can be brought into play. Remarkably little range of traction is available if the sideshift is maintained, which makes it very specific to a small number of segments.

21.32 ▲ Traction unilaterally supine Sit at the head of the table and fix the head to the pillow with the wrist, forearm and lateral border of the hand. Slip the other hand under the head and hook the fingers under the occiput or around the spinous process of a vertebra. Maintain the pressure with both hands and pull gently in the long axis of the spine.

Tips: Note that some rotation and slight side-bending has been introduced to focus the movement to a specific area on the lower side.

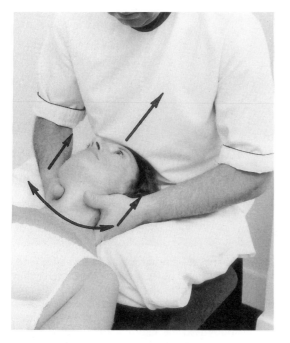

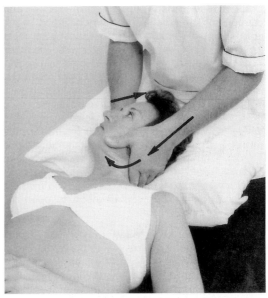

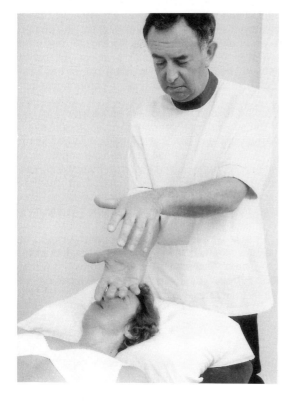

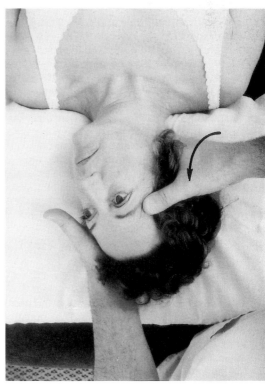

21.33 ◄ (see previous page, top left) **Traction and sidebending articulation combined** Stand at the head of the table and fix the head against your upper abdomen. Apply a slight lifting force with the index fingers to produce a small anterior shifting movement. Keep the arms fairly rigid and pivot your body into sidebending from side to side while leaning back slightly. The sum effect is to produce a sidebending and traction force that will vary in level according to how far down the neck you fix with the hands.

Tips: This can be rather hard work, but is capable of producing rapid changes in mobility, making it an extremely useful technique. Most useful in cases of brachial neuritis where the sidebending force will be introduced primarily in one direction to open the foramen on the convexity.

21.34 ◄ (see previous page, bottom left) **Thrust using cradle hold supine** (hand position) Stand slightly to the corner of the table on the side that the thrust is to be applied. Supinate the lower hand and pronate the upper one so that they form a mirror image of each other. Note that the fingers are slightly splayed to spread the force over a larger area. Note also that the elbows remain fairly close to the operator's sides.

21.35 ◄ (see previous page, top right) **Thrust into rotation, cradle hold supine** Use the hand position shown in photograph 21.34 and turn the head gently into the primary lever direction of rotation. There is unlikely to be a sense of barrier with this small amount of rotation, so add other components either individually or in combination to accumulate the most effective potential barrier. You need to constantly test the primary lever direction while adding the other components until the optimum barrier is sensed. Firm contact point pressure is important as it helps to further reduce the other components. Maintain all the secondary levers of sidebending, sideshifting, compression, anterior shifting and slight extension and apply the thrust into a small amplitude of rotation.

Tips: Note that the elbows are close to the sides, and the technique will be more efficient if you stand as upright as possible so that the arms move with the body. This technique is designed to slide the facet on the same side as the thrust is applied.

21.36 ◄ (see previous page, bottom right) **Thrust into rotation, cradle hold supine** This operator viewpoint photograph shows the underneath hand acting in compression against the thrusting hand. The vertex is maintained in the midline. Note that the wrist of the thrusting hand is in a neutral position. At the end of the thrust the hands accentuate their positions of supination and pronation respectively. This should slide the facet on the same side as the thrust.

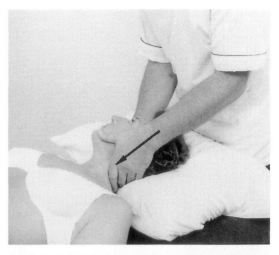

21.37 ▲ **Thrust using cradle hold into sidebending, supine** Stand at the head of the table slightly to the corner behind the head. Take up the hold with the underneath hand supinated to support the head. Apply the thrusting hand with the arm close to your body and the lateral aspect of the middle interphalangeal joint of the index finger slightly behind and to the side of the transverse process of the target segment. Keep gently testing the primary lever of sidebending while adding all the other available components until a sense of barrier accumulates. When the optimum barrier has been found, maintain the secondary components and apply a low amplitude thrust with the index finger directed toward the opposite shoulder.

The secondary components most often useful in this technique are contra-rotation, sideshifting, compression of the head between the hands, slight extension and localized pressure over the contact point with the finger. It is important that the underneath hand does not allow the head to move away from the barrier when the thrust is performed, as otherwise excessive torsion can result.

Tips: Most useful in cases of brachial neuritis on the side to which the neck is being rotated as the foramina on that side will be opened by this thrust. This thrust is designed to gap the facet on the opposite side to the thrusting hand.

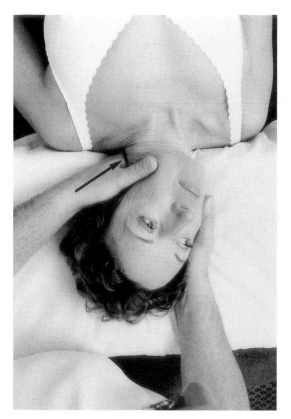

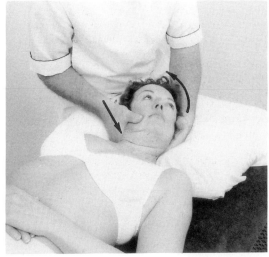

21.39 ▲ Thrust using cradle hold into sidebending This illustration is of the sidebending thrust applied to a lower cervical segment. The hold is taken up in the usual way, but instead of applying more levers, the head is being compressed between the hands so that the effect of the sidebending force is amplified. Note that the thrusting forearm is almost horizontal so that the neck is not being forced into a painful direction, and that the thumb is applied to the mandible to help block out upper cervical movement. This is designed to gap the facet on the opposite side to the thrusting hand.

21.38 ▲ Thrust using cradle hold into sidebending, supine This operator viewpoint photograph shows the hold described in photograph 21.37. Note the buckling of the neck over the operator's thrusting hand and that the vertex is almost in the midline. The hands are applying a compression toward each other to minimize the quantities of the other secondary levers. This should gap the facet on the opposite side to the thrust hand.

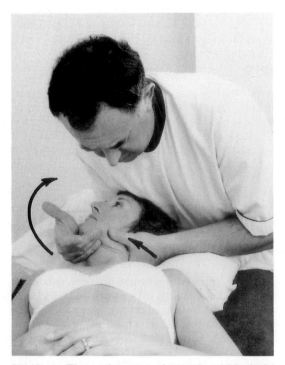

21.40 ▲ Thrust into rotation using chin hold
Stand at the head of the table, slightly at the corner
behind the head. Gently rotate the head to one side
and slide the chin hand under the side of the head
to take up the hold. Take a small step to the back
corner of the table and slide the thrusting hand into
place with the metacarpo-phalangeal joint of the
index finger applied behind the articular process.
Keep testing the primary lever direction of rotation
while adding the contra-sidebending and other
components until a suitable barrier has been
accumulated. Thrust with the hand behind the head
while stabilizing the head and chin with the other
hand. Note that the thrusting hand wrist should be
in line with the forearm, and both elbows close to
the sides. Note also that the forearm of the
thrusting arm is almost horizontal. The most useful
secondary components to focus this technique are
compression between the hands, slight sideshifting
in the opposite direction to the sidebending, and a
slight anterior shift of the whole assembly. This is
designed to slide the facet on the same side as the
thrusting hand.

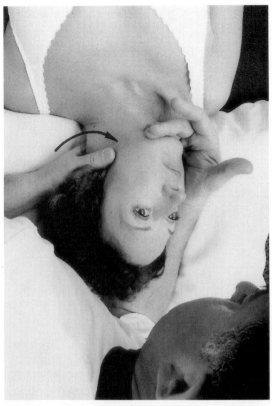

**21.41 ▲ Thrust using chin hold into rotation,
supine** This operator viewpoint photograph shows
the hold illustrated in photograph 21.40. Note the
midline position of the head, and the straight
position of the wrist of the thrusting arm. Note the
position of the supporting forearm under the head
is in front of the patient's ear. This technique is
designed to slide forward the facet on the side
being thrust.

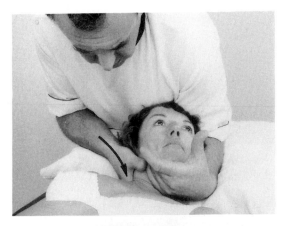

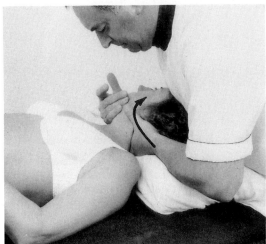

21.43 ▲ Thrust using chin hold into rotation of atlanto-axial joint Take up the chin hold in the manner previously described fixing behind the transverse process of the atlas with the thrusting hand. As the principal movement possible of this joint is rotation, only slight sidebending will be required. Introduce a very small extension to take the posterior tissues off tension, and apply the thrust in pure rotation through a small amplitude to gap the facet on the same side.

Tips: Most regions of the body can be treated in any order, but if it is necessary to thrust the atlanto-axial joint, it is often found to be best left to the last manipulation of a treatment session. This is not an absolute rule, but has sound reasoning. This joint is very susceptible to becoming hypermobile and therefore suffering recurrent lesioning. If it is manipulated first, it is liable to be stressed when any other thrusts are done in the area, thereby irritating it further.

21.42 ◄ Thrust using chin hold into sidebending This photograph shows the hold applied to a lower cervical segment from a different viewing angle. Take up the hold in the way previously described. Apply the lateral border of part of the index finger or metacarpal to the posterior part of the transverse process of the segment. Buckle the neck over the thrusting hand so that the sidebending and sideshifting occur at the same time. Introduce a small amount of controlled rotation with the other hand, and then balance all the secondary components against the primary lever of sidebending. At the optimum moment apply the thrust with one hand while maintaining the head position with the other. Note that the thrusting forearm is almost horizontal and that the vertex remains in the midline. This is designed to gap the facet on the opposite side to the thrust hand.

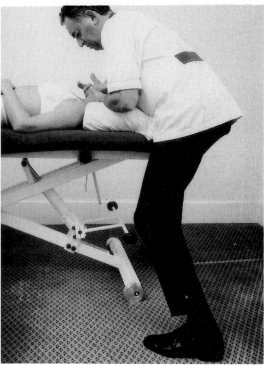

21.44 ▲ Thrust using chin hold into rotation or sidebending This photograph is to show the overall posture usually adopted for these types of techniques. Note that although the operator is bent from the waist, he has not flexed his spine. Note that the leg on the thrusting side is behind the other so that the operator's body is brought into the thrust. Note that the forearm of the thrusting hand is horizontal and that the patient's head has been left on the pillow.

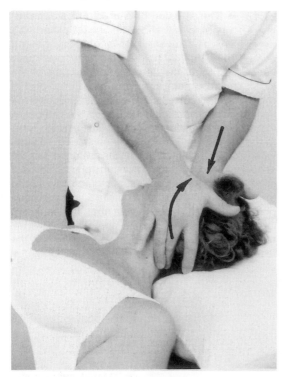

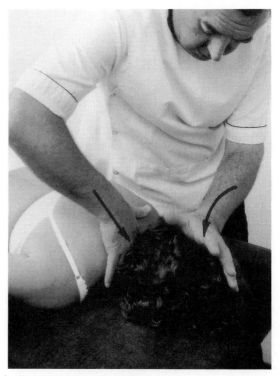

21.45 ▲ **Thrust using pulling hold supine** Stand to the side of the table and grip around the transverse process of the target segment with the middle phalange of the index or middle finger of the thrusting hand. Balance the forces with the other hand applied to the side of the forehead closest to you. Introduce part of the primary lever of rotation and slowly oscillate in the primary lever direction while adding the secondary levers until a satisfactory barrier accumulates. Maintain the secondary levers, and apply the thrust with a short sharp pulling action with the thrusting hand into rotation.

Tips: Some operators find that pulling techniques are easier for them than pushing ones. This technique is most useful in these cases. It is also useful where the operator has a problem in using one particular hand for any reason. The left side of the neck is usually thrust with the left hand of the operator, but with this technique the right hand is thrusting the left side of the patient's neck.

21.46 ▲ **Thrust into rotation prone** Stand to the side of the prone patient and stabilize the head with the upper hand. Use the thrusting hand as a fulcrum to sidebend the neck. Maintain the head in the midline and carefully push the lateral side of the index finger into the neck against the posterior aspect of the articular process of the target segment. The primary lever of rotation is going to be a force directed in the line of the forearm as shown. Maintain the position with the stabilizing hand and apply the thrust behind the articular process through a very small amplitude.

Tips: Note that there is a tendency to introduce extension, and that this is potentially dangerous and must be avoided. Although a sidebending thrust could be applied with this hold, it is even more likely to produce an unwanted hyperextension. If a table with a breathing hole is being used, either plug it up for this technique, or have the patient move slightly to one side so that the chin can act as a pivot directly on the table. Least useful for patients over 40 years of age.

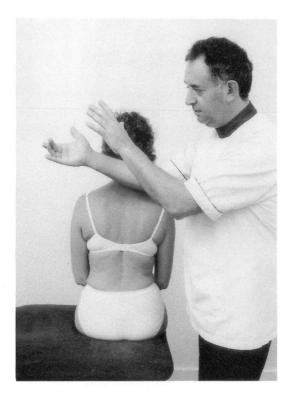

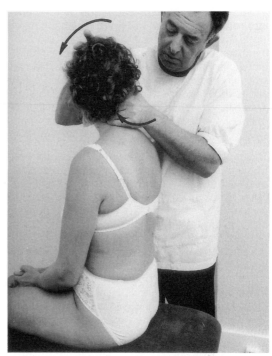

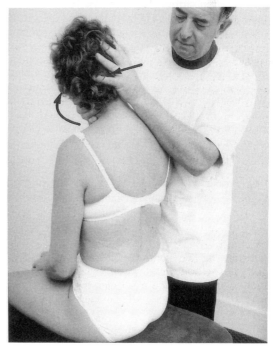

21.47 ▲ **Thrust into rotation sitting** Have the patient sit across the table toward one end. Stabilize the head with the front hand, and apply the pads of the fingers behind the articular process of the target segment with the other. Introduce sidebending toward the thrusting hand, and rotation away. Keep testing the primary lever of rotation while adding the secondary components of the composite lever until a suitable barrier accumulates. Maintain the secondary levers and apply a short sharp thrust into rotation with the hand applied to the neck.

Tips: This is a rather difficult technique to control as the neck tends to try to escape from the tension induced unless it is very carefully managed. Many operators may find it difficult to generate the sharpness needed to break facet fixation with this hold. It is, nevertheless, useful as some patients will not relax well in a supine position, and may find this hold more comfortable.

21.48 ◄ (see previous page, top right) **Thrust into rotation sitting (hand hold)** The hand reaching in front of the patient is supinated, and either the index or the middle finger is flexed to make it more prominent and ready to apply behind the articular process. The other hand is spread slightly and is applied to the nearside of the head to act as a stabilizer for the thrusting hand. Note that the operator's elbows are close to his sides.

21.50 ► **Thrust into rotation sitting (hand hold)** The patient sits across the table near the end. Stand at the end of the table and reach around the neck with the front hand so that the lateral border of the hand can pull forward on the far side articular process. Place the thumb of the pronated posterior hand on the far side of the spinous process of the next lower vertebra. Maintain a small amount of sidebending away from you by firm pressure against the side of the spinous process. The thrust will be applied with both hands. One is pulling forward from behind the articular process, and the other pushing the spinous process toward you. This will produce a contra-rotation force between the adjacent vertebrae.

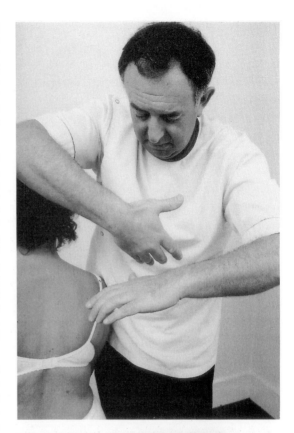

21.49 ◄ (see previous page, bottom right) **Thrust into rotation sitting** The hold described in photograph 21.48 is applied. Rotate the head using both hands until it is approximately in mid rotation. Apply some sidebending to the opposite side. Maintain the rotation and opposite sidebending and circumduct the patient's body through a small arc keeping the vertex directly over the sacrum. When tension accumulates in the target segment, apply the thrust with a short sharp pulling action with the front hand while aiding it with the other. Note that firm compression between the hands is a critical part of this technique.

Tips: It sometimes helps to ask the patient to exhale just before the thrust to produce an optimum state of relaxation. Another useful relaxation aid is to ask the patient to let the shoulders drop; as they do this, there will be an interval of 2 or 3 seconds when the thrust is more easily performed.

21.51 ► (bottom right) **Thrust into rotation sitting** Take up the hold with the grip described in photograph 21.50. Produce a buckling into sidebending at the target segment, and pull back slightly on the clavicle with the posterior hand while prising the spinous process toward yourself. The secondary components of sideshifting, antero-posterior shifting and compression are balanced. At the optimum barrier, the thrust is applied by a stabilizing force with the posterior hand and a rotation force with the anterior hand.

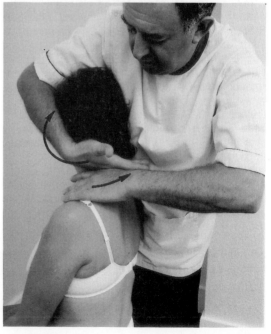

The occipital and upper cervical regions are areas where extreme caution is necessary in preliminary assessment before techniques are applied. Care is required in all areas, but in the occipital region this is even more critical. There is the possibility of damage to the vertebro-basilar system if instability is present. Precautions need be undertaken before performing any thrust technique that is in any way liable to put the area under mechanical stress. As in the rest of the neck, the patient is often fearful of manipulation, and as light a force as will achieve the required result is essential. It is often difficult for students to achieve the required acceleration and subsequent braking force necessary in thrust technique in this area, and there is no substitute for practice and practical experience.

The reader is referred specifically to the section on contra-indications. However, suffice it to say that anything that can compromise the integrity of the ligamentous structures of the area requires extreme caution in the choice of technique. Some will say that all thrust technique should be avoided in the area if there is so much potential danger. However, this would be to deny the possibility of aid in many cases where almost nothing else will work as well.

Occipital thrust techniques performed without excessive force require a well-developed barrier sense. The angles through which any given technique will succeed are very small. Slightly too much leverage will block the techniques and more force is then often mistakenly applied to counteract the lack of ability to focus accurately. Maximum safety is paramount and too much force jeopardizes this. If a given technique is not working, try reducing levers and forces rather than increasing them. It may seem paradoxical, but this often works much better. It is often necessary to make many subtle changes in direction or plane to find the optimum for each technique. Every patient will differ, and changes in table height, operator position in relation to the patient, and quantities of the varied components of a composite lever vary. Many cases will respond well to general mobilizing and articulation. Some, however, will only achieve full and lasting relief from treatment when a specific thrust is successfully performed to fully liberate a facet fixation.

Although specific positions of lesion fixation are often described, the techniques shown here are simply designed to break fixation. If positional correction is deemed necessary, the fixation is dealt with first, and then the joint is coaxed into the direction required afterwards with articulatory technique.

If a barrier does not seem to accumulate in one direction, another is sought. This removes some of the fear of many students that they may be performing the technique in the 'wrong' direction. If this does not satisfy the purist in relation to lesion directions, then several of the techniques shown can be applied in a 'correction' direction if required. I have included the details of these under the 'Extra considerations' headings.

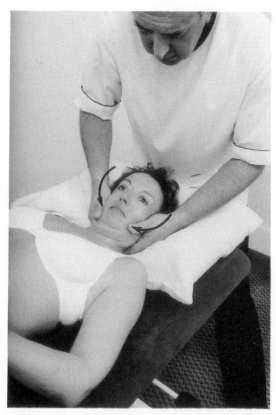

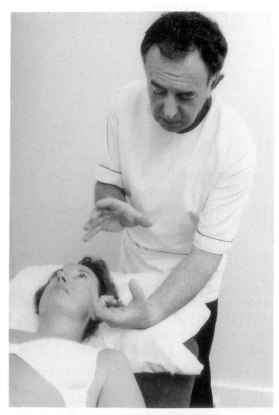

22.1 ▲ **Articulation into flexion supine** Push the head into flexion with your thumbs on the mandible while you pull under the occiput with your finger-tips.

Tips: Try adding traction to the movement. Try adding sidebending to the movement. Ensure the patient has time to breathe between repetitions as the flexed position may obstruct the ability to breathe.

22.2 ▲ **Articulation supine (hand hold)** Form a pivot with the pad of thumb and index or middle finger. Rest the back of the hand on the pillow. Apply the other hand to the forehead of the patient to be able to tip the head into all the directions that the technique allows.

22.3 ▶ **Articulation into extension supine** Apply the hand hold shown in photograph 22.2 and tip the head into extension with the forehead hand while pivoting it over the occiput hand. Once the head is in extension it can be rolled into sidebending to either side to focus the force to each condyle of the occiput.

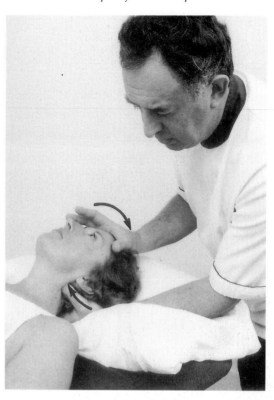

22.4 ▼ (bottom left) **Articulation into flexion supine** This operator viewpoint photograph shows the hold from photograph 22.3 in use for flexion. Note that the pillow is retained, partly to allow it to be used as a fulcrum, and partly as most patients seem to prefer the security and familiarity of a pillow.

Tips: Allow the patient time to breathe between pressures as the trachea can be obstructed in extreme passive flexion!

22.5 ▼ (bottom right) **Articulation into extension supine** In this operator viewpoint photograph the head is pushed up with the lower hand while tipping it into extension with the frontal hand. Note that this is an extension focused to the occiput rather than an extension of the whole neck.

Tips: Try alternating this movement with flexion and sidebending to focus forces to one specific condyle of the occiput. Try varying the spacing of the lower hand to find the optimum for efficiency and comfort.

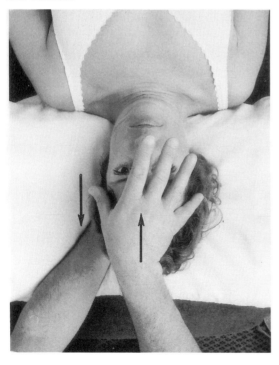

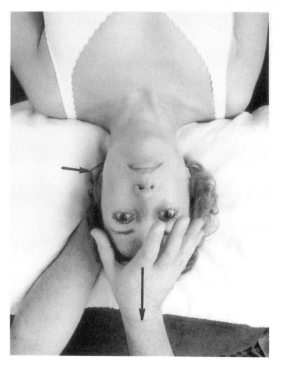

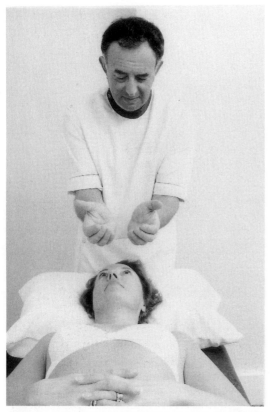

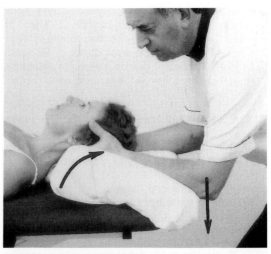

22.7 ▲ Traction to occiput supine Apply the hand hold shown in photograph 22.6. Lower your elbows over the end of the table to form a fulcrum, and fix your hooked fingers under the occiput. As you lower your elbows, the traction force accumulates automatically. Although this would not seem to be very powerful, it does reach very specifically to the occiput and can be very useful if localized traction is desired.

22.6 ▲ Traction to occiput (hand hold) The operator has his fingers close together and is hooking them so that they can pull cephalically under the occiput into localized traction. The backs of the forearms will be applied to the pillow with the elbows over the end of the table. This will allow him to produce traction partly by pulling, and partly by levering his forearms against the end of the table.

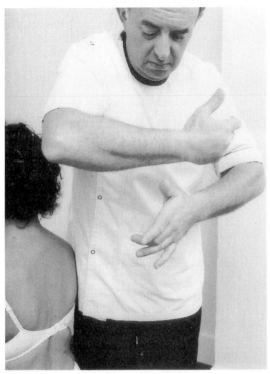
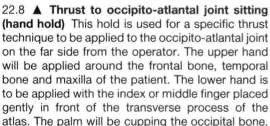
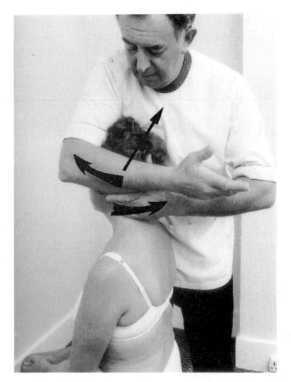

22.8 ▲ Thrust to occipito-atlantal joint sitting (hand hold) This hold is used for a specific thrust technique to be applied to the occipito-atlantal joint on the far side from the operator. The upper hand will be applied around the frontal bone, temporal bone and maxilla of the patient. The lower hand is to be applied with the index or middle finger placed gently in front of the transverse process of the atlas. The palm will be cupping the occipital bone.

22.9 ▶ (top right) Thrust to occipito-atlantal joint sitting The hold illustrated in photograph 22.8 has been applied. Stand to the side and slightly behind the seated patient. Fix the frontal bone with your biceps avoiding the eyes. The forearm of the upper arm lies around the temporal bone and the inside of the elbow is in contact with the maxilla. The technique will not work effectively if the hand of the upper arm is in contact with the patient. The grip is only performed with the medial aspect of the forearm. Your lower hand grips gently around the anterior aspect of the transverse process of the atlas with the pad of the index or middle finger. Pull carefully backwards on the atlas while performing a bowing movement with your body. As the head is in contact with your chest this bowing action will form a sidebending action of the neck so that the atlas is driven slightly toward you.

You must simultaneously supinate your upper forearm. The patient's body is now in sidebending away from you, and you can rock into circumduction from your ankles. As the barrier accumulates, increase the compression of the head toward you, and momentarily grip the atlas firmly as you adduct both arms. The cumulative effect of this is to produce a rotation of the head toward you, and of the atlas away.

Tips: Most useful in cases where it is best to avoid excess rotation of the head on the neck. This technique works with the head in any degree of rotation so it is hardly necessary to torsion the neck at all. It is probably the safest of the thrust techniques that can be applied to this joint. Least useful if the atlas is extremely sensitive to touch as the pressure may be unacceptable. **Extra considerations**: Ensure that firm compression of the head into your body is maintained throughout. Only pull back on the transverse process of the atlas for as short a time as possible to avoid excess discomfort.

22.10 ▶ Thrust to occipito-atlantal joint sitting (rear view) The technique described in photograph 22.9 is set up. Note that the patient is sidebent toward the operator at the pelvis, and away at the neck. Note the supinated upper arm that is maintaining the compression. Note that the upper arm hand is not in contact with the patient. Note that the patient's head is in a position of almost no rotation but a contra-rotation force is, nevertheless, being applied to the occipito-atlantal joint.

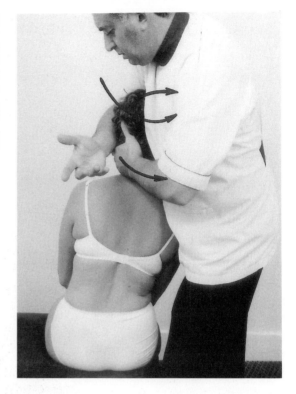

22.11 ► Thrust using minimal leverage to gap occipito-atlantal joint supine This technique is designed to gap the occipito-atlantal joint on the side where the thrust is applied. It is a minimal leverage technique as the neck is not taken to full rotation, but merely placed in an available position so that the contact point is available for the thrust. Some small quantities of levers are used, but the emphasis is mostly on carefully applied compression, and high velocity with very short amplitude. Keep the vertex of the head in the midline and take up the chin hold with one hand. Keep the head resting on the forearm applied anterior to the ear. Ensure that the head is against your upper arm and thorax so that it is firmly controlled, cradled and supported. Place the applicator, the first metacarpophalangeal joint of your thrusting hand, on the posterior aspect of the arch of the atlas. Keep the vertex midline and press firmly into the atlas to take up the slack in the soft tissues. Apply the thrust with a rapid force toward the patient's opposite eye and a simultaneous force of the other forearm against the side of the head.

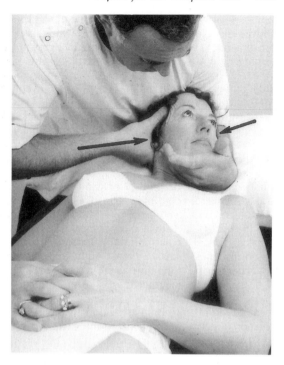

The total of these forces should keep the head still while the atlas is driven forwards underneath the occiput. This is not a torsional force of the head on the neck, but a force of the atlas under the occiput to break fixation on the side of the thrusting hand. If excessive head movement is allowed, the occipito-atlantal joint on the other side will be strained, with a sidebending force. There will also be a tendency to strain the atlanto-axial joint into excess rotation. **Note**: this is an extremely difficult technique to perform well as there is no sense of accumulating barrier. The control of acceleration and braking and accurate directions of force are the governing factors. If it is performed as described here there is little chance of trauma but if torsion is added instead of the method described it is then no longer a minimal lever technique and tissue stress is more likely.

Tips: Most useful where torsion is best avoided and fixation is not too severe. Least useful if the operator is not able to develop the skill to apply the necessary ultra-high velocity, and the strict control of the braking force. **Extra considerations**: Try asking the patient to look over the shoulder of the side to which the head is being rotated. This will increase the effect of the small amount of levers applied as the eye torsion tenses the cervical musculature. Conversely, try asking the patient to turn the eyes to the other side if the tension accumulates too fast as this will have the effect of reducing neck tension.

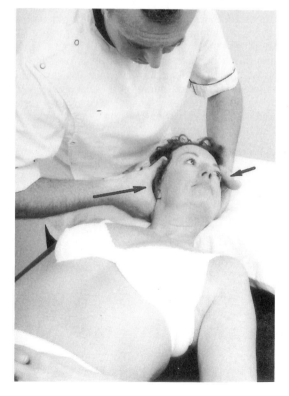

22.12 ◄ (see previous page, bottom right) **Thrust atlanto-axial joint cradle hold supine** As the main movement of the atlanto-axial joint is into rotation, thrust techniques normally used are rotatory types. This technique is designed to break fixation on the side of the thrusting hand. Apply the proximal metacarpo-phalangeal joint of the thrusting hand behind the arch of the atlas. Support the head in the palm of the underneath hand and apply a compression force toward the thrusting hand to absorb the slack into compression to avoid excess torsion. Keep the vertex in the midline and gently rotate the head to about 50% of its available range. Apply a small amount of sidebending opposite to the rotation and a very small extension of the head on the neck to take the posterior tissues off tension. This will make room for the applicator to reach the atlas. Slowly increase the compression while gently oscillating the head into rotation until a sense of barrier accumulates under the thrusting hand. Apply a short amplitude and high velocity force to the atlas to break fixation in a forward or rotation direction of the atlas on the axis.

　Tips: Most useful in older necks as the compression force helps to minimize the torsion necessary. Least useful if the operator is not able to develop the speed necessary to break fixation in this type of technique. **Extra considerations**: This hold makes several variations of the technique available. It is possible to thrust into sidebending to gap the other side of the occipito-atlantal joint. It is possible to thrust on the occiput itself to gap the occipito-atlantal joint on the same side. It is possible to thrust on the posterior aspect of the atlas while holding the head still to gap the occipito-atlantal joint of the same side.

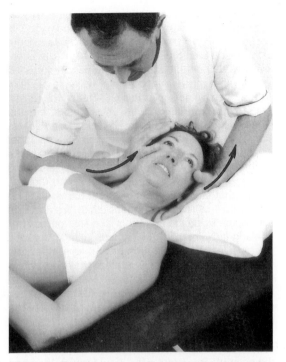

22.13 ▲ **Thrust to occipito-atlantal joint supine** This hold is useful if a traction component is found to be necessary to gap the joint. It is also useful if a sidebending component is necessary. Pronate the arm of the thrusting hand and apply it behind the occiput on one side of the head. Rotate the head to the other side and fix the head against your chest and the pillow with the underneath hand. Rotate the head to about 50% of the neck range and apply a traction force with the underneath hand. Compress the head between the hands and push firmly up into the occiput with the pisiform of the thrusting hand. Apply very slight extension and sidebending toward the thrusting hand to take the tissues off tension and allow the thrusting hand to reach the target tissues. Perform the thrust as a traction with the underneath hand and a rapid adduction with the pisiform.

　Tips: Most useful in cases where there is a sidebending component in the lesion complex. Least useful where operator arm strength may not be sufficient or where the patient may have an extremely large head. **Extra considerations**: A sidebending, rotation or traction force can be used according to which gives the optimum barrier.

22.14 ▶ Thrust to occipito-atlantal joint supine
This technique is useful for breaking fixation in a sidebending or rotation direction. Leave the head on the pillow and take a small step to the corner of the table. Slip your upper hand under the occiput so that the fingertips just curl under the base of the skull. Pull gently upwards under the occiput on the lower side as you apply the other hand to the maxilla and mandible on the upper side. Use a small compression between the hands to hold the head firmly, but avoid excessive pressure on the mandible as otherwise the temporo-mandibular joint can be strained. Tip the head into very slight extension to take the posterior tissues off tension, but not enough to reach the end of range of movement in the occipito-atlantal joints.

Increase the rotation to about 50% of full range and then balance all the components together until tension accumulates on the occipital condyle nearer the table. Apply a short amplitude thrust into sidebending with the maxilla hand while tugging upwards with the occiput hand. Note that this thrust can also become a rotation thrust with the maxilla hand around the fixed axis of the underneath hand. This will have the effect of gapping the upper condyle rather than the lower as in the sidebending thrust.

Tips: Most useful in cases of sidebending restriction. Least useful in patients who have a very mobile mid cervical spine as the force will too easily dissipate there and not accumulate at the occipito-atlantal joint. **Extra considerations**: Try using this position as a firm articulation procedure, but do not carry it on for very long as the forces generated are very strong and will provoke discomfort.

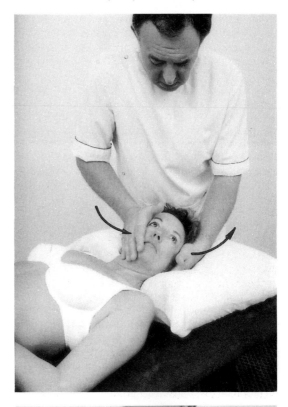

22.15 ▶ Thrust to occipito-atlantal joint 'fly-wheel' technique (hand hold) This technique is a complex one where both hands work in opposition to hold the axis and rotate the occiput on it. The axis hand is to be placed with the thumb gently applied in front of the transverse process and the reinforced middle finger posterior to the transverse process on the other side. The chin hand will be rotating the head to one side as the atlas is held to the other. Even though momentum is used, the head should not reach full rotation even at the end of the technique. It is the effect of the one hand pulling back on the atlas as the head is rotated which causes the joint to gap, not full rotation of the head on the neck.

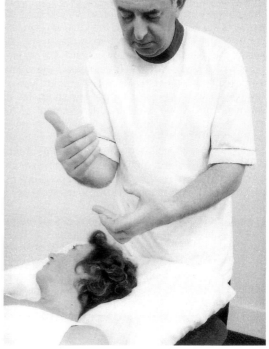

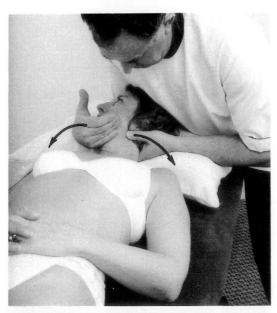

22.16 ▲ Thrust to occipito-atlantal joint 'fly-wheel' technique Stand to one corner at the head of the table. Take up the chin hold with one hand while using the other to take a hold on the atlas. The atlas hand is applied with the thumb placed just in front of the transverse process. The reinforced middle finger is placed on the other side just behind the transverse process of the atlas. As you drop the elbow of the atlas hand toward the table while pulling carefully back on the transverse process you will rotate the atlas slightly back toward the neutral position. As you rotate the head toward the pillow, you will tend to carry the atlas with the head. Make a few gentle rotation movements with both hands moving in the same direction of movement of the chin toward the pillow. At the optimum moment accelerate the chin hand to rotate the head sharply toward the pillow. At the same time grip for as short a time as possible on the atlas to hold it from joining the head rotation. Release the atlas immediately the technique is completed as the transverse process is usually very tender to pressure.

Tips: Most useful in fairly flexible necks where the mobility makes normal locking techniques difficult. Least useful in stiff necks with degenerative changes as the torsional forces, however carefully applied, can be potentially problematical. **Extra considerations**: Try tipping the head into very slight extension to take the posterior tissues off tension and make the atlas more accessible. At the moment of thrust try pushing the head into the pillow to add a compression component that may help in localization.

The nasal sinuses are a common site of congestion, infection and inflammation and osteopathic intervention using vibration and frictional techniques can play a part in treatment in some cases. Rarely will these be a complete answer, and other methods from hot or cold packs through to antibiotics are all appropriate in certain cases. The osteopathic input can, however, add a dimension to treatment which may not have been considered by other practitioners. Some apparently simple manoeuvres can have a very profound effect on drainage, and produce benefit out of all proportion to the time and effort used. Some of these techniques can also be taught to the patient for their own use if appropriate.

Special precautions are mostly those relating to the possibility of spreading infection when the 'mask' area of the face is being worked. The lack of valves in the veins draining the face, and the chance of infection backtracking into the skull and brain must always be borne in mind.

The temporo-mandibular joints are a site of symptoms and dysfunction in some patients, and can be somewhat improved in their function by osteopathic intervention. Hypermobility is clearly not going to respond well to mobilizing techniques; however, when that hypermobility is due to over-stress produced by the opposite side being too tight, suitable mobilization of the restricted side can be useful. The dental surgeon has a role in assessing the occlusion of the teeth and making any suitable adjustments here, but gentle stretching of over-tight muscles and capsule can be valuable.

There are few special precautions here except to consider the indications as much as the contra-indications, and to be aware that poor results in treatment are often due to the wrong choice of treatment as much as the wrong choice of technique.

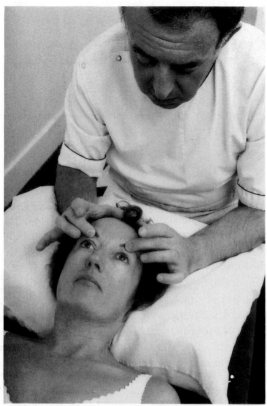 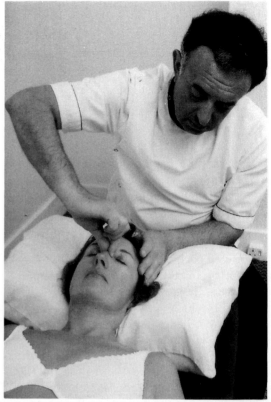

23.1 ▲ Friction or vibration frontal sinus supine
Direct friction over the emission of the supra-orbital nerve as it emits from the ridge of the frontal bone is being used here. The operator's fingers are directly applied to the notch, and either circular friction or vibration can be performed.

Tips: Most useful in conjunction with other friction and vibration points and particularly when the frontal sinus is involved. Least useful where acute sinusitis makes the friction points too tender. **Extra considerations**: Start slowly and superficially and gradually work deeper, repeating the technique intermittently during treatment rather than keeping up the contact for a long period.

23.2 ▲ Friction or vibration over nasal bones supine The nasal bones can be gently squeezed and massaged in this hold where the operator is steadying the head with one hand and applying the technique with the other.

Tips: Most useful in conjunction with other sinus friction and vibration techniques. **Extra considerations**: Start gently and gradually increase pressure and perform the technique for short periods during the treatment session, repeating this several times.

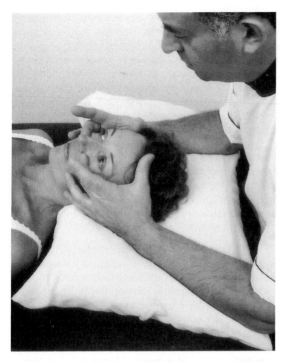

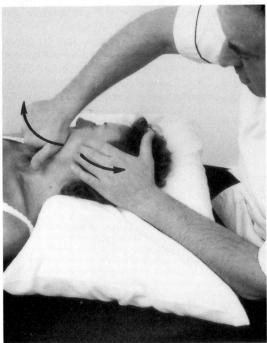

23.3 ◄ Friction and vibration maxillary sinus supine The operator is sitting at the head of the table and has applied the tips of middle fingers to the maxilla so that direct pressure can be used over the emission of the nerve. Vibration can be applied over the maxillary sinus in this position also. The patient's head is stabilized by the heels of the operator's hands.

Tips: Most useful where maxillary sinus is involved. Least useful where acute sinusitis makes pressure extremely uncomfortable. **Extra considerations**: Start gently and gradually increase pressure, perform technique for short periods and return several times during treatment session.

23.4 ▼ (bottom left) Springing temporo-mandibular joint supine While sitting at the head of the table, the operator is holding back on the temporal bone with one hand and applying a repetitive force along the ramus of the jaw with the other. It is possible to make small adjustments to the angle of that force so that the articulation can be stressed in different ways according to the restriction of motion encountered. It is necessary for the patient to let the jaw sag to make the joint accessible; when the masseter is tense, the technique will not produce any effect.

Tips: Most useful in cases of unilateral temporo-mandibular joint dysfunction and intra-articular disc derangements. Least useful in cases of bruxism where it is more important to work on the muscles and occlusion than the joint. **Extra considerations**: While under stretch try antero-posterior movements and lateral movements to find the optimum.

23.5 ► (see next page, bottom left) Articulation temporo-mandibular joints supine From the head of the table the operator can gently grip both sides of the mandible between fingers and thumbs and apply a direct distraction force to the joints on one or both sides. It is necessary for the patient to relax the jaw so as to take the muscles off tension to make this effective. The whole mandible can also be taken into a forwards or backwards direction as required, and if the patient slowly opens and closes the jaw while the distraction force is applied, adjustment of the 'tracking' during this action can be brought to their attention as this often is an essential part of any treatment to these joints.

Tips: Most useful in cases of mal-occlusion and bilateral joint dysfunction where the traction component is helpful. Least useful where muscle tissue is very tight and prevents effective traction. **Extra considerations**: Extreme tenderness at the angle of the jaw can be an indication of occipito-atlanto dysfunction.

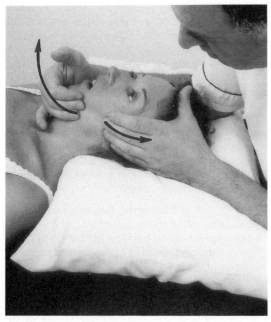

23.6 ◄ Traction and articulation temporo-mandibular joint supine The operator is holding directly over the joint and palpating for sense of tension as the other hand pulls on the mandible to distract the joint in a variety of directions as necessary. It is also possible to hold over the articular disc, and sensing when the joint is on optimum tension, apply a force directly over it which may give an opportunity for the disc to relocate if it is mal-aligned in the joint. As in most temporo-mandibular joint techniques it is necessary for the patient to relax the jaw muscles during these procedures.

Tips: Most useful where muscle stretch is needed and intra-articular disc dysfunction exists. **Extra considerations**: Add antero-posterior and lateral movements for optimum tension.

23.7 ▼ Traction temporo-mandibular joint supine A suitable wooden rod is interposed between the teeth as far back as possible to form a fulcrum, and the operator is carefully closing the jaw as distally as possible. This causes a direct traction force to be generated in the temporo-mandibular articulation on the side of the fulcrum. Traction can be a useful force as it is an accessory movement to the joint and can thus produce mechanical changes that primary movement under the control of the patient's own muscles cannot achieve.

Tips: Most useful where muscle stretch rather than articular work is required and where patient has own teeth. Least useful with dentures. **Extra considerations**: Pad wooden rod if necessary and vary the thickness to find the optimum tension.

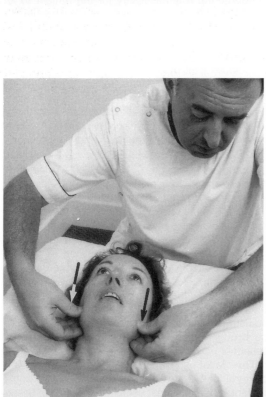

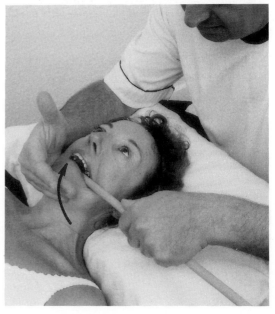

The clavicle is mentioned often in early osteopathic literature, yet relatively little attention seems to have been given to it in modern times. Although the nomenclature given to lesion positions was attractive, and gave specific directions of force to be applied to reverse the positions, it also limited thinking into certain directions only. Some specific directions of fixation are common, but modern thinking is much more directed toward function, and techniques designed in such a way that they can restore perceived deficits of function.

The clavicle can be thought of in isolation, or as a structure influenced by trauma, posture and occupational disorders. It can be considered as a bone with a pair of joints attaching it to the sternum and the scapula. Whatever the type of thinking, the main object of osteopathic technique is to restore normal mobility where it has been lost. This aims to re-introduce integrity of function to the pectoral girdle that may have diminished if the clavicle is not working properly.

Precautions are minimal, except that hypermobility of the joints can occur, and then techniques applied will be irrelevant and indeed may worsen the situation. Some techniques use the arm as a lever, but possible shoulder conditions may need protection, or alternative techniques sought in these cases.

The clavicle acts as a prop to join the arm to the body and to protect the vessels and nerves underneath it. It is essentially a stable unit, but when the stability is lost, disproportionate symptoms and dysfunction of the arm may occur. This in turn can make restoration of function of the clavicle an important part of any syndrome affecting the upper thoracic or shoulder area. Many 'difficult' upper thoracic cases will respond well if clavicular dysfunction is attended to as a major part of the treatment approach.

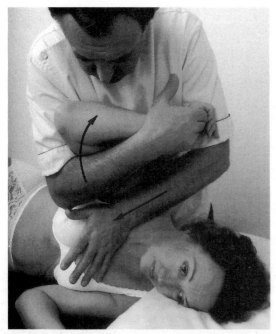

24.1 ▲ Articulation of clavicle sidelying Stabilize the scapula with your body and while you hold the clavicle down circumduct the shoulder. Varied degrees of abduction will influence the sterno-clavicular or acromio-clavicular joints or simply place the main emphasis on the shaft of the bone.

Tips: Most useful when the muscles attaching superiorly to the clavicle are involved. Least useful when the use of the shoulder as a lever would be a problem. **Extra considerations**: Try using different phases of respiration.

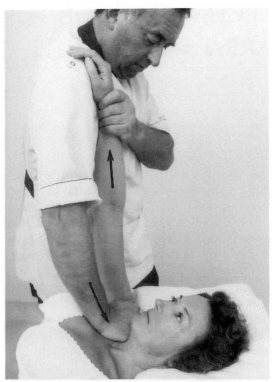

24.3 ▲ Articulation of clavicle supine Hold the patient's wrist and forearm firmly against you so that as your hand applied to the clavicle fixes toward the table, a small straightening of your knees will perform the articulation. The opposite can be applied if you gently lift the clavicle with your fingertips and apply a downward pressure through the patient's arm.

Extra considerations: Try using varied angles of rotation of the shoulder.

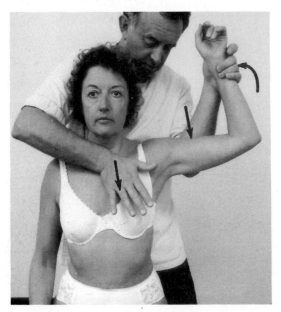

24.2 ◄ Articulation of sterno-clavicular joint sitting Stabilize the scapula with your body and hold down on the medial end of the clavicle. Abduct the patient's arm and extend and externally rotate it to apply a pull along the length of the clavicle. Due to the shape of the joint, the most common dysfunction is a riding upwards and medially of the sternal end of the clavicle. In a true subluxation, this technique may produce a realignment of the joint but it will not last, as the capsule and ligaments will have been disrupted, probably permanently.

Tips: Most useful where for any reason the recumbent patient position is a problem. Least useful in very mobile subjects where it would be difficult to achieve a localization. **Extra considerations**: Try using different phases of respiration.

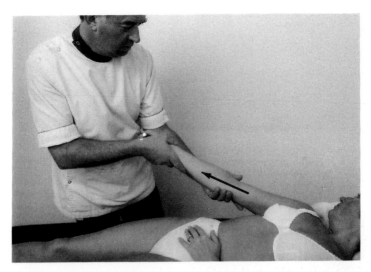

24.4 ▲ Thrust to acromio-clavicular joint supine Fixation in the acromio-clavicular joint is most usual on the anterior aspect and can be addressed well with this technique. To avoid excessive tension on the brachial plexus when the tug is applied, the patient's head is sidebent and rotated to the same side. Pull steadily on the distal part of the forearm and above the elbow with the other hand. Make small circumduction movements and vary the angles of flexion and abduction of the shoulder until tension is felt to accumulate in the acromio-clavicular joint. Apply the thrust without releasing the previously applied tension as otherwise a whipping action will occur which makes the technique ineffective.

Tips: Least useful when gleno-humeral dysfunction is present.

24.5 ▶ Thrust to a cromio-clavicular joint sitting The final position for this technique is shown here. The operator has applied an external rotation, flexion and traction to the patient's shoulder while firmly holding back on the clavicle so that forces accumulate at the acromio-clavicular joint. As a preliminary the patient's arm is taken from a position with the back of her hand facing forwards at, or behind her waist and then thrust out sharply forwards while supinating her forearm. This puts a gapping force on the acromio-clavicular joint.

Tips: Least useful in very flexible subjects as the force will tend to dissipate. **Extra considerations**: Try using different phases of respiration and varying the flexion angle of the shoulder.

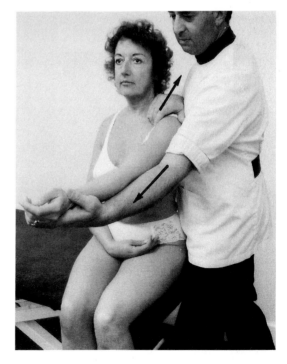

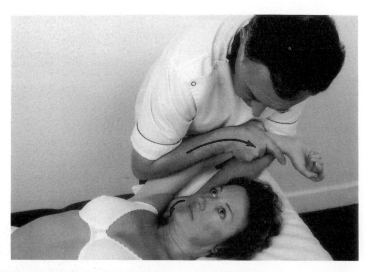

24.6 ▲ Thrust to acromio-clavicular joint supine Start with the patient's arm by the side and firmly fix the distal third of the clavicle with the pad of your thumb. Bring the patient's arm into elevation and rotate it gently until tension accumulates at the acromio-clavicular joint. An articulatory force can be used, or if tension is suitable, a small thrust can aid in breaking fixation in the joint. Care must be taken to apply the thumb to the plateau on the top of the clavicle to keep the discomfort of the pressure to a minimum.

Tips: Least useful where there is gleno-humeral dysfunction making this range of movement impossible.
Extra considerations: Try sandwiching the patient's wrist between your hand and forearm and then moving your whole body and arms together.

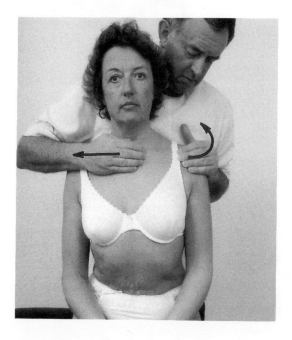

24.7 ◄ Articulation of sterno-clavicular joint sitting Hold tension with both hands in opposite directions and fix the patient's scapula with your thorax, then twist into rotation both ways to produce a mobilizing force on the sterno-clavicular articulation and first rib anteriorly.

24.8 ▶ **Thrust to sterno-clavicular joint supine**
Use crossed hands to put a longitudinal force
through the shoulder and, therefore, the clavicle
while holding back against the sternum with the
ulnar border of the sternal hand. When tension
accumulates, the sternal hand maintains the pressure and the pisiform pushes toward the table and
along the clavicle by means of the hand deviating
into an ulnar direction. It may be necessary to
rotate the patient's head to one side or the other to
optimize the accumulation of tension in the joint.

Extra considerations: Try varying the range
of abduction and adduction in the shoulder to
optimize the tension.

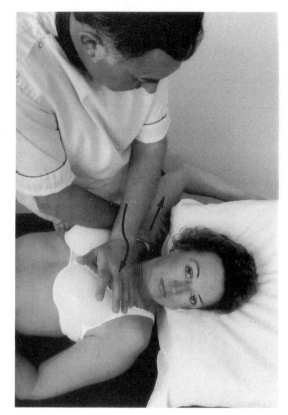

Patients often present in osteopathic practice with dysfunctions and disorders of the gleno-humeral articulation and the shoulder area generally. The shoulder can be described as a structure that is slung from the occiput, and tethered to the pelvis, so, like all other areas of the body, cannot be considered in isolation. The joint itself can manifest mechanical derangement as well as pathological conditions, particularly those involving the capsule and the surrounding muscles and tendons.

Special precautions that must be considered when working on the shoulder with manual techniques include the possibility of bone-weakening conditions such as osteoporosis, as some of the levers used will be long and potentially strong, and excess force could possibly compromise bone strength. In practice the amount of force used should never be enough to cause bone damage even in a diseased state. However, it may not always be realized how much leverage is being applied. From the point of view of indications, accurate diagnosis of the cause of any particular syndrome is not always easy. Pain due to inflammatory disorders and secondary protection of hypermobility may not be responsive to physical treatment and much wasted time, discomfort and expense can be avoided by recognizing this. As the joint is a ball and socket, thrust techniques directly applied to the shoulder do not play a large part in the treatment of dysfunctions.

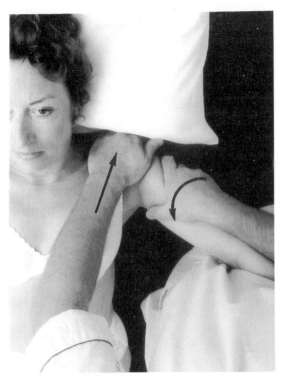

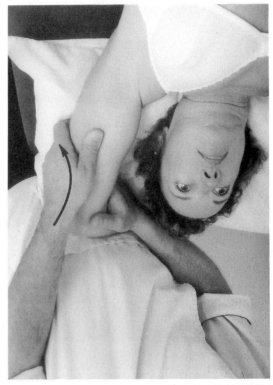

25.1 ▲ Kneading shoulder muscles supine This is an operator view of the technique. It shows the hands applied with the use of a 'wringing' action to the soft tissues to work either the anterior, superior or even the posterior aspects of the joint. Varying degrees of abduction, compression and rotation can be used to aim the forces to the tissue or area desired. The technique can be applied with the medial hand while the other one remains still, or the medial hand can remain still while the operator's body and other hand move in varied directions together. There are many more variations of this hold than would appear at first glance, and a little experimentation will reveal some interesting changes in target tissue with only small adjustments of hold and pressures.

Tips: Most useful in cases where shoulder dysfunction permits a reasonable degree of abduction. Least useful in acute capsular conditions where abduction beyond a small range is impossible. **Extra considerations**: As with all techniques that are designed to work on soft tissues, the duration of the hold is an important element. A finite quantity of time of several seconds with the tissues under slight sustained pressure is necessary to produce a significant change. Simply stretching and immediately releasing the tissues will produce a less efficient result as fluid interchange will not have had time to take place.

25.2 ▲ Kneading upper arm muscles supine This operator's viewpoint photograph shows cross-fibre kneading being applied to the triceps. If the hands were changed over, the biceps and brachialis could be worked in the same way. Similar work on the muscles can be performed with the arm in a neutral position. In the position shown the muscles and fascia are on some tension that can allow more efficient combined technique with stretch as well as cross-fibre work.

Tips: Most useful in cases where the belly of the upper arm muscles rather than the tendons is the target. Least useful in cases of articular dysfunction where the muscles may be less important. **Extra considerations**: Varying the degree of abduction or adduction will change the initial tension on the muscles to make the technique a combined kneading and stretch procedure.

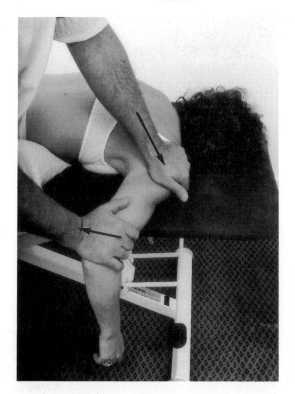

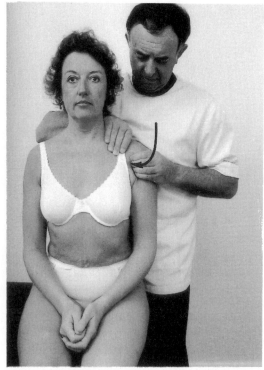

25.3 ▲ **Kneading shoulder prone** The posterior parts of the shoulder and muscles are more accessible in this position. Control the arm with your hand so that you can vary the angle at which the shoulder is held to reach the particular tissue desired.

Tips: Most useful where the posterior muscles and the scapula are involved. Least useful where the patient finds prone lying a problem for any reason. **Extra considerations**: Varying the position of head rotation can change the effect of the technique.

25.4 ▲ **Articulation of shoulder sitting** Induce antero-posterior and supero-inferior movement in this position. The long head of the biceps is available for friction in cases of tendonitis, as is the rotator cuff tendon behind the shoulder that you can work with your thumb.

Tips: Most useful in any patient who finds a recumbent position difficult. Least useful where shoulder movement of any amplitude must be introduced to make the technique reach the target tissue. **Extra considerations**: Introduce a traction component with the patient holding a small weight as the technique is being performed.

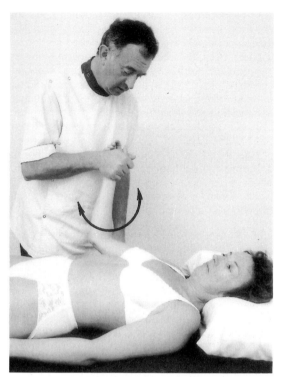

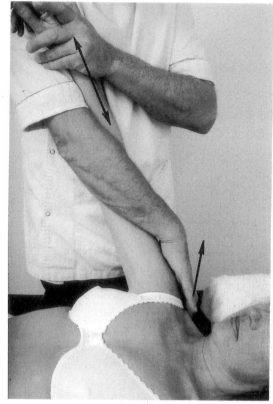

25.5 ▲ Harmonic technique hold for shoulder supine Clasp the patient's hand between your hands and induce a harmonic oscillation into a pendulum-like movement of the arm into abduction, adduction and internal and external rotation. Flexion or extension can be introduced as well, or combinations of several components are possible. An appropriate rhythm for this technique would be slightly different in each subject but would vary between fifty and a hundred oscillations per minute. The correct rhythm is determined by finding the rate that can be maintained with least effort by the operator.

Tips: Refer to earlier section specifically relating to harmonic technique.

25.6 ▲ Traction of shoulder supine Fix the patient's arm between your upper arm and hand while you apply the other hand behind the head of the humerus. Lean back and allow the fingertips to fall into the space produced by the traction. These fingers monitor the force necessary and can add a small tugging motion to the joint.

Tips: Most useful in mild inflammatory disorders where this gentle oscillation allows circulatory interchange. Least useful in cases of specific individual muscle disorders where this technique is non-specific. **Extra considerations**: Try varying the angle of rotation of the arm and the abduction and flexion angles as well for optimum effect.

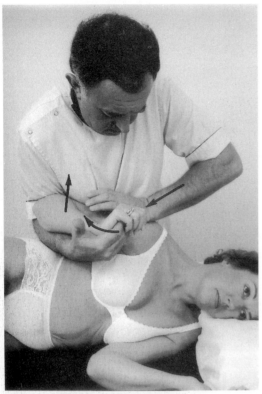

25.7 ◄ Traction of shoulder sidelying Fix the patient's forearm between your flexed wrist and biceps and keep the elbow well flexed so that as you lean back, the forearm and upper arm is carried into traction. Apply the other hand just below the acromium to produce a traction and distraction force at the shoulder. Varied degrees of abduction and rotation and flexion, extension can be induced to maximize the effectiveness and reach different parts of the capsule.

Tips: Most useful where rotation in traction is indicated rather than pure rotation. Least useful where there is any dysfunction in the elbow or wrist. **Extra considerations**: Try applying the traction with alternating hands.

25.8 ▼ (bottom left) **Articulation of shoulder sitting** The sitting position allows you to treat the shoulder by your body movement while the shoulder is held still rather than the shoulder being moved on the body. Fix the scapula to your sternum and rotate or sidebend yourself, thereby influencing different parts of the shoulder joint complex. You must maintain a firm grip so that you and the patient move as a unit.

Tips: Most useful where the long muscles affecting the shoulder inferiorly are involved. Least useful in very mobile subjects. **Extra considerations**: Take care to avoid the patient's trachea.

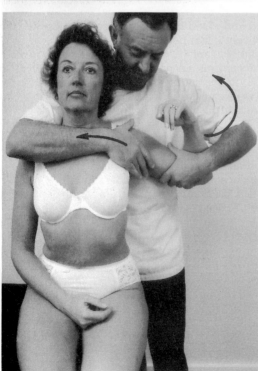

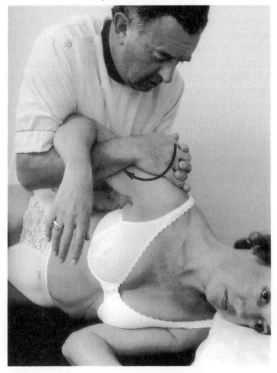

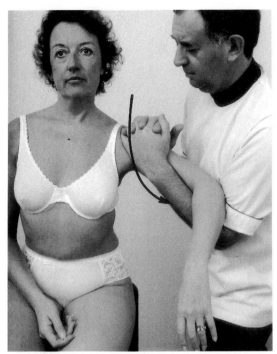

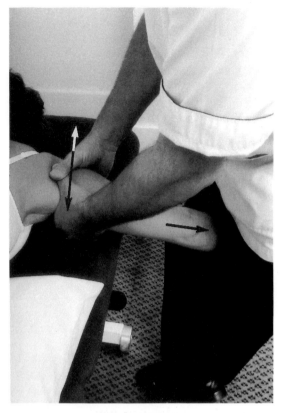

25.10 ▲ Traction to shoulder sitting Place your interlocked fingers just below the acromium and apply a traction and distraction force. While this force is maintained take the shoulder through a variety of movements while the body is torqued into the opposite directions. This will have the effect of influencing the shoulder directly and the long muscles acting on it.

Tips: Most useful where for any reason the recumbent position may be a problem and where good abduction range is possible. Least useful in very flexible subjects where spinal movement will absorb the levers. **Extra considerations**: An initial force applied diagonally toward the opposite hip first, before the traction, is useful.

25.11 ▲ Traction and articulation to shoulder prone Clasp the patient's forearm between your thighs and grip the shoulder between your hands. Rest the back of your fingers on the table and while you hold the shoulder firmly in position straighten your knees to produce the traction. You can move the hands into a variety of directions.

Tips: Most useful where accessory movements of antero-posterior and supero-inferior movement are required. Least useful where lying prone for any reason is a problem. **Extra considerations**: An adjustable table is essential to allow the patient to be lowered so that the arm is horizontal.

25.9 ◄ (see facing page, bottom right) **Traction and articulation to shoulder sidelying** Place your interlocked fingers just under the acromium and apply a force toward the axilla so that you produce a distraction and traction to the joint. Some variation of angles of rotation can be introduced to affect different parts of the capsule.

Tips: Most useful where it is necessary to avoid putting forces through the elbow or wrist. **Extra considerations**: Firm pressure toward the table is an essential component.

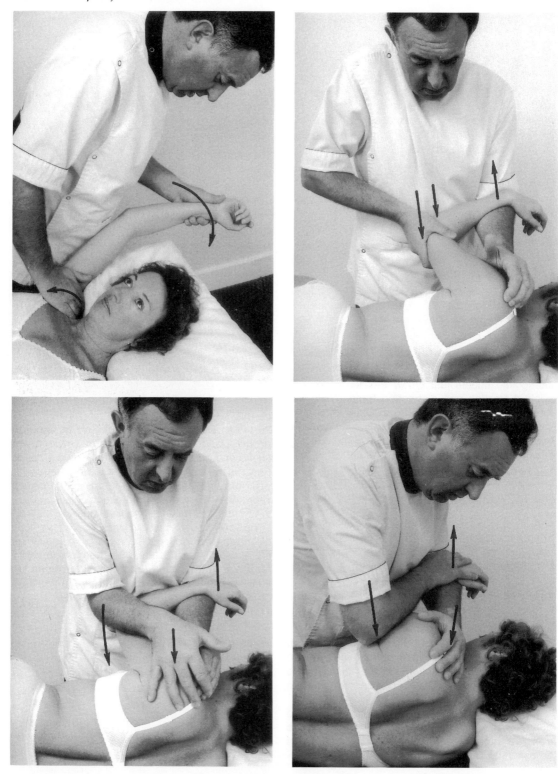

25.12 ◄ (see facing page, top left) **Articulation of shoulder supine** Hold the acromion and the clavicle into the table and pull them slightly caudally while your other hand elevates the arm until resistance is felt. Different degrees of rotation and more or less abduction can be introduced to focus to particular parts of the joint.

Tips: Most useful where it is desired to isolate the clavicle from shoulder movement. Least useful in very kyphotic subjects as this range of movement can be very limited as the anterior tissues will be rather shortened.

25.13 ◄ (see facing page, bottom left) **Articulation of shoulder into external rotation sidelying** Use your cephalic forearm to act as a fulcrum while that hand fixes the acromion and clavicle, and palpates the shoulder joint. The other hand ˙introduces external rotation with varying degrees of flexion while your body assists the movement. The greater the degree of flexion in the shoulder the stronger this articulation will be.

Tips: Most useful where a strong mobilizing force is required. Least useful where there is any suspicion of lack of bone strength as this is a long lever on the humerus. **Extra considerations**: Try holding the joint on tension and rocking the whole body backward and forward into rotation.

25.14 ◄ (see facing page, top right) **Articulation into external rotation of shoulder sidelying** In this hold, both of your hands are applied to the shoulder and your caudal elbow induces the rotary movement. This has the advantage that compressive force can be applied more firmly to the shoulder. This limits the range of motion from the joint itself which will therefore have a greater influence on the soft tissues.

Tips: As photograph 25.13.

25.15 ◄ (see facing page, bottom right) **Articulation into external rotation of shoulder sidelying** Fix the lateral border of the scapula with your caudal hand and use your cephalic hand to hold the scapula firmly against the posterior wall of the thorax. Apply the external rotation force with your upper abdomen pressing down on the patient's elbow.

Tips: As photographs 25.13 and 25.14 but most useful in very flexible subjects to avoid scapulo-thoracic movement and focus into the shoulder itself.

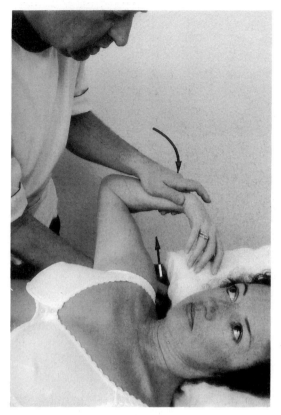

25.16 ▲ **Articulation into external rotation of shoulder supine** This very strong long lever articulation needs great care, but with your caudal hand you apply a postero-anterior force so that the shoulder can be externally rotated. The other hand is used rhythmically, to increase range of motion.

Tips: Most useful where a strong lever is required. Least useful where there is any fear of lack of bone strength. **Extra considerations**: Vary the angle of shoulder abduction to find the optimum.

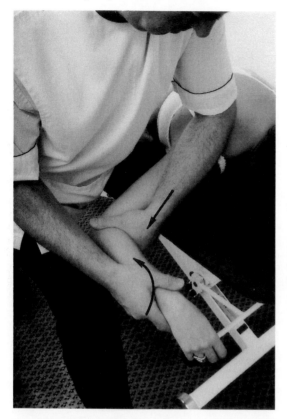

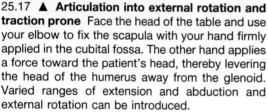

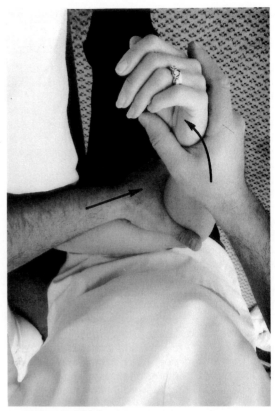

25.17 ▲ Articulation into external rotation and traction prone Face the head of the table and use your elbow to fix the scapula with your hand firmly applied in the cubital fossa. The other hand applies a force toward the patient's head, thereby levering the head of the humerus away from the glenoid. Varied ranges of extension and abduction and external rotation can be introduced.

Tips: Least useful in patients where lying prone is a problem for any reason.

25.18 ▲ Traction and external rotation articulation to shoulder supine Face the head of the table and apply traction by placing your hand in the cubital fossa while the other hand applies the external rotation force.

Tips: Most useful as the scapula is held by the table and strong traction and external rotation can be applied. Least useful where the biceps tendons are sensitive as pressure on them will be a problem. **Extra considerations**: Vary the angle of abduction and flexion to find the optimum.

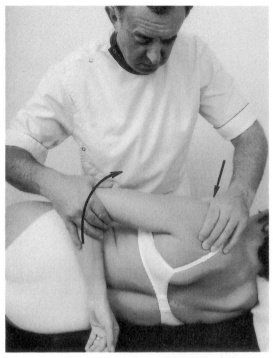

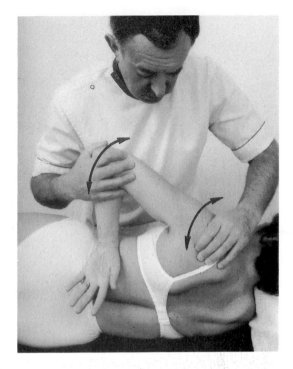

25.19 ▲ Articulation into internal rotation of shoulder sidelying From in front of the patient you fix the shoulder with your cephalic hand while the caudal hand applies the internal rotation force.

Tips: Most useful where a strong force is required. Least useful in cases of severe movement restriction as the position will be difficult to attain. **Extra considerations**: Try applying a traction force at the same time.

25.20 ▲ (top right) **Articulation into internal rotation of shoulder sidelying** Abduct the shoulder just sufficiently so that the patient's wrist is fixed behind the lower ribs. The internal rotation force will be much stronger in this position. The cephalic hand can either hold back on the scapula and clavicle or assist the rotary movement by pulling on the head of the humerus.

Tips: As photograph 25.19.

25.21 ▶ Articulation into internal rotation of the shoulder sidelying Fix the scapula from behind with your torso and introduce the rotary movement by holding firmly with your cephalic hand while carefully pushing your caudal hand anteriorly.

Tips: Most useful where the scapula tends to wing excessively. Least useful in cases of severe movement restriction where the position may be difficult to attain. **Extra considerations**: Try using traction in addition to rotation.

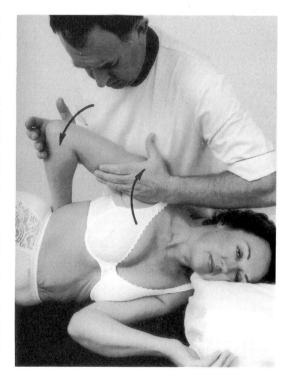

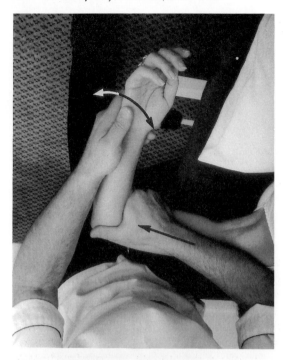

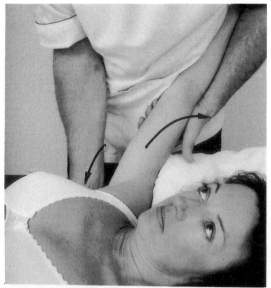

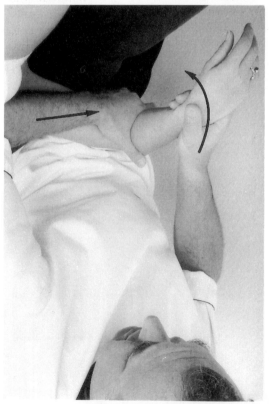

25.22 ▲ (top left) **Articulation into internal rotation of shoulder prone** In this operator viewpoint photograph you face the foot of the table and while fixing the scapula with your elbow, you apply a traction force through the patient's cubital fossa. Your other hand carefully raises the patient's hand toward the ceiling while maintaining pressure on the distal end of the forearm toward the table to induce traction.

Tips: Least useful where the patient may find prone lying a problem for any reason.

25.23 ◄ **Articulation into internal rotation and traction of shoulder supine** In this operator viewpoint photograph you face the foot of the table and fix the shoulder to the table with your elbow while the hand in the cubital fossa acts as a fulcrum for the other hand. Push, at the same time, toward the table for the traction and toward the floor for the internal rotation.

Tips: Most useful where a strong force is required. Least useful where there is any elbow dysfunction. **Extra considerations**: Vary the angles of abduction and flexion for optimum results.

25.24 ▲ (top right) **Articulation of shoulder supine** Fix the lateral border of the scapula with one hand while firmly gripping the lower end of the humerus with the other hand which can induce rotation movements, elevation and traction as required. The fixation of the scapula causes the movement to be localized to the shoulder joint itself rather than the scapulo-thoracic articulation and naturally less range of motion will be achieved.

Tips: Most useful where there are adhesions in the inferior aspect of the capsule. Least useful in acute cases where this much abduction would be a problem.

Mechanical dysfunctions in the joints of the elbow are not uncommon. Their importance in painful syndromes and disturbances of usage varies, but is often a factor that can be addressed by osteopathic treatment. From a mechanical viewpoint the elbow poses various problems. There are rather small but important ranges of accessory movement and it is necessary to use these in treatment techniques. They may be difficult to control. Other problems are posed by the fact that the joints will tend to escape from corrective forces if the grip is not firm enough. However, an excessively firm grip will produce pain and even more resistance. A balance between force, direction and amplitude is critical. The joint complex must be considered as a whole; the elbow, radio-humeral articulation, and distal articulation at the wrist all work together. Often individual joint dysfunction will not be corrected until a suitable balance is obtained between all the relevant joints and soft tissues. The fascial state is also important as poor circulation, healing and myofascial tone may be part of the equation.

Special precautions need to be considered to exclude the possibility of myositis ossificans, which sometimes affects the brachialis muscle in the presence of a haematoma after trauma. The ulnar nerve is vulnerable to damage on the medial side of the ulna. An ulnar neuritis takes a very long time to heal when traumatically induced. It would be very hard to do this in treatment, but an existing condition could be irritated by injudicious technique. It is essential to avoid excessive force, particularly into extension as there is a possibility of damage to the floor of the olecranon fossa.

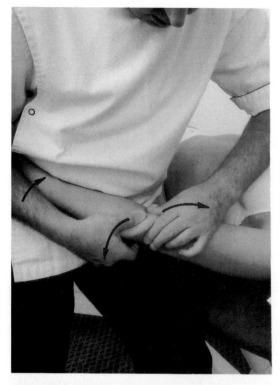

26.1 ◄ **Kneading of lateral tissues supine** Clasp the arm between your body and forearm and knead the extensor muscles on the lateral side of the arm. The hands share the pressure in opposite directions to reduce the amplitude of movement necessary in each.

Tips: Try varying the angle of shoulder abduction and rotation; this will change the initial tension in the muscles before they are kneaded. If there is extreme tenderness, try holding the muscles on some tension and moving the arm back and forth rather than the muscles themselves.

26.2 ▼ (bottom left) **Kneading of medial and anterior tissues supine** Fix the patient's forearm to your side with your forearm and then apply a kneading and stretching to the medial compartment muscles with both thumbs. It is possible to reach deep into the cubital fossa with this hold.

Tips: Take care to protect the brachialis and brachial artery from excessive pressure.

26.3 ▼ (bottom right) **Kneading of lateral compartment muscles supine** Sit on the edge of the table. Put some tension on the muscles with the proximal hand and then, while maintaining this pressure, pronate the forearm with your other hand to generate the kneading force.

Tips: Try varying the angle of elbow flexion and adding components of traction or circumduction to the hold. As an alternative, the operator can perform this technique standing.

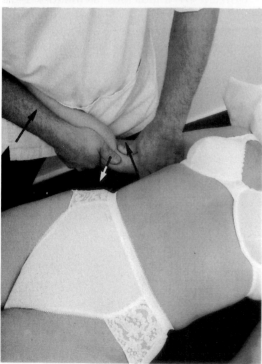

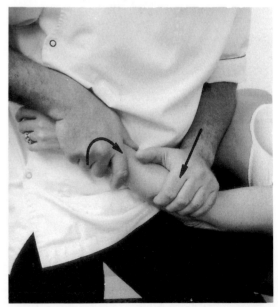

26.4 ▶ **Stretching of medial compartment supine**
Fix the arm to the table with your proximal hand and
apply some compression to the medial side of the
elbow. Apply a stretching force with the other hand
by pulling the forearm into your side. Keep your arms
against your sides and rotate away from the table.

Tips: Try varying the pronation and supination
during the technique to reach different parts of the
muscles.

26.5 ▼ (bottom left) **Stretching of intra-osseous
membrane supine** Grip the forearm between your
hands and apply opposite movements with each
hand of traction and compression as well as
antero-posterior shearing.

Tips: Try varying the angle of flexion before
applying the other levers.

26.6 ▼ (bottom right) **Traction supine** Fix in the
ante-cubital fossa with your pronated proximal
hand and grip the forearm with the other. Compress the forearm against your abdomen and turn
away from the table to pivot round the fixing hand
to apply traction.

Tips: Most useful where there has been a
longitudinal compression force injury and it is
necessary to disengage the joints.

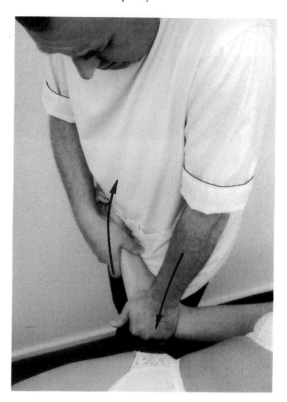

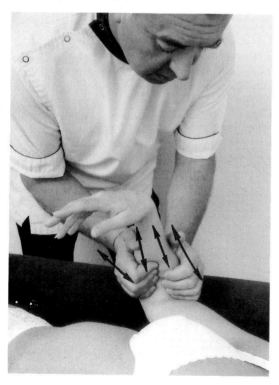

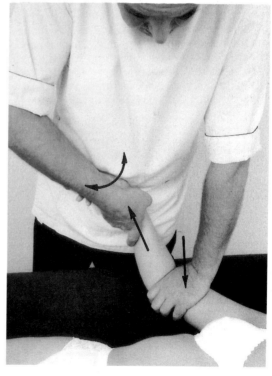

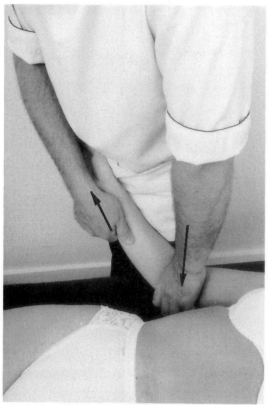

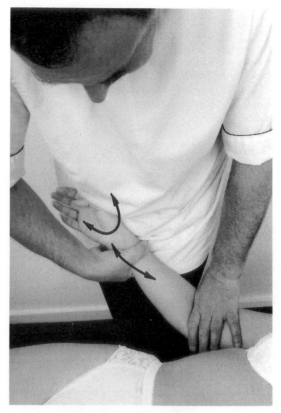

26.7 ▲ **Traction to ulna supine** Fix the upper arm to the table with the pronated proximal hand. Grip the ulna with the other hand and compress the forearm against your abdomen. Pivot around your fixing hand to apply a specific traction to the ulna.

Tips: Try adding a small circumduction force to the traction.

26.8 ▲ **Traction to radius supine** Fix the upper arm to the table with your pronated hand and reach around the forearm with the distal hand to grip the radius. Apply traction and mobilize in pronation and supination.

Tips: Most useful in cases of 'tennis elbow' where there tends to be an element of compression in the radio-humeral joint. Least useful where the forearm is very large and it would be difficult to reach around the ulna to the radius.

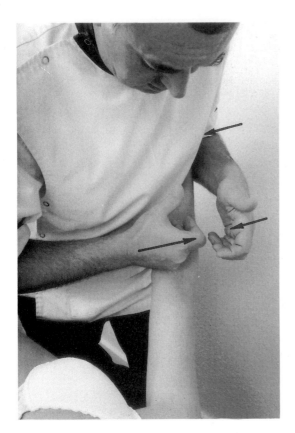
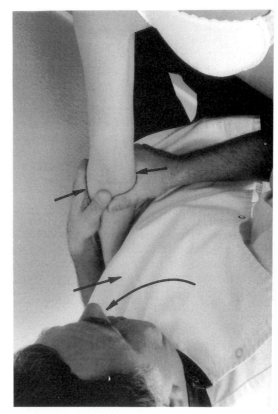
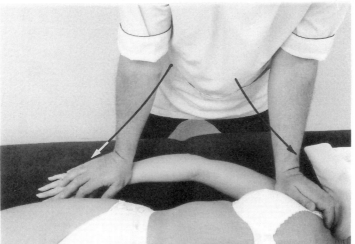

26.11 ▲ Thrust to radio-humeral joint supine The patient is lying supine but slightly turned toward the affected arm. Apply your hands to the slightly flexed arm. Contact the shafts of the radius and ulna and the upper part of the humerus. Compress with both hands toward the table and apply a gentle rocking force from side to side until tension accumulates in the radio-humeral joint. The thrust is applied without releasing this preliminary tension by dropping some weight onto both hands.

Tips: If preferred, use crossed arms to apply the hold.

26.9 and 26.10 ◄ (see previous page, top left and top right) **Thrust to radio-humeral joint supine** Fix the patient's forearm to your side and clasp around the slightly flexed elbow, applying the web of your thumb to the medial aspect of the joint. Compress the elbow between your hands and circumduct through a small range to find the optimum point of tension. The tip of the index finger of either hand palpates for this tension and applies a local compression to the radio-humeral joint. The thrust is performed with an increase of compression between the hands, an increase of fixing of the arm to your side and a short, sharp rotation of your body away from the table.

Tips: Note the angle of the thrusting arm is not directly across the joint but is directed slightly anteriorly, as the radio-humeral joint is anterior to the humero-ulnar joint. This technique may require several priming forces of gradually increasing amplitude until the optimum tension accumulates.

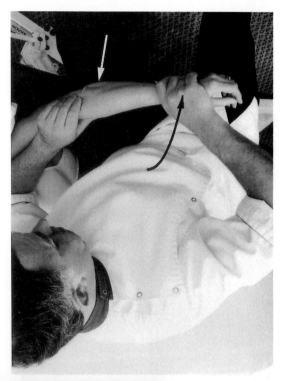

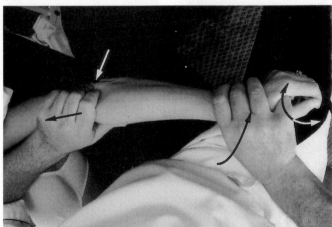

26.12 and 26.13 Thrust to radio-humeral joint supine These operator viewpoint photographs show a complex technique for gapping the radio-humeral joint. Sit on the edge of the table and place the internally rotated arm across your lower thigh. Fix the medial epicondyle against your thigh and hold back on the distal end of the humerus. Your other hand grips the distal end of the radius and applies a force directly toward the floor. Vary the pronation and supination until tension is felt to accumulate. The thrust is performed by an accentuation of all three forces, the operator's thigh and upper and lower hand simultaneously.

Tips: Try placing the fifth finger in the palm of the patient's hand to allow better control of the pronation and supination. This also allows control of the flexion and extension of the wrist to help focus the forces in the elbow. If a stronger effect is needed, instead of using more force, try introducing ulnar deviation of the wrist with the distal hand. If an even stronger effect is needed, place the patient's thumb in the palm of their hand to place the extensor muscles on stretch, and then apply ulnar deviation. **Note**: The internal rotation of the arm is essential if this is not to become an extension thrust. It is often very difficult to maintain this internal rotation. Ensure that the medial and lateral epicondyles are vertical before performing the technique.

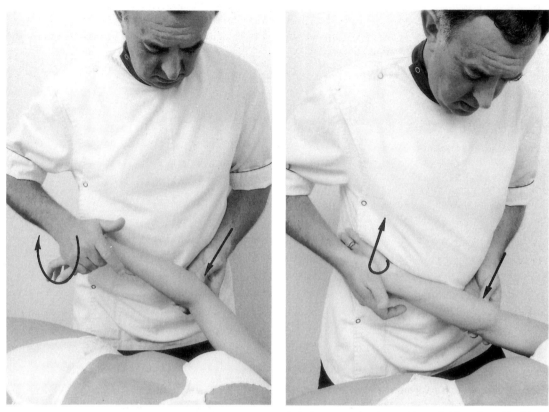

26.14 and 26.15 Thrust to radial head supine Place your thumb behind the radial head and hold the distal end of the forearm against your abdomen. Maintain slight flexion of the elbow throughout the whole technique. Sharply pronate the forearm, flex the wrist and extend the elbow to slap the forearm against your abdomen. This **'Mills procedure'** is often performed with hyperextension, which is not only painful, but can be potentially dangerous as the proximal end of the ulna can be driven through the floor of the cubital fossa. Hyperextension also means that the force will be unlikely to reach the radial head so the technique will be ineffective for the purpose intended!

Tips: Try compressing the radial head between thumb and fingers of the proximal hand to help localize the levers.

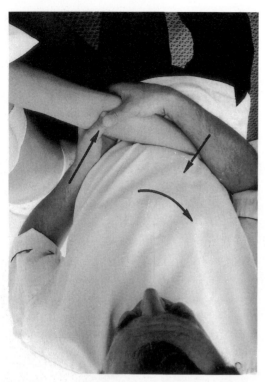

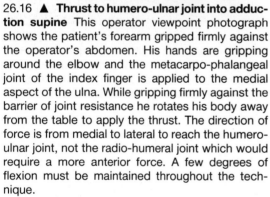

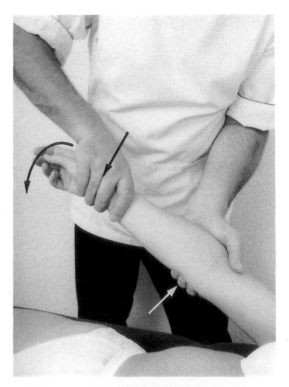

26.16 ▲ Thrust to humero-ulnar joint into adduction supine This operator viewpoint photograph shows the patient's forearm gripped firmly against the operator's abdomen. His hands are gripping around the elbow and the metacarpo-phalangeal joint of the index finger is applied to the medial aspect of the ulna. While gripping firmly against the barrier of joint resistance he rotates his body away from the table to apply the thrust. The direction of force is from medial to lateral to reach the humero-ulnar joint, not the radio-humeral joint which would require a more anterior force. A few degrees of flexion must be maintained throughout the technique.

Tips: This technique would be used where there is an increased carrying angle or a perception of an inability for the head of the ulna to locate in the fossa on full extension.

26.17 ▲ Thrust to humero-ulnar joint into adduction supine Stand outside the slightly flexed arm and pull with your proximal hand on the medial aspect of the ulna. Push the distal end of the forearm in the opposite direction to produce a force designed to reduce the carrying angle.

Tips: Try adding varied amounts of wrist deviation to help focus the technique. This hold can be used to perform the opposite function of increasing the carrying angle where necessary, by reversing the hand directions.

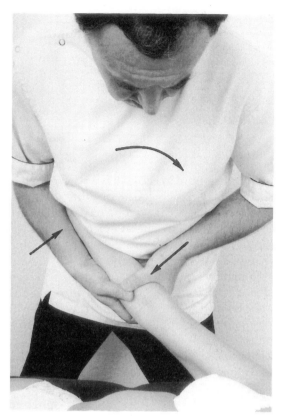

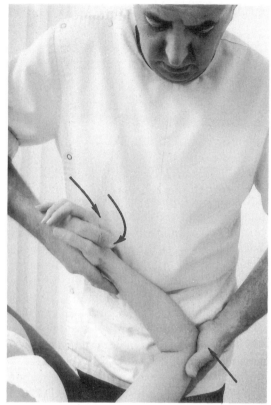

26.18 ▲ Thrust to humero-ulnar joint into adduction supine Fix the forearm against your side and grip firmly around the elbow with both hands. Apply the metacarpo-phalangeal joint of your index finger of the proximal hand to the lateral aspect of the upper end of the ulna. Maintain slight flexion in the elbow and apply the thrust with your proximal hand and a small rotation of your body.

26.19 ▲ Thrust for 'pulled' radius supine Shake hands with the patient and fix behind the elbow with your other hand. Apply a small compression force between the hands and gently pronate and supinate the elbow until the radial head is felt to relocate within the annular ligament.

Tips: This technique should only be necessary in children and any suspicion of a 'pulled' radius in an adult should alert the operator to the possibility of a fracture or dislocation. Dislocations of the ulna must NEVER be reduced using pronation and supination as there is a danger of the coronoid process damaging the brachial artery!

TECHNIQUES FOR THE FOREARM AREA

The forearm transmits torque between the elbow and hand by way of the fascia, bones and muscles. Bones in life are somewhat malleable, and torque on these tissues can cause mechanical problems. The state of the fascia that encloses the muscles and vessels is particularly important here, and myofascial techniques are extremely useful in contributing to improvement in function. Tension states in the muscles of the forearm can have an adverse influence on wrist and elbow function and may be maintaining factors in dysfunction at those sites.

Muscle energy techniques are useful here and are based on anatomical knowledge of muscle planes and attachments. Deep frictional cross-fibre massage has a part to play in specific soft tissue states of adhesions and local irritability. This can be of particular use over the medial or lateral epicondyles of the humerus in states of 'golfer elbow' and 'tennis elbow', respectively.

Rehabilitation of post fracture cases can also often be helped by direct work on the muscles and fascia of the forearm. Particular care should be applied where there is a true neuritis as this can be aggravated by physical treatment applied over the nerve itself. No technique holds have been illustrated for this section as the principles are similar to those in the upper arm or the calf holds shown in the relevant sections.

The wrist is an extremely delicate structure that requires mobility and yet stability. Sometimes this balance goes wrong, and then osteopathic intervention is appropriate. Techniques can be general or specific, and although general techniques can often be effective in restoration of function, specific manipulative skill is sometimes essential. Some apparently pathological conditions can be influenced by osteopathic treatment such as carpal tunnel syndrome, and osteopathic management including direct work on the wrist and hand can be valuable.

Special precautions need be considered in relation to the true cause of symptoms. In many cases there is hypermobility, and although this will manifest as subjective stiffness, accurate motion testing should reveal the real nature of the problem. Undiagnosed fracture of the scaphoid, for example, is well documented in books on fractures and traumatology and should never be overlooked. Inflammatory disorders such as rheumatoid arthritis need special care, and although gentle short treatment can be helpful, excessive mobilization is not wise.

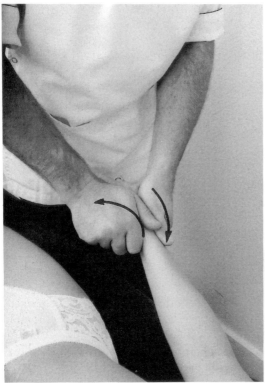

28.1 ◄ **General mobilization** The patient is lying supine and the operator is performing alternating ulnar and radial deviation with his hands, gripping around the wrist. This will produce a shearing force that will reach many of the carpal articulations.

Tips: Try fixing with one hand and moving the other or using both hands. This hold can be applied to the palmar or dorsal surface of the wrist.

28.2 ▼ (bottom left) **Shearing of carpal rows** The operator is standing by the side of the supine patient and is introducing a direct dorsal and palmar force with the wrist maintained in a neutral position.

Tips: Try moving both hands distally to focus on the inter-carpal articulations rather than the true wrist joint. Try squeezing or spreading the patient's hand with the distal operator's hand or applying traction between the operator's two hands.

28.3 ▼ (bottom right) **Kneading thenar eminence** In this operator viewpoint photograph, the lateral border of the hand is being held stable while the operator's thumb is applying kneading to the thenar eminence.

Tips: Use care and a gradual introduction of force as these muscles are often extremely tender initially. Try adding circumduction articulation simultaneously.

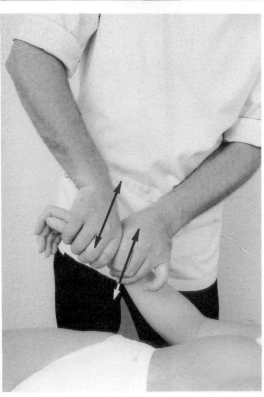

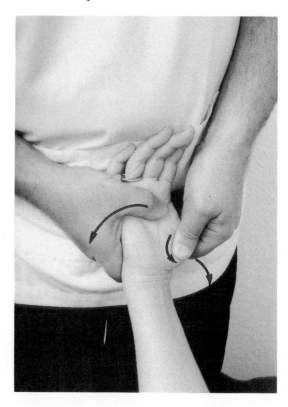

28.4 ► **Stretching palmar surface** In this operator viewpoint photograph the hand is being stretched laterally between the operator's hands.

Tips: Most useful in cases of carpal tunnel syndrome where shortening of the flexor retinaculum may be a maintaining factor. **Extra considerations**: Try inducing an ulnar and radial deviation of the operator's hands when tension has been applied to reach different parts of the flexor structures.

28.5 ▼ (bottom left) **Stretching proximal part palmar surface** The operator is gripping over the hammate and scaphoid to produce a strong stretch on the flexor retinaculum.

Tips: Most useful in cases of carpal tunnel syndrome. **Extra considerations**: Try sustained stretch for several seconds and then adding a diagonal torsion to reach the proximal and distal parts of the retinaculum.

28.6 ▼ (bottom right) **Stretching palmar surface** This operator's viewpoint photograph shows the hand held against the operator's abdomen and his hands applying a diagonal stretch to the ulnar border of the patient's hand.

Tips: Most useful in carpal tunnel syndrome and Dupetrens contracture if slowly applied and maintained for several seconds.

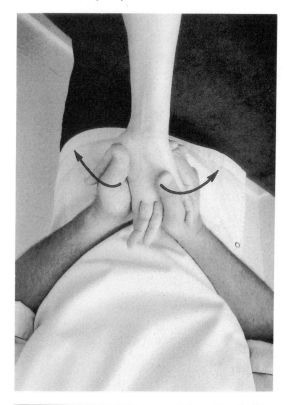

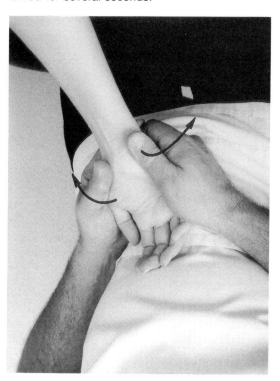

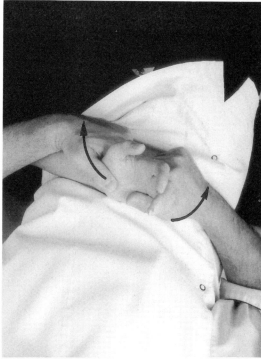

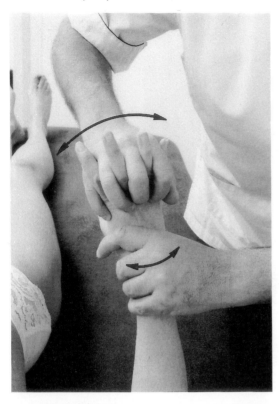

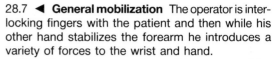

28.7 ◄ **General mobilization** The operator is interlocking fingers with the patient and then while his other hand stabilizes the forearm he introduces a variety of forces to the wrist and hand.

Tips: Try each range of possible movement including combinations, not forgetting traction and compression.

28.8 ▼ (bottom left) **Specific articulation carpometacarpal joints** This operator viewpoint photograph shows the distal hand pulling on a metacarpal bone while the proximal hand fixes on the appropriate part of the wrist to introduce a traction articulation. Other vectors can be used, such as rotation, circumduction and abduction/adduction, as the restriction demands.

Tips: Most useful in cases of carpo-metacarpal dysfunction rather than the actual wrist itself.

28.9 ▼ (bottom right) **Specific articulation carpometacarpal joints** This operator viewpoint photograph shows the patient's pronated hand being fixed against the table while the operator's distal hand grips one of the metacarpals. Traction, with or without other ranges of movement, can be introduced.

Tips: Most useful in impaction injuries where the metacarpal may be driven into the related carpal bone.

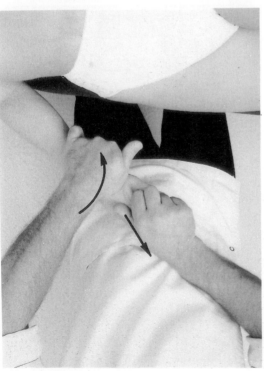

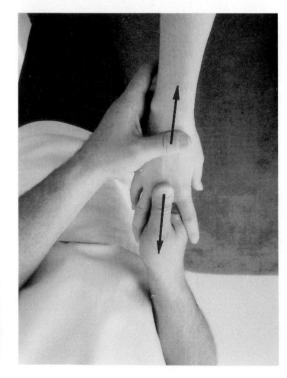

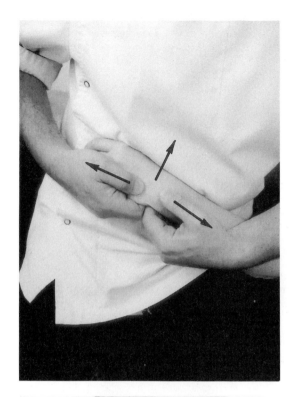

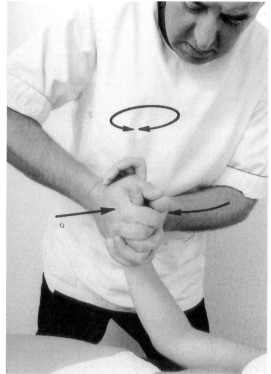

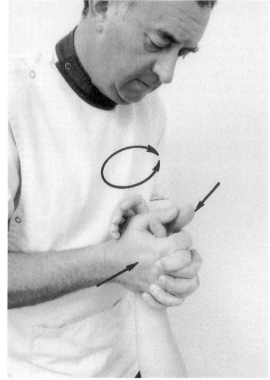

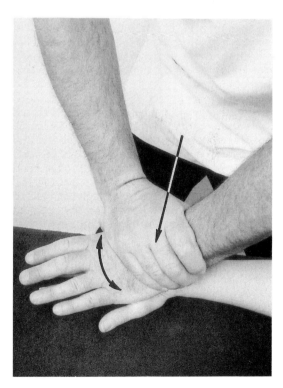

28.10 ◄ (see previous page, top left) **Articulation carpo-metacarpal joints lateral border** The operator clasps the wrist of the supine patient to his abdomen by turning his back to the table. He holds firmly on the relevant metacarpal and carpal bone and then turns his body to produce the traction and mobilizing effect. Many different vectors of force can be introduced while the traction is applied, to effectively address the restriction of movement.

28.11 ◄ (see previous page, bottom left) **Circumduction articulation/thrust** The operator is very firmly clasping the patient's hand between the heels of his hands. He applies a circumduction motion and, within the movement, an arc of effective resistance will be felt. If this is a soft resistance, increased pressure between his hands may create a suitable thrust barrier, where he can perform a short, sharp force against the restriction.

Tips: Try varying the part of the applicator performing the compression, thus directing the force to different parts of the wrist (see photograph 28.12). **Extra considerations**: This technique requires fairly high compression force that must be varied to reduce operator strain and patient discomfort.

28.12 ◄ (see previous page, top right) **Circumduction articulation/thrust** See description for photograph 28.11, but note that in this hold the operator is applying the force with his hypothenar eminences to the proximal part of the patient's wrist. He is also in a different arc of the circumduction cycle.

28.13 ◄(see previous page, bottom right) **Thrust mid carpus pronated** This operator viewpoint photograph shows the patient's hand pronated and the operator is pressing firmly with his pisiform directly over a chosen articulation. His other hand is reinforcing the pressure and he maintains this pressure while slightly deviating the thrusting hand into ulnar or radial deviation to find the optimum tension. Without releasing the tension a very small amplitude thrust is applied.

Tips: Most useful where it is necessary to reduce the angle of the curve of the wrist and stretch the anterior structures while specifically manipulating any restricted joint.

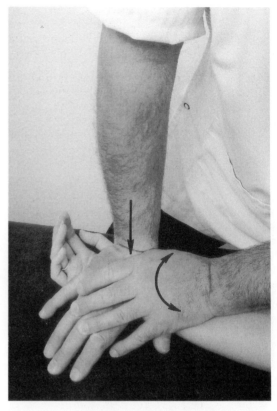

28.14 ▲ **Thrust mid carpus supinated** This operator viewpoint photograph shows the patient's hand supine and the operator is applying a direct force between the scaphoid and the hammate to open out the wrist curve, The other hand is reinforcing. He slowly twists his applied hand until tension accumulates in the wrist and then a very small amplitude thrust is introduced. **Note**: for clarity, this illustration shows the initial contact; at the point of thrust the fingers will be in the same direction as those of the patient.

28.15 ▶ Thrust specific articulations dorsal surface This operator viewpoint photograph shows the patient's pronated hand held between the operator's hands. He crosses his thumbs over the dysfunctional articulation on the dorsum of the wrist. He circumducts the wrist while introducing small changes in ulnar and radial deviation and if tension accumulates efficiently he can apply a very short amplitude thrust with the thumbs.

Tips: This can be a very uncomfortable technique unless the amplitude is kept extremely small. Try making the thrust more of an increase of compression rather than dorsi-flexion.

28.16 ▼ (bottom left) Thrust metacarpo-phalangeal joints This operator viewpoint photograph shows the operator is fixing and pulling back the metacarpal while applying a traction and flexion force to the phalange.

Tips: Least useful in inflammatory disorders such as rheumatoid arthritis.

28.17 ▼ (bottom right) Thrust interphalangeal joints This operator viewpoint photograph shows the patient's pronated hand gripped at the wrist. The operator's finger and thumb of the other hand are applying a medial and lateral gapping force to the interphalangeal joint.

Tips: Keep the interphalangeal joint slightly flexed to reduce strain on the capsule and to take the lateral ligaments off tension. This technique may require several priming movements until the tension accumulates efficiently.

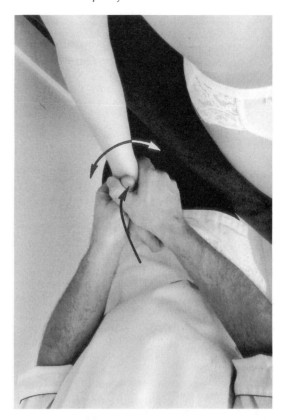

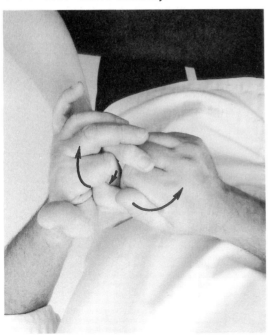

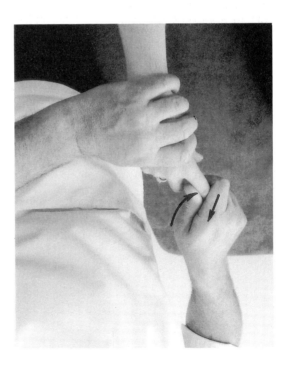

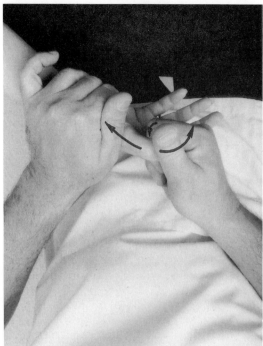

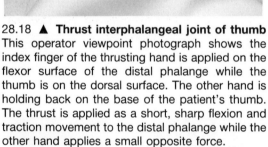

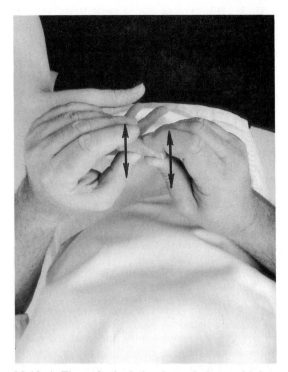

28.18 ▲ Thrust interphalangeal joint of thumb
This operator viewpoint photograph shows the index finger of the thrusting hand is applied on the flexor surface of the distal phalange while the thumb is on the dorsal surface. The other hand is holding back on the base of the patient's thumb. The thrust is applied as a short, sharp flexion and traction movement to the distal phalange while the other hand applies a small opposite force.

Tips: Not all interphalangeal joints can be gapped due to their inherent joint configuration and excessive attempts to do so are unwise.

28.19 ▲ Thrust/articulation interphalangeal joints
This operator viewpoint photograph shows an articulatory force into direct medial and lateral gliding being performed. If a thrust is necessary a small component of flexion will be required to produce the optimum barrier sense in the joint.

Tips: Least useful in inflammatory disorders where the joint structure may be weakened. **Extra considerations**: Several priming movements are often necessary before applying a thrust to these joints.

The hip joint can be a source and site of symptoms in itself although in most cases pain originating in the hip will be referred along the third lumbar nerve root down the medial side of the thigh to the knee. Hip disease, whether of an acute or chronic nature, can produce a characteristic discomfort deep in the groin, but not usually where the patient perceives the hip to be. Restoration of even a small part of lost mobility can be very successful in relieving many of the symptoms of hip disorders, even if the progress of the degenerative state has not been changed at all. Technical problems occur mostly due to the deep nature of the joint, and the need to use quite long levers to reach it. There is, therefore, a possibility of inducing a strain of the knee in the process. Harmonic techniques are particularly useful here in re-establishing normal movement patterns.

Precautions relate particularly to the possibility of undiagnosed fracture of the neck of the femur, which even though still allowing the patient to have movement, shows on X-ray as severe damage. Unexpected hip fracture in an inappropriate age group can be due to a secondary deposit from a cancerous growth elsewhere, and clearly the indications for osteopathic treatment must be carefully considered. The full implications of the possible ill-effects of treatment on possible diseased bone are considerable.

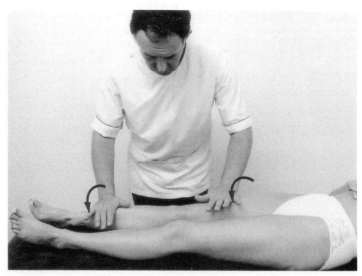

29.1 ▲ Harmonic technique into rotation supine Roll the lower extremity harmonically into rotation as a unit. See earlier section referring to harmonic technique.

   Tips: Most useful in cases where there is considerable stiffness and loss of 'dynamism' in the limb.
Extra considerations: Try using varied degrees of preliminary abduction to produce the most useful angle of the hip.

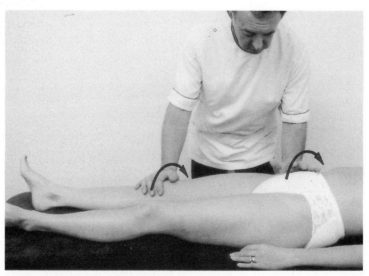

29.2 ▲ Harmonic technique pelvic hold supine Choose whether to fix on the pelvis and roll the leg, or fix on the leg and rock the pelvis. This hold will allow the peri-articular tissues of the hip to be reached. See earlier section relating to harmonic technique.

   Tips: Harmonic technique is rarely going to be a complete treatment by itself, but is often a useful preliminary to other procedures to loosen the tissues.

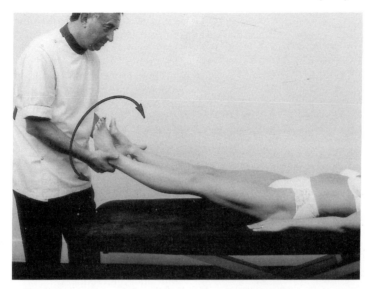

29.3 ▲ Harmonic technique both legs supine Roll both legs into rotation and apply alternating traction and abduction/adduction as required. See earlier section relating to harmonic technique.

Tips: This hold is useful in cases of bilateral dysfunction. Alternating traction and compression will also address a lumbar dysfunction that is restricting sidebending.

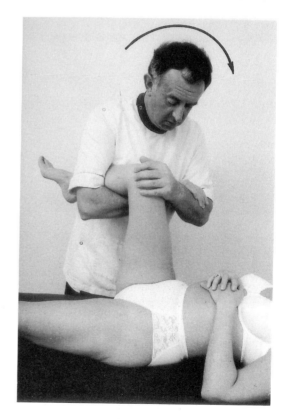

29.4 ▶ Articulation into internal rotation supine Interlock your arms and hold over the knee to avoid straining it. Apply a rhythmic internal rotation movement to the hip as you vary the range of flexion and abduction/adduction according to the needs of the case.

Tips: Most useful where strong mobilizing is required. Least useful in cases of extreme movement limitation as the position may not be attainable. This hold may be unacceptable in cases of severe knee disorders as the strain may be excessive.

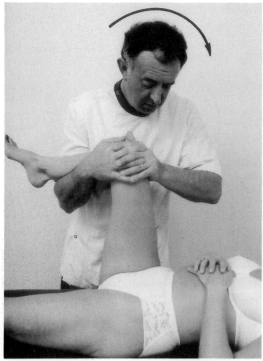

29.5 ◄ **Articulation into internal rotation supine** Grip around the knee and you can partly protect the knee joint while you apply an internal rotation force to the hip.

Tips: Most useful where the knee joint may require some protection. Least useful where strong mobilizing is necessary as the lever is not very powerful. **Extra considerations**: Try using varied angles of flexion or abduction/adduction as necessary to reach the part of the hip capsule desired.

29.6 ▼ (bottom left) **Articulation into abduction and adduction sidelying** Fix firmly above the greater trochanter to limit the movement to the hip joint and prevent movement into the lumbar spine. Hold the lower medial side of the thigh with the other hand to produce the abduction force. Varied degrees of flexion, extension and rotation can be introduced as required.

Tips: This position can also be used for muscle energy technique holds. To reduce any discomfort in this technique try varying the angle of flexion of the lower leg in the initial set-up of the technique. This will allow the lever to change the effect on the pelvis and lumbar spine.

29.7 ▼ (bottom right) **Articulation in external rotation and abduction sidelying** This hold is similar to that in photograph 29.6 except that you can hold further round the thigh and it is easier to introduce the strong external rotation possible with this technique.

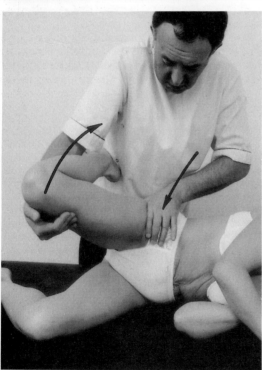

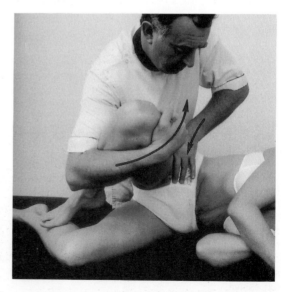

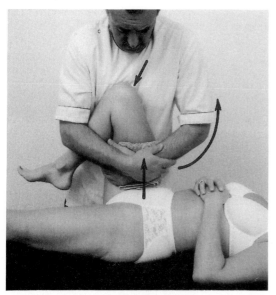 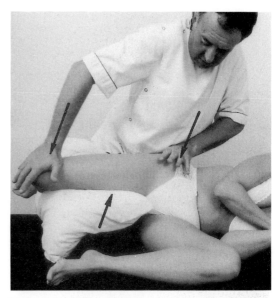

29.8 ▲ Traction to hip supine Pull laterally against the padded upper, inner thigh at the same time as you create a fulcrum with your chest against the lateral aspect of the knee. The sum of these two forces will be to produce a true traction force that will tend to separate the head of the femur from the acetabulum.

Tips: Most useful in cases of degenerative hip disease where traction can allow greater circulatory interchange. The actual stretch on muscles is very small, but this technique can produce considerable symptomatic improvement. **Extra considerations**: Try varying the angle of flexion of the hip to find the optimum for the case.

29.9 ▲ Traction sidelying Use a pillow over your anterior thigh to act as a fulcrum over which you place the patient's upper thigh. Fix down toward the table with the cephalic hand, and push toward the table with the caudal hand to produce a true traction effect on the hip. Note that the other leg has been flexed well out of the way.

Tips: Most useful in cases of degenerative disease where fairly strong traction may be needed. **Extra considerations**: Extension movement may be a problem in many cases of hip degeneration so that some flexion may be necessary to make the technique feasible.

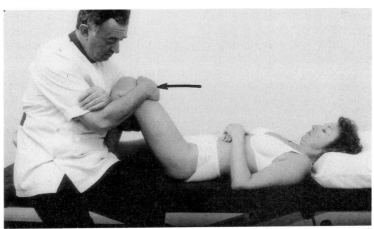

29.10 ▲ Traction and distraction supine Fold your arms and interlace your forearm under the patient's knee. The traction is produced simply by leaning back.

Tips: Most useful in cases of severe degenerative disease as the knee and hip are in considerable flexion, reducing the strain on them, but still allowing the effect to reach the hip. **Extra considerations**: Try varying the abduction and flexion range to find the optimum.

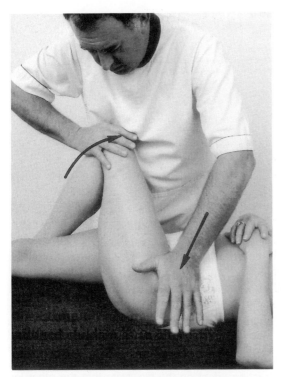

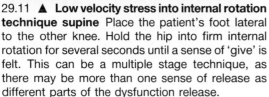

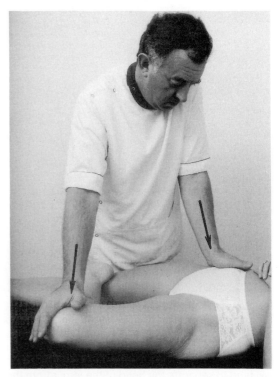

29.11 ▲ **Low velocity stress into internal rotation technique supine** Place the patient's foot lateral to the other knee. Hold the hip into firm internal rotation for several seconds until a sense of 'give' is felt. This can be a multiple stage technique, as there may be more than one sense of release as different parts of the dysfunction release.

Tips: Most useful in almost all cases of hip dysfunction providing the patient can achieve the position; if not, place the foot medial rather than lateral to the other knee. This will, however, reduce the lever somewhat. **Extra considerations**: Try also varying the angle of hip flexion to find the optimum.

29.12 ▲ **Low velocity stress technique into external rotation supine** Place the foot of the affected side on the thigh of the other leg. Hold down on the knee with the hip well abducted, while fixing on the other side of the pelvis to prevent lumbar rotation. After a few seconds there should be a sense of release in the hip. This may be a multiple stage technique. Release may be only partial if it is not repeated in slightly varied angles.

Tips: Most useful in almost all cases of hip joint dysfunction as stress techniques do not put undue strain on the articulation, but allow it to adopt its own path of free movement. **Extra considerations**: If the position is impossible due to severe limitation of movement, try placing the foot medial to the other knee. Try varied degrees of hip flexion to find the optimum for the case.

The thigh contains some of the strongest muscles in the body and can be very influential in postural problems. It is also the site of many sports injuries, and although not a very common presenting site of symptoms in most osteopathic practices, may well be involved in hip, knee and lower back problems.

Although it is possible to work on most of the muscles with conventional structural stretching and cross-fibre techniques, muscle energy and inhibitory pressure are often useful here.

Special precautions include the obvious one of the necessity to work sometimes in sensitive areas near the groin, but with suitable choice of technique position, and care in handling, this should not present too much of a problem. There is also the chance of interfering with an organizing haematoma, and the possibility of myositis ossificans, particularly in gracillis and to a lesser extent in the quadriceps, must be considered.

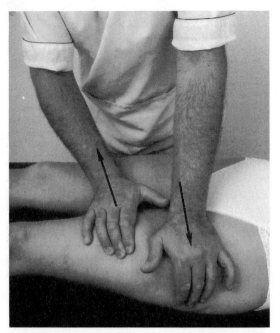

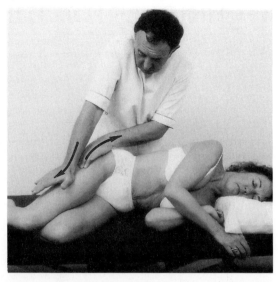

30.1 ▲ Kneading anterior thigh supine From the opposite or same side of the table the operator can apply a cross-fibre kneading to the quadriceps by concentrating either on the hand pushing away from himself, the hand pulling towards himself, or a bit of both according to the needs of the tissue. The more the work is shared by both hands, the less the amplitude of movement with each hand, and therefore the less discomfort for the patient.

Tips: Most useful where the muscles are not very well developed as it is possible to get into the belly of the muscle well. Least useful with large strong muscles and very tight fascia. **Extra considerations**: Deep and slow produces the best result as the muscle has time to relax, and fluid interchange takes place.

30.2 ▲ Stretching lateral aspect of thigh side-lying As it is impossible to adduct the thigh more than a small amount to stretch the lateral tissues, direct stretch with pressure is sometimes the only way to get to these tissues. Here the operator has adducted the patient's thigh as much as possible, and then while holding back on the superior part, is applying a longitudinal stretch with the other hand. As the ilio-tibial band is largely non-extensible, very little stretch can be produced, and this procedure can be very uncomfortable. This is one of the few osteopathic techniques where the use of a lubricant oil or cream may make the technique more effective.

Tips: Most useful in severe cases of osteo-arthrosis of the hip where it is not possible to mobilize the hip directly. Least useful when there are fibrous bands in the fascia lata which are very tender. **Extra considerations**: Change the angle of the hip flexion to find the optimum in each case.

30.3 ▶ Kneading lateral and anterior muscles of thigh From behind the patient the operator has grasped the muscles on the lateral side of the thigh and, while applying a pushing force with the thumbs, is pulling with the fingers to produce a cross-fibre kneading to the area. There are many variations of hand hold that can be used here.

Tips: Most useful where the patient can take direct kneading on the muscles and where the fascia is mobile enough to accept stretch in this way. Least useful where the patient has any problems with the other side making sidelying difficult. **Extra considerations**: Vary the angle of the hip for optimum tension, fix hands and use body movement rather than hand movement alone.

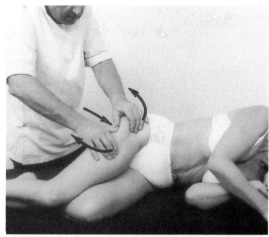

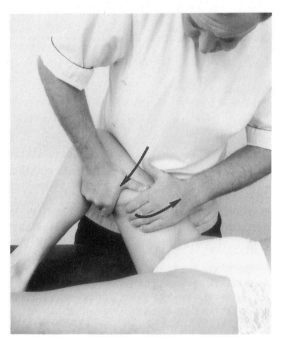

30.4 ▲ Kneading medial or posterior muscles of thigh supine With the patient's knee and hip flexed and firmly held against the operator's abdomen, a cross-fibre kneading action is being performed. The more the work is shared by both hands, the less the discomfort of the movement, and the deeper the technique can be applied to produce a better and quicker result. With the hip and knee flexed, the muscles are off tension and therefore easier to work in most cases.

Tips: Most useful in cases where the patient cannot extend the hip fully. Least useful when the patient is very ticklish. **Extra considerations**: It may be necessary to experiment to find whether it is better in a particular case to fix with one hand and move with the other or to work both hands.

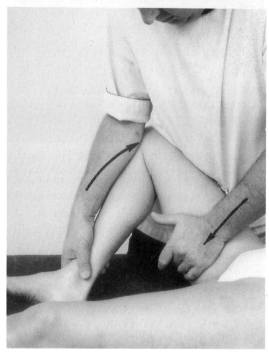

30.5 ▲ Kneading thigh supine Here the operator has fixed the anterior part of the thigh to himself, and is holding the patient's foot into the table at varied angles of flexion of the knee to optimize the technique. The other hand is applying the cross-fibre kneading to the adductor muscles. In this position it is possible to reach well up to the origin of the muscles.

Tips: Most useful where there are tight bands in the adductor muscles, particularly close to the pubis. Least useful when the patient may feel threatened by this position. **Extra considerations**: Sometimes the kneading hand can be held still and the operator and his other hand moved against it.

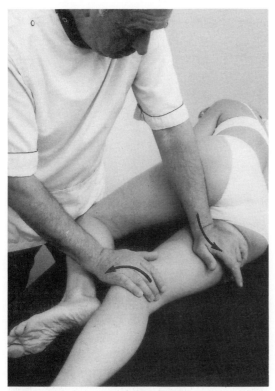

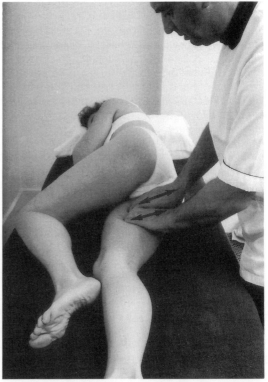

30.6 ▲ **Kneading thigh sidelying** The operator is in front of the patient and is working on the medial aspect of the leg on the table. Both hands are working in opposite directions to minimize the amplitude of force in each. In this position the upper thigh 'protects' the groin area and it is possible to reach very high up into the origins of the muscles; this also allows the pubic ramus to be reached without excessive embarrassment to the patient.

Tips: Most useful where it is necessary to apply the technique high in the adductors. Least useful where the patient has difficulty sidelying. **Extra considerations**: Changes in the angle of flexion of the knee and hip can make it possible to reach different parts of the muscles.

30.7 ▲ **Kneading thigh medial aspect sidelying** The operator is standing behind the patient and using the fingertips to work deep into the muscles. It is possible to get behind the quadriceps in this position, and right up to the adductor muscle origins to the pubis as the patient's other thigh 'protects' the groin area.

Tips: Most useful where it is necessary to reach deep into the muscles. Least useful where the muscles are extremely tender. **Extra considerations**: Find which works best in each case, either pushing or pulling.

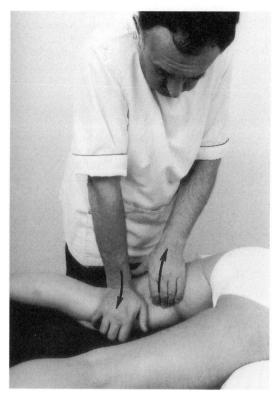

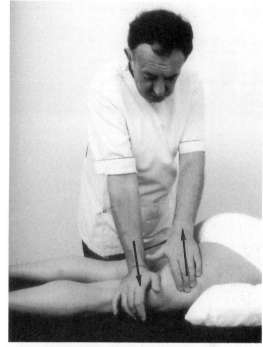

30.8 ▲ **Kneading thigh prone** The operator is standing on the same side as the leg being worked on. The medial and posterior aspects of the thigh can be reached in this position. According to the needs of the case and the preference of the operator this can be made into a pulling technique or a pushing technique as desired. As in all such techniques, the more the work is shared between the hands, the less amplitude need be applied with each one as the conjoint effort produces the result.

Tips: Most useful where muscles are fairly slack as it is possible to work deeply into them. Least useful where muscles are extremely tight, as the technique will be very uncomfortable. **Extra considerations**: Vary the angle of knee flexion if necessary, with a pillow.

30.9 ▲ **Kneading thigh prone** This position enables the operator to work on the posterior and lateral aspect of the thigh on the opposite side from where he is standing. As usual with this sort of technique, the hands are performing opposite actions so that the work is shared and this reduces the amplitude of the forces and the distortion of the tissues accordingly.

Tips: Most useful in smaller patients where leaning across the table is not too much of a stretch. Least useful in large subjects or where the patient finds lying prone difficult. **Extra considerations**: Vary the angle of flexion at the knee and abduction at the hip for best results.

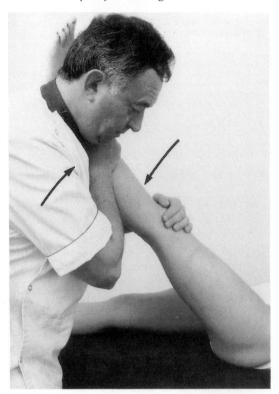

30.10 ◄ Muscle energy posterior thigh The lower extremity is taken to a point of tension in the posterior muscles and held there. The patient is asked to push the leg against the shoulder for about six seconds, and then after relaxing, a new motion barrier is found at a greater angle of flexion of the hip. After a few seconds this is repeated, usually three times to achieve a state of enhanced stretch of the muscles and a new barrier to motion at a greater range of joint motion. As with all muscle energy procedures, the resistance need not be more than about 25% of muscle force.

Tips: Most useful in chronic contracture where direct work on the muscle may be too uncomfortable. Least useful in acute muscle strains as it may be too painful. **Extra considerations**: See the earlier section on principles of muscle energy technique.

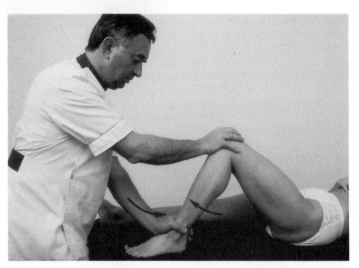

30.11 ▲ Muscle energy technique thigh supine The operator is holding the patient's foot against the table and the patient is asked to push against the hand either into flexion of the knee or extension as necessary for the case. The other hand is stabilizing the knee. As in most muscle energy techniques, the force applied by the patient is about 25% of muscle action, and the position is held for about 6 seconds, repeated usually three times with short rest periods between.

Tips: Most useful in small, light subjects where the operator can resist easily. Least useful in large or strong subjects where it may be difficult to keep a true isometric contraction controlled. **Extra considerations**: See earlier section on muscle energy technique.

The knee is both a simple and a very complex joint. Osteopathic thinking embraces the concept of mechanical dysfunction with or without positional displacement. The bones making up the joint can be working in one of several different disturbed positions. This is not so much a positional finding as a lack of function in various possible directions. Techniques are designed to restore function generally, or to mobilize in a particular direction to restore normal relationships. Function is seen to be more necessary than symmetry and position. Nevertheless, in some cases, directions of force are chosen for specific reasons. These usually relate to perceptions of mechanical dysfunction manifesting as apparent malpositioning.

Precautions include the need to avoid excessive force and pain, as in all other areas, but also include the need to avoid excessive pressure over any varicose veins. Some knee syndromes are manifestations of hyper-mobility masked by muscle protection. If this is the case, mobilizing techniques are not indicated, so careful assessment should precede treatment. If a knee is degenerative it will generally tend to have lost some of its normal hyperextension, and excessive attempts to restore this are doomed to failure and will only provoke more pain and problems.

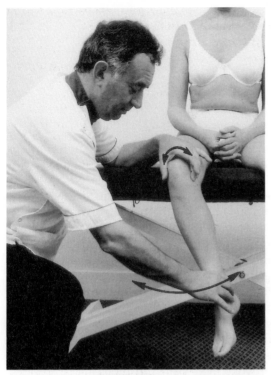

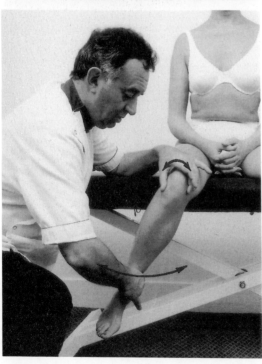

31.1 and 31.2 ◄ Harmonic technique into circumduction sitting The patient sits with her leg over the side of the table. Hold the superior aspect of the tibia with one hand and rock the leg from side to side with the other. At the same time circumduct the foot to induce a rhythmic oscillation in the knee. See earlier section relating to harmonic technique.

Tips: Most useful in cases where rhythm and spring has been lost in normal knee movement. Harmonic technique is particularly useful as a preliminary procedure to structural mobilizing to loosen the tissues and help re-establish circulatory function. **Extra considerations**: Light patient resistance can be introduced into this movement as a 'muscle re-training' procedure.

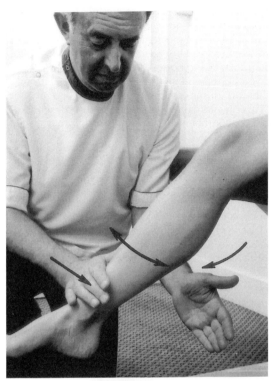

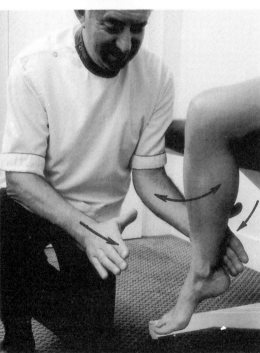

31.3 and 31.4 ◄ **Harmonic technique into flexion and extension sitting** The patient sits with her legs over the side of the table. Instruct her to resist your movements with a light pressure only. Rock the leg forward and back to flex and extend the knee. Vary the start and finish point so that the flexion and extension movement will be through a larger and smaller arc. This has the effect of 're-training' the proprioceptive feedback from the joint. See earlier section relating to harmonic technique.

31.5 ▼ **Articulation patello-femoral joint supine** This hold allows mobilization of the patella through all possible ranges. The accessory ranges of diagonal movement in particular can be addressed as release of these often improves overall function.

Tips: Most useful in the majority of cases of knee dysfunction as the patello-femoral joint may be involved and can often be a neglected element. To avoid discomfort, preliminary work on the surrounding soft tissues is helpful to release the area prior to this technique.

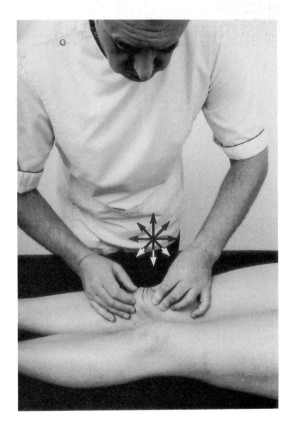

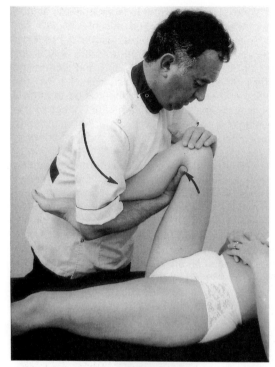

31.6 ◀ Articulation flexion supine Flex the knee over your hand placed in the popliteal space. Use your other hand to monitor the tissue tension to avoid excessive strain. Hold the leg firmly between your forearm and body. Circumduction movements can be added so that the flexion becomes one part of the arc of movement.

Tips: Avoid excessive flexion in the presence of any effusion unless it is very slight.

31.8 ▼ Articulation extension supine Grip the knee firmly and hold it against the table while your other hand braces the foot and lifts the heel. This hold has the advantage over the one shown in photograph 31.7, in that the gastrocnemius is placed on some tension and will be stretched if desired.

Tips: Try varying the amount of dorsiflexion in the foot to assess at what point the limitation of extension manifests. The earlier this occurs, the more the gastrocnemius will be involved in the lack of extension.

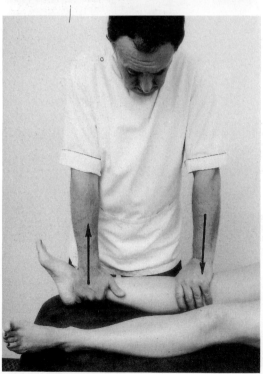

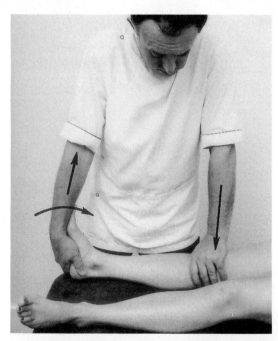

31.7 ◀ Articulation extension supine Grip the knee firmly and hold it against the table while your other hand lifts the lower end of the tibia.

Tips: Many knee dysfunctions manifest as a lack of hyperextension, particularly internal derangements. This movement is as much an assessment of successful restoration of function as it is a treatment.

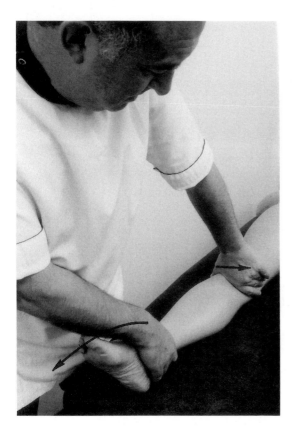

31.9 ◄ **Traction supine** Hold back on the femur with your fully pronated hand avoiding the patella. The other hand applies the traction and can vary rotation, abduction and adduction of the tibia as necessary.

Tips: Many internal derangements of the knee seem to have some sort of internal entrapment involved. Traction can be very helpful in these instances.

31.11 ▼ **Articulation rotation and flexion supine** Hold directly over the joint line with your upper hand and introduce internal and external rotation with varied degrees of flexion with the other.

Tips: Most useful in cases of meniscal dysfunction where there is often a limitation of full flexion and rotation combined, at one specific point in the range of movement. **Extra considerations**: In many cases of meniscal dysfunction it is useful to break fixation in flexion before trying to re-establish full extension.

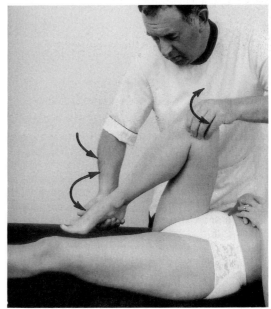

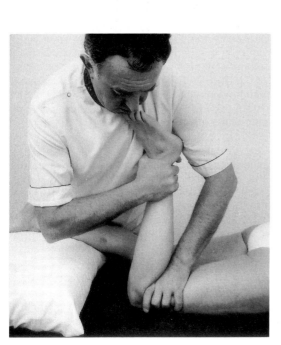

31.10 ◄ **Traction prone** Fix the femur into the table. Lift the leg, from above the ankle, with the other hand while introducing different ranges of flexion and rotation. This can be applied to the near or far leg. It has the advantage over supine methods in that it can be performed in flexion and can be made into a circumduction movement at the hip to be more rhythmic.

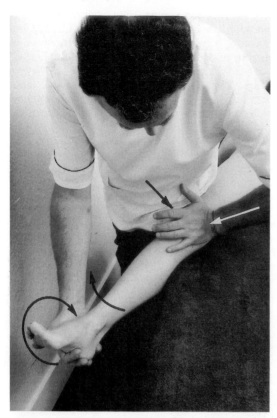

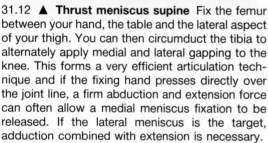

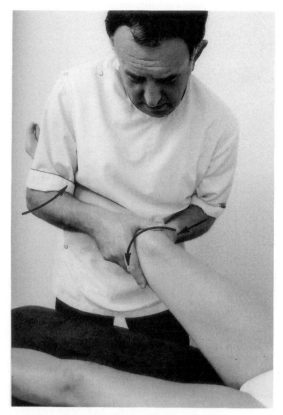

31.12 ▲ **Thrust meniscus supine** Fix the femur between your hand, the table and the lateral aspect of your thigh. You can then circumduct the tibia to alternately apply medial and lateral gapping to the knee. This forms a very efficient articulation technique and if the fixing hand presses directly over the joint line, a firm abduction and extension force can often allow a medial meniscus fixation to be released. If the lateral meniscus is the target, adduction combined with extension is necessary.

Tips: As the hand pressure increases over the joint the available ranges of abduction and adduction will reduce to a specific small arc. Within this arc will be found the appropriate barrier to apply the final very short amplitude force.

31.13 ▲ **Thrust medial meniscus supine** Firmly clasp the ankle between your body and forearm. Grip around the leg just below the knee and introduce a circumduction movement. Within this circumduction there will be a point of tension. This point usually occurs with a combination of abduction and external rotation of the tibia. At this point apply a force combining further abduction, external rotation and extension. It is more of a flick than a thrust.

Tips: Visualize a piece of string with a weight attached tied around the knee and hanging down on the lateral side. Try to flick the weighted string over to the medial side sharply. This gives an image of the direction and type of force necessary.

31.14, 31.15 and 31.16 **Thrust to medial meniscus supine** This series of photographs shows the sequence of moves normally used in this technique. Flex and externally rotate the knee to break fixation in the medial meniscus. Gently repeat this a few times until nearly full flexion is attained. Maintaining the external rotation and some abduction of the knee, extend it until the position shown in photograph 15. At this point the final part of the technique takes over which is an extension, traction and internal rotation movement. At the end of the technique it is important to hold the knee firmly into extension, to avoid reflex muscle contraction into flexion that may dislodge the meniscus again.

Tips: Least useful where there is a suspected tear in the meniscus and the extension movement would be very painful. **Extra considerations**: It may take several attempts to produce sufficient flexion to unlock the joint. It may be very uncomfortable at the position shown in photograph 31.15 where the patient loses active control of the joint. It is important to pass through this point fairly quickly.

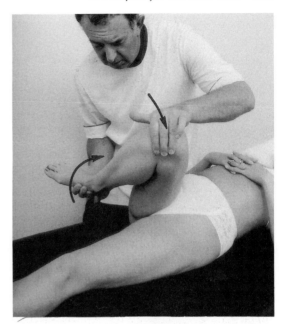

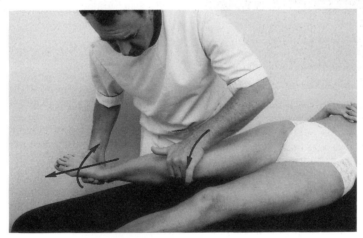

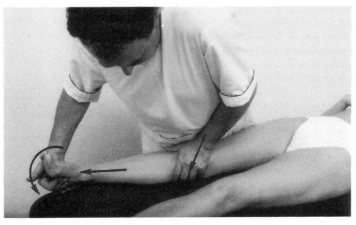

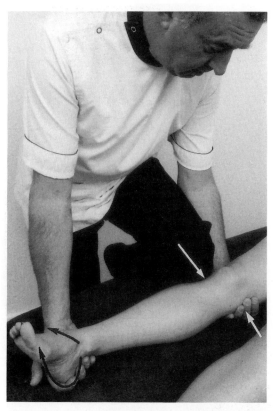

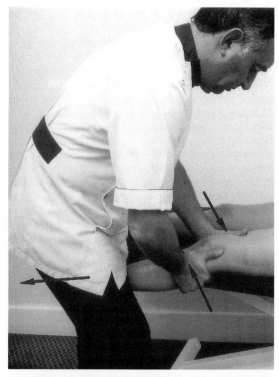

31.17 ▲ Thrust for lateral shift of tibia supine Internally rotate the patient's thigh slightly and place your infra-patella tendon against the small plateau on the antero-lateral part of the tibia. Your upper hand is placed under the knee maintaining a small amount of flexion and holding the femur over the medial condyle. The lower hand clasps the heel. Focus the forces by pulling the femur toward the fulcrum of your applied knee while circumducting the ankle and tibia. The thrust is a combination of a small push with the knee and a pull toward you with both hands.

Tips: Because the operator is pivoting on the middle part of his tibia against the side of the table, it is important to adjust the patient's position accordingly. If the patient's leg is not externally rotated sufficiently, painful pressure occurs on the head of the fibula. Have the patient close enough to the edge of the table so that your tibia can be nearly vertical at the start of the technique.

31.18 ▲ Thrust lateral shift of tibia supine Fix the patient's leg between your crossed thighs. Apply your staggered hands to the medial aspect of the femur and the lateral aspect of the tibia with firm compression. Circumduct the knee using both hands and as the point of tension builds, sharply increase the pressure with both hands while straightening your knees to produce a traction effect.

Tips: As this position is inherently unstable for the operator it may help to lean against the side of the table. Keep the patient's knee slightly flexed throughout.

31.19 ▶ Thrust for medial shift of tibia supine
Fix the patient's leg between your crossed thighs. Apply your staggered hands to the medial aspect of the tibia and the lateral aspect of the femur. Use firm compression and circumduct your hands until tension accumulates and then apply the thrust with both hands at the same time as straightening your knees to produce the traction.

Tips: Maintain a small amount of flexion to prevent the patient's knee from locking.

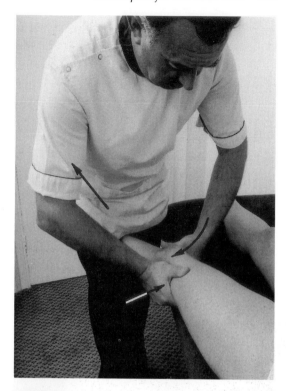

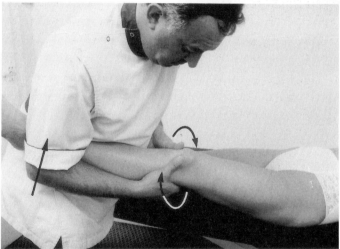

31.20 ▲ Thrust for medial shift of tibia and lateral meniscus Fix the abducted leg between your body and forearm and grip the knee firmly just below the joint. Maintain a small amount of flexion and firm compression and apply a rapid circumduction and lateral gapping force by rotating your body away from the table. A direct lateral force will tend to correct the tibial shift whereas an abduction force will reach the lateral meniscus.

Tips: Visualize a piece of string with a weight attached tied around the knee, with the weight hanging down medially. The movement of this technique is to flick the weight from the medial side over to the lateral side.

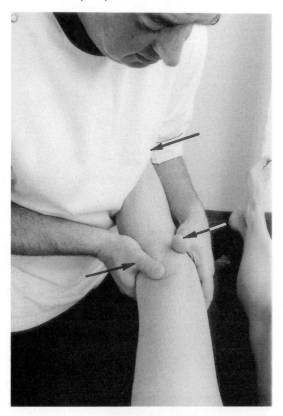

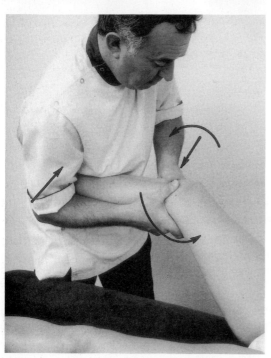

31.21 ◄ **Thrust for lateral shift of tibia and medial meniscus** Place the leg between your body and forearm and clasp the knee firmly between your hands. Use several small oscillating movements to prime the joint and then apply a small rotation of your body toward the table to open the medial side of the joint. This can be a circumduction movement or a medial gapping movement.

Tips: This technique can be suitable for correcting an internal rotation restriction of the tibia if the tibia is held firmly with both hands and externally rotated at the same time as the gapping force is applied.

31.23 ▼ **Thrust for internal rotation fixation of tibia** Firmly clasp the upper end of the tibia between your hands and hold the lower end between your forearm and body. Adduct the thigh to produce a torsional force into external rotation of the knee. Apply a small extension force to break fixation into an external rotation direction.

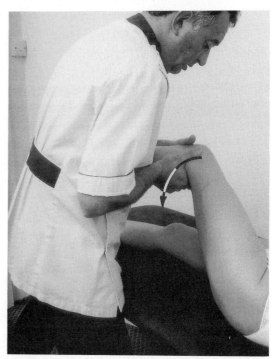

31.22 ◄ **Thrust for external rotation fixation of tibia** Grasp the tibia firmly between your hands and against your body with your forearm. Abduct the thigh and flex the knee slightly and then apply an internal rotation force by using your grip and by sidebending your body toward the table. A small final extension force may be necessary.

Tips: Use the weight of a more abducted thigh as a resistance to the internal rotation force.

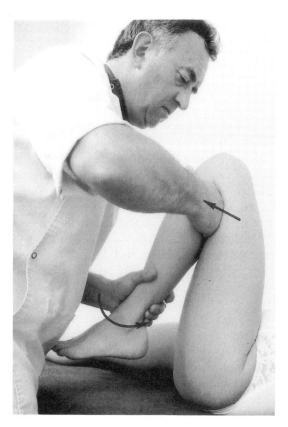

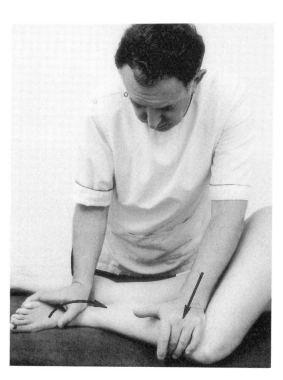

31.24 ◄ **Thrust superior tibio-fibula joint supine**
Place the metacarpo-phalangeal joint of your index finger behind the fibular head. Adduct the thigh and externally rotate and flex the leg until you feel the fibular head gripping your hand. Apply a small flexion force to the leg while prising the fibular head toward you.

Tips: Least useful in the presence of degenerative disease in the knee that may make extreme flexion painful. **Extra considerations**: Try varying the distal hold to grip under the foot if preferred.

31.26 ▼ (**Thrust superior tibio-fibular joint side-lying** Dorsiflex the foot slightly with your thigh while holding the inferior end of the fibula back. Your other hand applies a compression and forward movement to the upper end of the fibula. The thrust is applied to the upper end while the lower part is held stable or the lower lever is slightly increased.

Tips: Least useful where the operator may find the thrust with the abducted arm difficult.

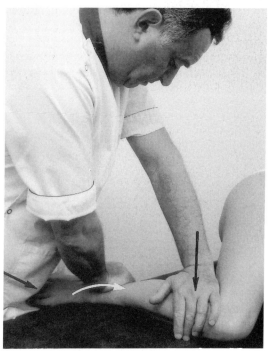

31.25 ◄ **Thrust superior tibio-fibular joint side-lying** Stand behind the patient and apply a forward force against the head of the fibula of the flexed knee. Hold back on the distal end of the fibula with varied degrees of dorsiflexion of the foot to find the optimum tension. Hold the foot firmly and then apply the thrust against the fibular head.

Tips: Most useful where full flexion of the knee may be a problem.

The calf area is often involved in conditions of dysfunction in the foot and the knee. Conditions of the calf muscles themselves such as muscle tears and direct trauma sometimes need addressing. Contracture due to postural conditions and occupational disorders can also occur.

Particular care should be taken in phlebitis or varicose vein cases where there is the possibility of thrombosis, haemorrhage and haematoma formation. If a clot is present, there is a distinct possibility of it being shifted and subsequently lodging in heart, lung or brain with potentially disastrous results.

Technique to be used on the soft tissues can be cross-fibre, stretching or muscle energy.

It is performed with the knee extended to reach the gastrocnemius, and flexed to take the gastrocnemius off stretch and make it easier to reach the deeper muscles. Calf muscles are closely concerned with posture, which means that there may be only partly reversible contracture and fibrosis present. Techniques should usually be slow and deep to produce the best result. Control of rhythm is also important. There may be remote causes of calf muscle hypertonicity, such as nerve root pressure in the lumbar spine or circulatory deficit in the arterial supply. Initial attention to these extraneous causes should be considered to get the best result from any later work on the calf.

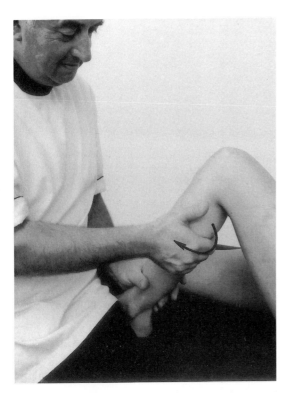

32.1 ◄ Kneading of lateral calf supine Sit on the end of the table, stabilizing the patient's foot by resting your thigh on it. Hold the ankle to prevent movement of the leg. Apply deep cross-fibre kneading to the calf muscles with the pads and tips of the fingers.

Tips: Most useful where it is necessary to reach the lateral muscles of the calf. **Extra considerations**: Try varying the angle of knee flexion and rotation.

32.3 ▼ Kneading of medial part of calf supine Sit on the table stabilizing the patient's foot with your thigh. Hold against the knee with your stabilizing hand. The medial aspect of the calf is available to the fingertips of the kneading hand.

Tips: Most useful when working on the musculo-tendinous junctions deep in the calf. Try varying the angles of knee flexion and rotation to achieve the optimum for the technique.

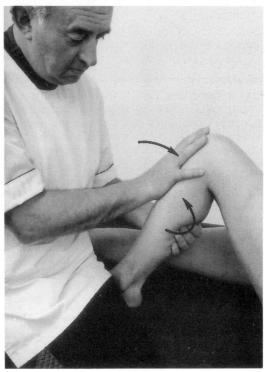

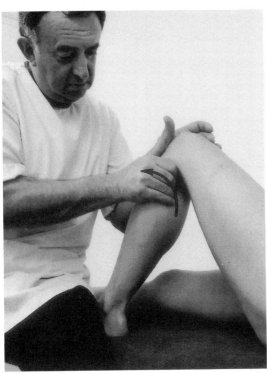

32.2 ◄ Kneading of lateral calf supine Sit at the end of the table. Stabilize the patient's foot with your thigh. Fix the knee with one hand and knead the muscles around the fibular head with the other.

Tips: Most useful when it is necessary to stabilize the knee when working on the upper part of the calf. **Extra considerations**: Try varying the angles of flexion and rotation of the knee to vary the tension on the muscles before the technique is applied.

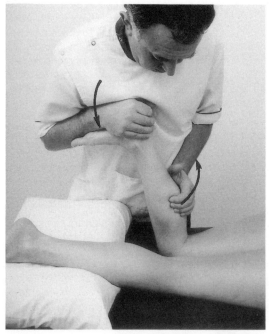

32.4 ▲ Kneading and stretching calf prone
Stretch the muscles by applying a dorsiflexion force to the foot. Use a pulling or pushing force on the bellies of the muscles with the other hand.

Tips: Most useful where it is necessary to get very deep into the muscle tissue. Try circumducting the knee to reach different parts of the muscle. Try changing the order of the stretch and kneading to produce the best combination of comfort and effectiveness.

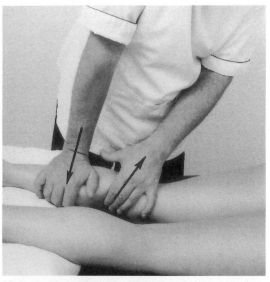

32.5 ▲ Kneading of calf prone Support the tibia on a small pillow and then apply a cross-fibre kneading to the calf muscles with both hands working in opposite directions.

Tips: Try using varied sizes of pillow or no pillow at all, if it is desired to make the principal effect on the gastrocnemius.

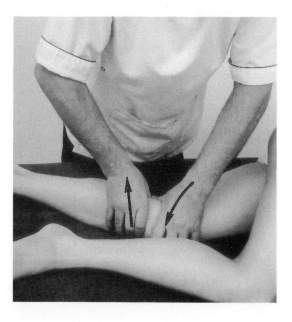

32.6 ▶ Kneading of calf sidelying Stand behind the patient and apply opposite forces with both hands, using the thumbs to knead the muscles of the calf.

Tips: In this hold it is possible to work the whole length of the calf of either leg with the thumbs. If use of the fingertips is preferred to use of the thumbs, work from the other side of the table.

Some osteopaths neglect foot technique in patient care as they find the techniques difficult to master, and sometimes uncomfortable on the hands. Many cases of foot dysfunction receive benefit from general mobilization and some practitioners are happy to use such methods rather than specific techniques. However, specific techniques can often be a short cut to good results, and save not only time and effort, but can produce a better and longer-lasting relief from mechanical dysfunction problems. The foot is the foundation of posture, and to neglect it is to leave out a very important part of patient care. Clearly a poor foundation is not going to help in resolution of mechanics in other parts of the body if a practitioner is trying to restore good function. There are also local problems of pain and disturbed mechanics in the foot that can often be suitably addressed by osteopathic treatment.

As in all areas of the body, particular care must be taken in cases of potential bone weakness as techniques may induce quite strong effects on bone. However, the chance of damage is quite small, as the stresses used are liable to be less than those in normal locomotion. Infection, cellulitis and inflammatory disorders are common in the foot, and will need careful pre-treatment assessment. By its very nature osteopathic treatment is designed to increase mobility. Many cases of disturbed foot mechanics are due to excess mobility or hypermobility and, therefore, further mobilization may be unwise. In some cases, relative hypomobility in one part of the foot will cause relative hypermobility in another. This is where very specific treatment to the hypomobile section will help to 'unload' the excessively mobile articulations. Hypomobility also seems to have reflex effects in maintenance of hypermobility in adjacent areas. If a hypomobile joint is satisfactorily mobilized, there is often an immediate restoration of ligamentous tone in adjacent, previously diagnosed, hypermobile joints. This is too rapid to be simply a balancing of mechanics, and seems to be due to fascial tension alteration and some proprioceptive feedback mechanism.

Most positions used traditionally for thrust techniques are perfectly suitable for articulation procedures. This is not mentioned each time in the descriptions appended to the photographs to avoid repetition. Where a technique is declared a thrust, a repetitive articulation is usually performed as a preliminary, and if tension accumulates to a suitable sense of barrier, the thrust can be performed. If it does not, repeated articulation may deal with the dysfunction adequately. A suitable thrust barrier has a potential for the short amplitude movement that implies a quite characteristic 'crispness'. Without this the thrust is not liable to succeed as a specific technique and is best avoided, as the tissues may become traumatized. A successful short amplitude thrust performed well is rarely traumatic in the foot. An unsuccessful one may be uncomfortable, although rarely damaging.

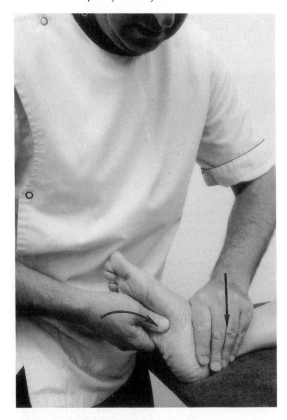

33.1 ◄ Kneading of sole supine Stabilize the foot with the cephalic hand and use your thumb to work on the soft tissues of the sole.

Tips: Many patients are ticklish and the grip should be firm but not painful. Kneading is more likely to be of benefit than stretching, as a normal standing posture stretches the tissues more than any technique is able to do. Try varied degrees of plantar flexion to reach different layers of tissue.

33.3 ▼ Thrust to tibio-talar joint supine Cup the calcaneum and pull the foot into a neutral point between plantar and dorsiflexion. Push the tibia with the cephalic hand toward the table and allow the natural recoil of the tissues to cause it to spring back. The plane of the joint is not directly antero-posterior and it will be necessary to slightly internally rotate the hip to produce the optimum resistance for a thrust. If there is a barrier, several priming movements will be necessary before the thrust can be executed.

Tips: Most useful where the patient mentions the symptom that they are unable to achieve comfort in the ankle in any position and feels that the joint needs to 'crack'. **Extra considerations**: When a satisfactory thrust is attained with this technique, the amplitude of movement within the thrust will often be greater than expected and possibly alarming to the practitioner!

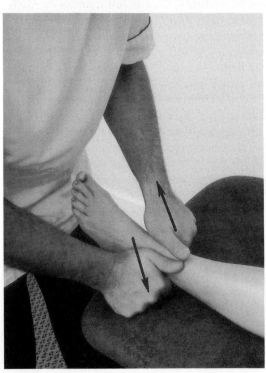

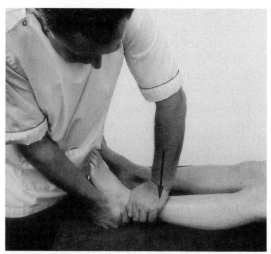

33.2 ◄ Articulation to distal tibio-fibular joint supine Stand at the foot of the table and grasp the tibia and fibula between the index finger and thumb of each hand. Introduce antero-posterior and slight supero-inferior movements.

Tips: Most useful in cases where fibular mobility is particularly relevant, that is most ankle dysfunctions and some knee conditions. **Extra considerations**: Try dorsi-flexing the foot with the operator's thigh to produce the optimum tension in the joints.

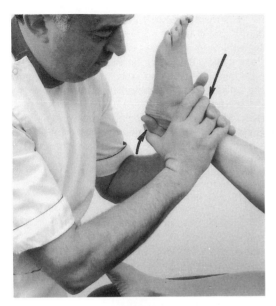

33.4 ◀ **Thrust to tibio-talar joint supine** Fix the calcaneum with your crossed thumbs, and grip firmly around the front of the ankle. This produces a dorsiflexion component and an antero-posterior component. As you lower the foot toward the table increase the firmness of the grip. You can then amplify the hold to apply a force in an antero-posterior direction to the tibia to separate the joint.

Tips: Least useful where the operator may have any weakness in the thumbs. It is also difficult in large feet to maintain the dorsiflexion necessary and to grip around the foot at the same time. **Extra considerations**: The thrust is performed by the operator adducting his arms at the same moment as the grip tightens.

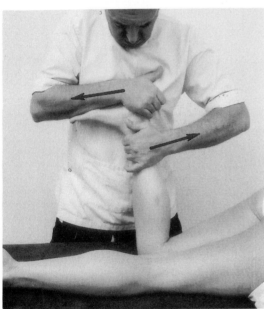

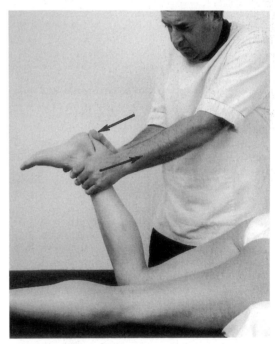

33.5 ▲ **Thrust to tibio-talar joint prone** Apply some pre-tension to the joint by gripping around the anterior aspect of the ankle while pulling forward on the calcaneum. Maintain a degree of dorsiflexion of the foot with your forearm and when the forces accumulate, execute a sharp adduction of your arms to cause a gapping at the joint.

Tips: Least useful for smaller operators, and for those where the necessary strength may be a problem. **Extra considerations**: Try circumducting the leg in the build-up to the technique, so that the perception of continuous tension for the patient is not too uncomfortable.

33.6 ▲ **Thrust to tibio-talar joint prone** Stand to the side of the prone patient facing toward the foot of the table. Grip round the front of the ankle as you push forward with your crossed thumbs behind the calcaneum. Rock the patient's leg forward and back. When tension accumulates emphasize the simultaneous pull and push to gap the joint.

Tips: The thumbs can also vary the dorsiflexion to focus the technique more accurately.

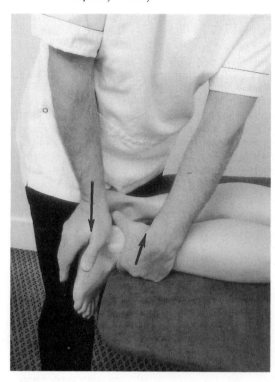

33.7 ◄ **Thrust to tibio-talar joint prone** Put the patient's foot over the end of the table and fix the tibia with your cephalic hand while taking up the slack with the other hand pushing down on the calcaneum. You can vary the dorsiflexion to achieve the optimum tension and then apply the thrust toward the floor.

Tips: Most useful for small operators as this technique relies on application of weight rather than use of levers and force. **Extra considerations**: Try using the operator's inner thigh to produce the relevant amount of dorsiflexion.

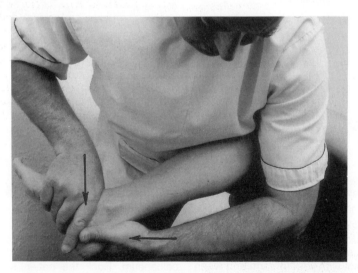

33.8 ▲ **Traction to tibio-talar joint supine** Brace your elbow against your flexed knee on the table under the patient's flexed knee. Use your lower forearm as a fixed lever while your upper hand pulls the foot into dorsiflexion and drives it straight down over the edge of the table. The larger the space between your elbow and the patient's knee the stronger the lever will be to open the tibio-talar articulation.

Tips: Try gently mobilizing the foot in circumduction while it is under traction.

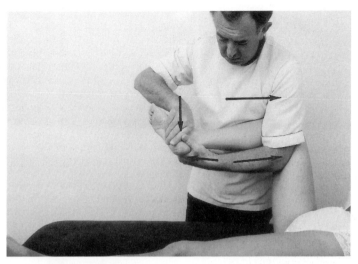

33.9 ▲ **Traction to tibio-talar joint supine** Brace your elbow against the back of the patient's flexed thigh. Cup the calcaneum in the same hand and fix the talus and the rest of the foot with the other hand. Traction is produced by maintaining these holds and simply leaning back. The push of the patient's flexing thigh against your elbow performs the technique.

Tips: Least useful where the operator's arm is very short and the patient's leg is very long. **Extra considerations**: Try abducting the hip further as necessary or placing a pad between elbow and thigh.

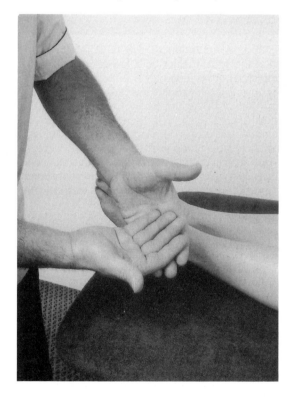

33.10, 33.11 and 33.12 ◄ (see also next page, top left and bottom left) **Articulation to sub-talar joints supine** This series shows the overlapping fingers hand hold in the shape of a letter 'W'; then the hands applied to the foot can produce inversion, eversion and circumduction to influence the sub-talar joints. The operator viewpoint photographs show the pressure being applied with one thenar eminence and the opposite hypothenar eminence. This is then reversed to gap the medial and lateral sides of the joint respectively.

Tips: Try varying the angle of dorsiflexion using the operator's abdomen against the sole of the foot. **Extra considerations**: This hold requires a firmer grip than may be apparent; it also requires a good control of rhythm.

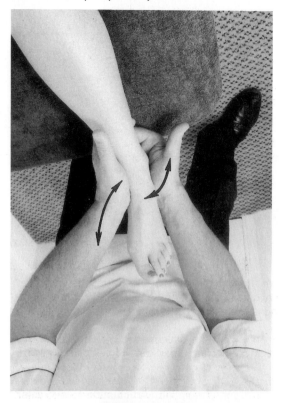

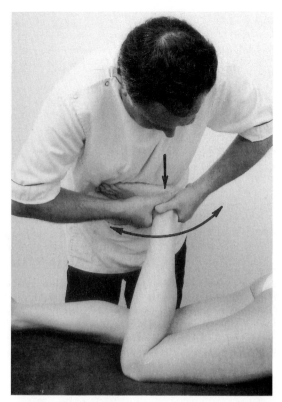

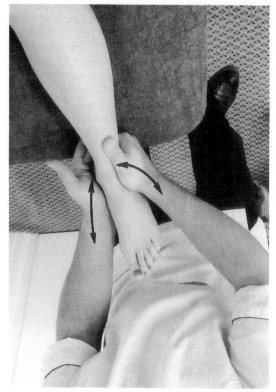

33.13 ▲ Articulation to sub-talar joints prone
Brace the foot against your lower chest. Fix the
fingers of both hands over the medial side of the
foot while gripping firmly under the lateral maleolus.
Rock forward over the foot to put tension on the
medial aspect of the joint. Then rotate your body to
alternate the stress applied to the anterior and
posterior parts of the joint.

Tips: Least useful for the smaller operator who
may find the reach a problem. **Extra considerations**:
A firm grip is necessary if this technique is to be
effective.

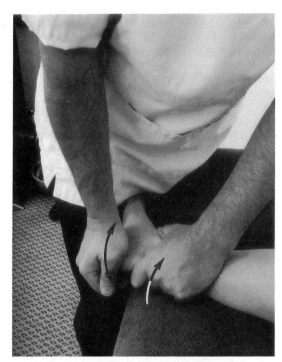

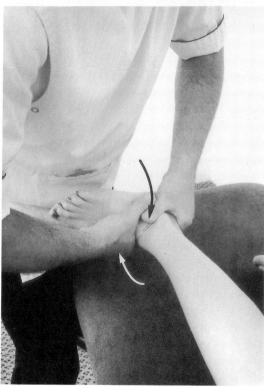

33.14 ◄ Articulation to sub-talar joint sidelying
The patient lies on the affected side and the operator fixes the dorsiflexed foot against his inner thigh. Hold it firmly against the table with the fixing hand and rock the calcaneum into inversion and eversion. Dysfunctional areas of the sub-talar joint are reached by varying the angles of movement.

Tips: This technique will only gap the medial aspect of the joint. **Extra considerations**: If the pressure on the table is uncomfortable, try interposing a pillow between foot and table.

33.15 ▼ (bottom left) **Articulation to sub-talar joint sidelying** In this operator viewpoint photograph the patient is lying on the unaffected side and the operator is gripping medially on the distal part of the calcaneum. Place your thumbs just under the lateral maleolus. Maintain a firm grip and lean forward until tension is felt to build in the joint. The medial side of the joint is being stretched.

Tips: Try varying the angle of dorsiflexion to reach different surfaces of the joint.

33.16 ► (see next page, top left) **Thrust to sub-talar joint sidelying** The patient lies on the affected side with the knee flexed. Fix the foot into dorsiflexion to stabilize the ankle. Fix the calcaneum to the table, and with your other hand invert the foot by fixing on the navicula and pushing up along the long axis of the tibia. Tension should accumulate in the sub-talar joint. Rock the foot between the hands until the optimum barrier is sensed. Maintain the pressure and thrust the whole foot toward the table thereby applying a gapping force to the target joint.

Tips: If the tension is correct the foot will rock back and forth like a saucer rocking from edge to edge. According to whether the anterior or posterior of the joint is dysfunctional, the tension will be felt better with the proximal or the distal hand. **Extra considerations**: If this position is very painful, try working from the lateral side of the foot as in next technique illustration.

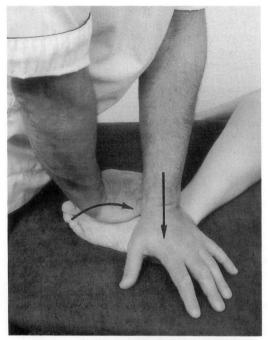

33.17 and 33.18 ▼ Thrust to sub-talar joint side-lying The patient lies on the unaffected side. Pull the medial side of the dorsiflexed foot into inversion with your distal hand. Maintain pressure toward the table with your other hand cupping the lateral maleolus. The calcaneum is, therefore, a fulcrum. This has the effect of putting a stress on the sub-talar joint on the medial aspect of the foot. Vary the degree of abduction with your distal hand until a suitable barrier is felt, and then apply a thrust with your proximal hand to gap the joint.

Tips: This may be useful when the opposite sidelying position is a problem. Note that the second photograph shows the distal hand in the final position. The wrist is now straight and the foot inverted and abducted. Firm compression is necessary if the force is not to be dissipated in the tissues generally. The sub-talar joint is extremely strong, and if the compression is not firm enough, the technique will be ineffective.

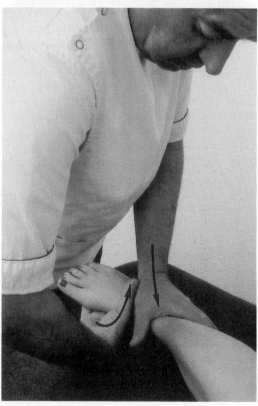

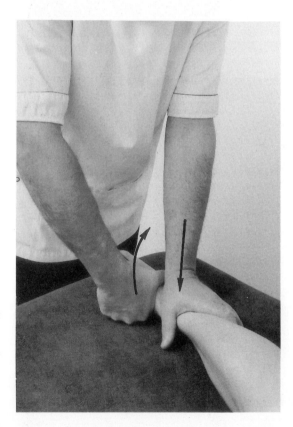

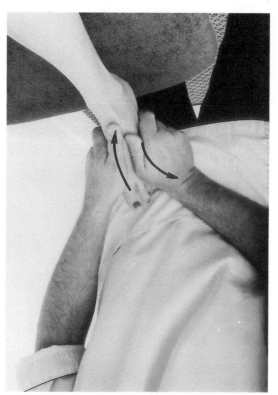

33.19 and 33.20 ◄ **Articulation mid tarsus supine**
These operator viewpoint photographs show a hold
for applying general mobilization to the mid foot.
The thumbs are aligned along the shafts of one or
more of the metatarsals. A torsional force is
introduced to direct the articulation forces to the
joint to be mobilized.

Tips: Try varying the spacing between the
thumbs or making them more proximal or distal to
reach different parts of the foot.

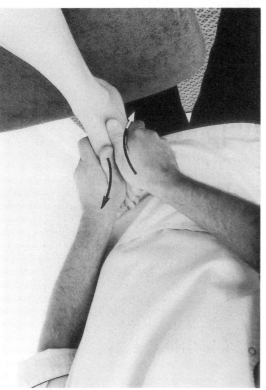

33.21, 33.22, 33.23 and 33.24 ▶ (see next page)
Articulation mid tarsus supine This series of
photographs show the so-called 'figure of eight'
technique in its various phases. Take the foot
through an imaginary figure of eight, in a variety of
planes, either vertically, horizontally or diagonally.
Tension accumulates at the cross-over in the
middle or at the outer edges of the figure as
directions change. Visualize the eight as having a
somewhat flat top and bottom.

Tips: Most useful in almost all cases of dysfunction causing restricted mobility in the foot. **Extra
considerations**: Quite firm compression is usually
necessary to the metatarsal heads by the operator's
lower abdomen to help focus the technique.

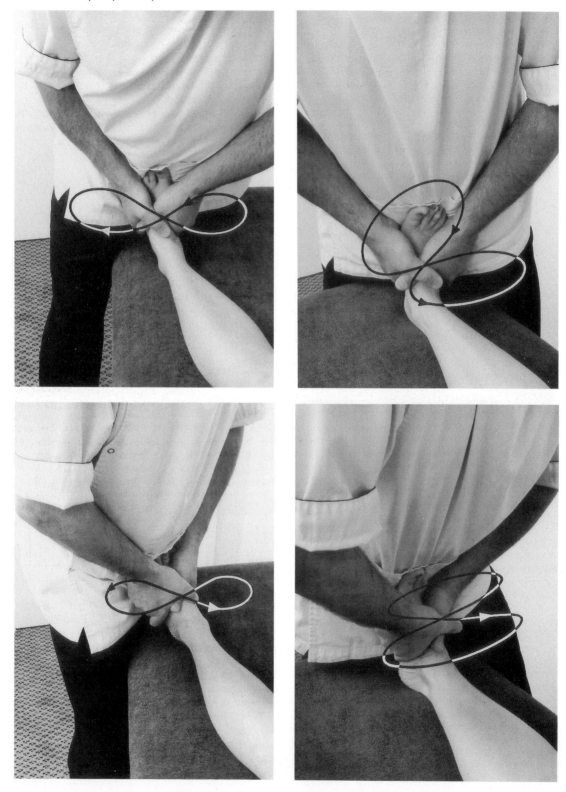

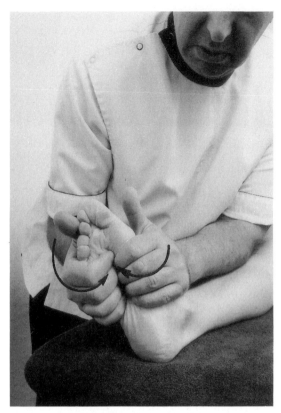

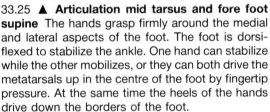

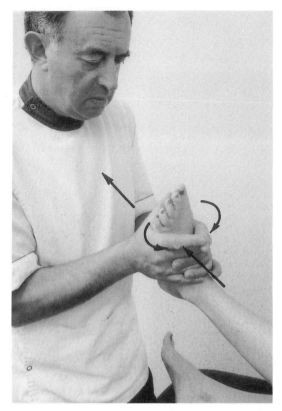

33.25 ▲ **Articulation mid tarsus and fore foot supine** The hands grasp firmly around the medial and lateral aspects of the foot. The foot is dorsi-flexed to stabilize the ankle. One hand can stabilize while the other mobilizes, or they can both drive the metatarsals up in the centre of the foot by fingertip pressure. At the same time the heels of the hands drive down the borders of the foot.

Tips: Try introducing twisting forces to direct the levers to different parts of the foot. With traction and firm moulding of the foot it is possible to reach most of the mid foot articulations.

33.26 ▲ **Thrust to mid tarsus supine** Fix over the target joint with the centre of your interlocked hands. Apply some traction to put the area on tension. Then spread the foot with the thumbs to allow some space for the bone you wish to manipulate. The mid tarsal bones are somewhat wedge shaped and need a space to 'fall into'. The thrust is performed with a short tug in the long axis of the tibia.

Tips: Try using slight variations of abduction and adduction while accumulating the optimum forces.

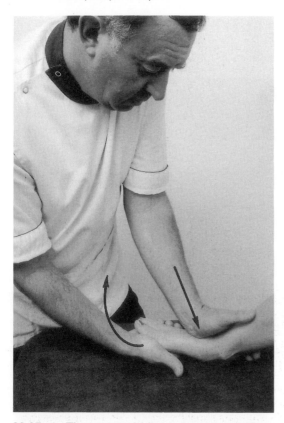

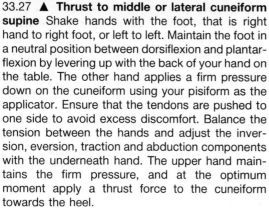

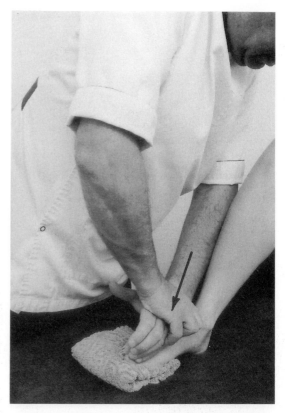

33.27 ▲ Thrust to middle or lateral cuneiform supine Shake hands with the foot, that is right hand to right foot, or left to left. Maintain the foot in a neutral position between dorsiflexion and plantar-flexion by levering up with the back of your hand on the table. The other hand applies a firm pressure down on the cuneiform using your pisiform as the applicator. Ensure that the tendons are pushed to one side to avoid excess discomfort. Balance the tension between the hands and adjust the inversion, eversion, traction and abduction components with the underneath hand. The upper hand maintains the firm pressure, and at the optimum moment apply a thrust force to the cuneiform towards the heel.

Tips: Try varying the knee flexion to find the optimum sense of tension in the foot. It generally helps to have the foot closer to the side of the table than the hip so that the leg does not fall into external rotation.

33.28 ▲ Thrust to middle and lateral cuneiforms supine This technique uses a similar principle to the one shown in photograph 33.27. The difference is that the operator is using a reinforced pisiform while a pad is performing the dorsiflexion resistance.

Tips: Most useful where the operator may not be able to develop the force sufficiently with the single-handed grip. The disadvantage is that part of the control of the inversion, eversion and traction is lost.

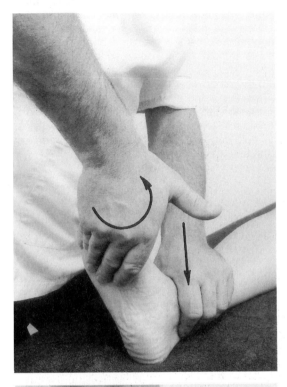

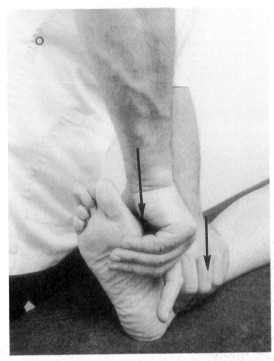

33.29, 33.30 and 33.31 **Thrust to middle or lateral cuneiform supine** These three sequence photographs show the foot pulled into dorsiflexion to lock the ankle. The upper hand then fixes the tibia to the table. The thrusting hand is then very rapidly pronated, and before the foot can drop into plantarflexion, it applies a force to the cuneiform with the thenar eminence. **Note**: This requires very fast movement by the operator to reach the cuneiform before the foot drops. Very few operators can achieve the amount of speed necessary, but if it can be developed, this is an extremely effective technique. If the thrust is performed on the cuneiform after the foot has dropped into plantar-flexion, it may be very uncomfortable on the tissues on the front of the ankle.

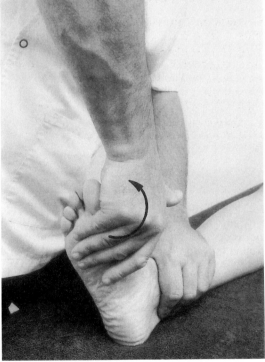

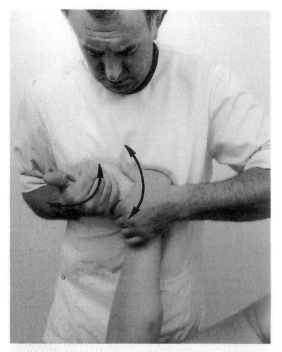

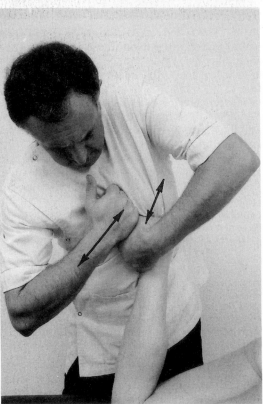

33.32 and 33.33 ◄ **Articulation of medial border prone** The foot is grasped with the target joint between the index finger of one hand and the fifth finger of the other. Fix the lateral border of the foot into your chest. Apply a dorsiflexion force with your distal hand, while holding a plantarflexion force with the other. Then reverse the movement.

Tips: Try using abduction or adduction, as well as traction, to amplify the primary levers. **Extra considerations**: If a suitable barrier accumulates, this hold can develop sufficient tension to perform a thrust.

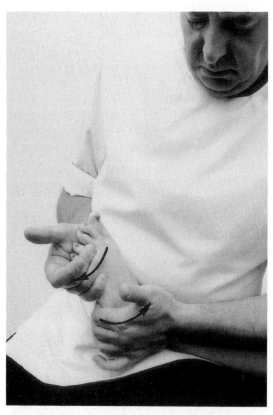

33.34 ▲ **Articulation of lateral border** Sit on the table and rest the patient's foot on your thigh. Fix the ankle with the inside of your wrist and clasp around the lateral border of the foot with the same hand. The other hand reaches under the foot and pulls the fourth and fifth metatarsals into plantar-flexion. The direction of forces of both hands can be reversed to produce the articulating force.

Tips: The sitting position cradling the foot can be quite a useful one for general mobilization as an alternative to standing.

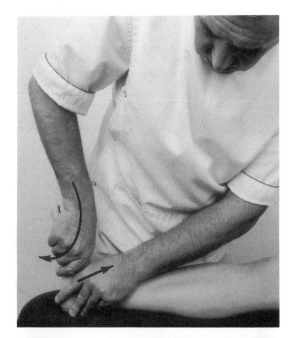

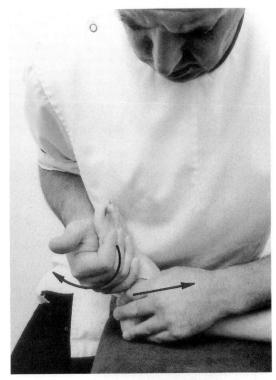

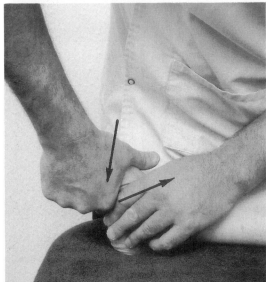

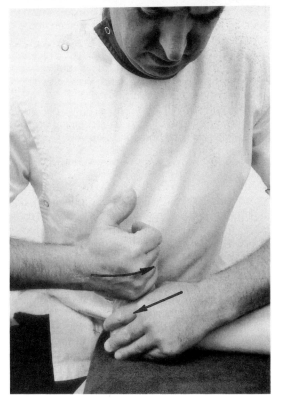

33.35 and 33.36 ▲ Thrust to medial border
Dorsiflex the foot to stabilize the ankle and fix the foot into the table with the stabilizing hand. Place the index finger of the stabilizing hand under either the talus, navicula or cuneiform according to which joint is being mobilized. Apply a buckling force toward the table with the thrusting hand and a combination of plantarflexion, eversion and abduction to focus at the target joint.

Tips: Several priming movements are often necessary to produce the optimum potential for the thrust.

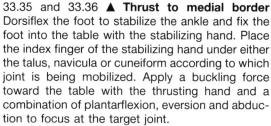

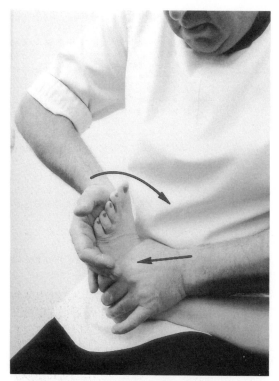

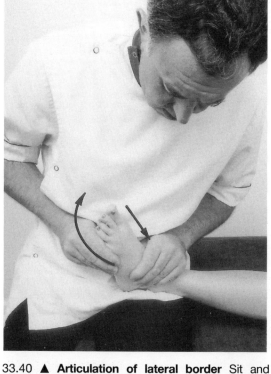

33.39 ▲ **Articulation of medial border** Sit on the table so that you can apply a very specific force to articulate the joints. The hand applied to the sole pushes the forefoot into dorsiflexion and varied degrees of inversion, eversion, abduction and adduction while the other hand fixes specifically, proximal to the target joint.

Tips: Although this hold does not allow a very powerful articulation it can be extremely specific. The sitting position can be a useful variation for the operator.

33.40 ▲ **Articulation of lateral border** Sit and stabilize the calcaneum or cuboid with the proximal hand. The distal hand articulates either the cuboid, or the fourth and fifth metatarsals on the cuboid. Form a fulcrum with the thumbs under the foot or the fingertips on the dorsum.

Tips: Try introducing traction and direct dorsal to plantar movement.

33.37 and 33.38 ◄ (see previous page, top right and bottom right) **Thrust to medial border** Stabilize the foot against the table holding the hind foot in dorsiflexion to lock the ankle. Supinate the other hand and pull the medial border of the foot into plantarflexion, abduction and eversion. Reverse the direction of forces and then, when a suitable tension is developed, execute the thrust with both hands. The stabilizing hand fixes on either the talus, navicula or cuneiform according to the target joint.

Tips: It may be easier to develop the eversion required with this hold than with some others, as the heel of the thrusting hand can be used.

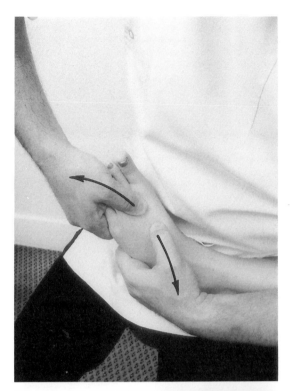

33.41 ◄ Articulation of mid tarsus supine Sit on the table and reach around the foot with both hands to fix the target joint between the clasping fingers and thumbs. Traction, circumduction, inversion, eversion, abduction and adduction are possible in this hold. Although this is not a very strong hold it is highly specific and can have a useful influence to re-introduce mobility in these otherwise inaccessible joints.

33.43 ▼ Articulation of lateral border supine Form a fulcrum either under the foot with the thumb or on the dorsum with the fingertips of the proximal hand. Apply traction, compression, abduction, adduction or circumduction to the third, fourth or fifth metatarsals with the distal hand. This will articulate the lateral cuneiform, cuboid and some of the mid tarsal joints.

Tips: Least useful with large feet as the reach may be a problem.

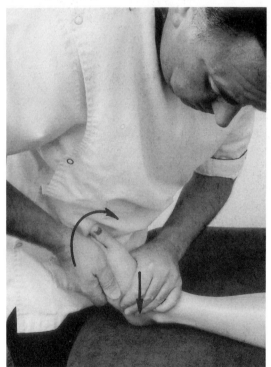

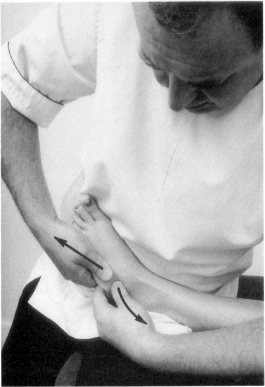

33.42 ◄ Articulation of cuboid supine Sit and clasp either the calcaneum or the cuboid to apply traction and adduction with different degrees of dorsiflexion and plantarflexion. Fix the foot against your abdomen to help block movement in the rest of the foot.

Tips: Most useful in very mobile feet where it may be difficult to isolate the cuboid.

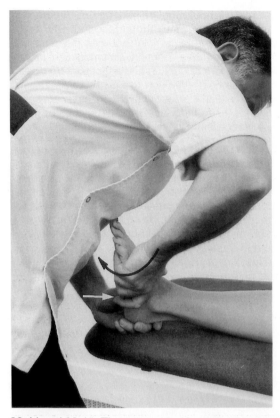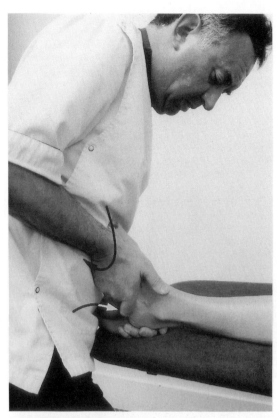

33.44 and 33.45 Thrust to cuboid supine Pull up on the fourth and fifth metatarsals with your fingertips. Apply the pad of the other thumb under the medial border of the cuboid. The thumb becomes a fulcrum over which you can plantarflex, invert and slightly adduct the foot. As tension accumulates you can amplify these components and add a compression force toward the table. The thumb forming the fulcrum should remain in as little abduction as possible to avoid straining it. Although the thumb applies a slight increase of force the thrust comes principally from the other hand. At the end of the thrust both elbows should be close to the operator's sides.

Tips: Least useful where operator thumb strength may be suspect. The technique could be modified so that the thenar or hypothenar eminences could be substituted. **Extra considerations**: If it proves impossible to build a suitable barrier, try lifting the whole leg off the table then bring it down sharply and, as the heel hits the table, execute the thrust. The momentum component may allow the barrier to be accessed more effectively.

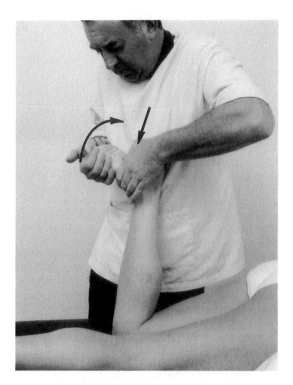

33.46 ◄ Thrust to cuboid prone Pull the foot into dorsiflexion with the distal hand and fix the other thumb toward the table on the medial border of the cuboid. Keep the arm close to the side, shrug the shoulder of the distal hand to produce an inversion of the lateral border of the foot with the heel of your hand.

Tips: Least useful where thumb strength is a problem but try substituting the thenar or hypothenar eminences. **Extra considerations**: Try circumducting the operator's body and the patient's lower extremity until the optimum thrust point is sensed.

33.47 ▼ (bottom left) **Thrust to cuboid prone** Cross the thumbs under the cuboid and dorsiflex the foot. Maintain the thumb pressure and plantarflex, invert and adduct the foot with some compression. This hold can be applied to most of the mid tarsal joints by changing the position of the crossed thumbs.

Tips: Ensure the ankle is maintained in dorsiflexion throughout as otherwise the force will dissipate through the ankle joint and the mid tarsal joints will tend to lock in plantarflexion.

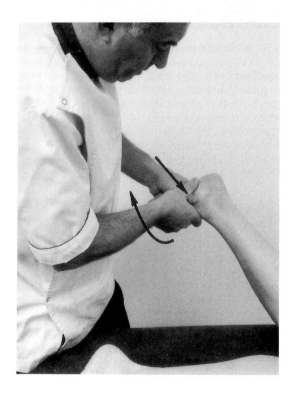

33.48 and 33.49 ▶ (see next page, top left and bottom left) **Thrust to cuboid prone leg over side** Cross the thumbs and apply them under the cuboid. Overlap the fingers on the dorsum of the foot and push with both thenar eminences against the sole to maintain dorsiflexion at the ankle. Keep dorsiflexion constant, and flex and extend the patient's hip and knee. Maintain the tibia in an almost horizontal position and push the leg away and allow it to recoil. Midway through one of these recoil movements drive the thumbs against the cuboid while the fingers produce inversion, adduction and compression.

Tips: Least useful in patients who may find the position a problem. **Extra considerations**: The coordination necessary for this technique is rather difficult. Note that it is applied as the tibia comes towards the operator, not away. If it is applied as the tibia moves away it becomes an undesirable plantarflexion thrust. It is possible to perform this thrust in simple plantarflexion but there are several disadvantages in this; greater force will be required, it will not be as specific, and the ankle will come under some strain.

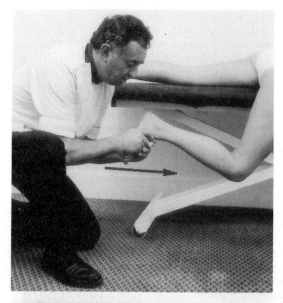

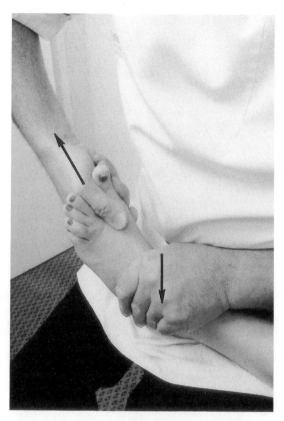

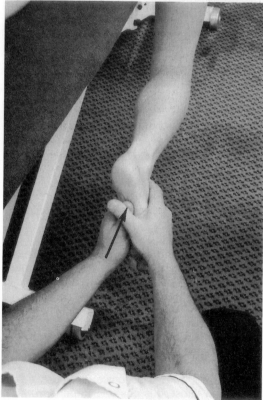

33.50 ▲ Articulation to metatarso-phalangeal joint of hallux supine Sit and rest the foot across your thigh. Fix the foot, particularly the first metatarsal, with your proximal hand and apply a traction and circumduction force to the first metatarso-phalangeal joint.

Tips: By gripping the distal end of the first metatarsal rather than the phalange the traction force will reach into the medial border of the foot.

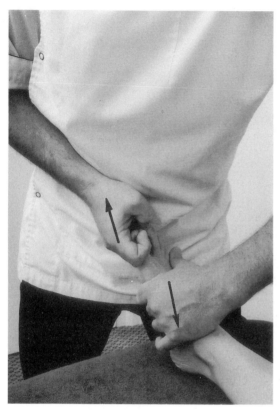

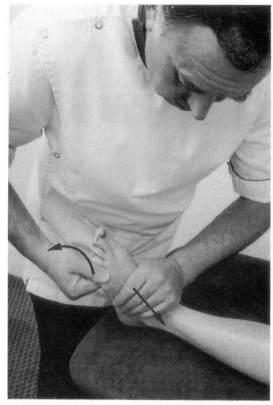

33.51 ▲ **Traction to hallux supine** Grip the first toe between your flexed fingers and hold back on the rest of the foot. This hold permits the use of traction, circumduction and rotation.

Tips: This grip allows a more comfortable hold than a simple clasping of the toe with finger and thumb.

33.52 ▲ **Thrust to metatarso-phalangeal joints supine** Fix on the body of the foot and apply a traction, then plantarflexion force to the toe. Small amounts of circumduction and rotation help localize the force.

Tips: Try using the finger under the toe as a fulcrum rather than just using traction or flexion.

RECOMMENDED READING

Bogduk, N. *et al.* (1985) Theoretical pathology of acute locked back: a base for manipulative therapy. *Manual Medicine*, **1**, 78–82.

Bourdillon, J.F. (1982) *Spinal Manipulation*, 3rd edn, Appleton-Century-Crofts, East Norwalk, CT.

Bowles, C.H. (1956) *A functional orientation for technique I*, Yearbook, New England Academy of Applied Osteopathy, Academy of Applied Osteopathy, pp. 107–14.

Bowles, C.H. (1956) *A functional orientation for technique II*, Yearbook, New England Academy of Applied Osteopathy, Academy of Applied Osteopathy, pp. 107–14.

Bowles, C.H. (1957) *A functional orientation for technique III*, Yearbook, New England Academy of Applied Osteopathy, Academy of Applied Osteopathy, pp. 53–5.

Bowles, C.H. (1981) Functional Technique, a modern perspective. *Journal of the American Osteopathic Association*, **80**, 326–31.

Chaitow, L. (1988) *Soft Tissue Manipulation*, Thorsens, Wellingborough, Northants.

Chaitow, L. (1980) *Neuro-muscular Technique*, Thorsens, Wellingborough, Northants.

Chaitow, L. (1993) *Palpatory Literacy*, Thorsens, Wellingborough, Northants.

Fryette, H.H. (1954) *Principles of Osteopathic Technique*, American Academy of Osteopathy, Carmel, CA.

Greenman, P.E. (1989) *Principles of Manual Medicine*, Williams & Wilkins, London.

Grieve, G.P. (1981) *Common Vertebral Joint Problems*, Churchill Livingstone, Edinburgh.

Grieve, G.P. (1990) Contra-indications to Spinal Manipulation and Allied Treatments. *British Osteopathic Journal*, **IV**, 23–4.

Haas, M. (1990) Physics of spinal manipulation. *Journal of Manipulative and Physical Therapeutics*, **13**, 204–6; 253–6; 305–8; 378–83.

Johnson, W.L. and Friedman H.D. (1994) *Functional Methods – A Manual for Palpatory Skill Development in Osteopathic Examination & Manipulation of Motor Function*, Osteopathic Supplies, Hereford.

Johnson, W.L., Robertson, J.A. and Stiles, E.G. (1969) Finding a common denominator for the variety of manipulative techniques. *Yearbook of the Academy of Applied Osteopathy*, American Academy of Osteopathy, Carmel, CA, pp. 5–15.

Jones, L.H. (1981) *Strain and Counterstrain*, American Academy of Osteopathy, Colorado Springs, CO.

Kimberley, P.E. (1976) Formulating a prescription for osteopathic manipulative treatment. *Journal of the American Osteopathic Association*, **75**, 486–99.

Kimberley, P.E. (1980) *Outline of Osteopathic Manipulative Procedures*, 2nd edn, Kirksville College of Osteopathic Medicine, Kirksville, MO.

Korr, I.M. (1976) Proprioceptors and somatic dysfunction. *Journal of the American Osteopathic Association*, **74**, 638–49.

Korr, I.M. (ed.) (1978) *The Neurologic Mechanisms in Manipulative Therapy*. Plenum, New York.

Lederman, E. (1992) Harmonic Technique. *British Osteopathic Journal*, **IX**, 11–13.

Lederman, E. (in press) *Physiological Basis of Manual Therapy*, Churchill Livingstone.

Lewit, K. (1986) Postisometric relaxation in combination with other methods of muscular fascilitation and inhibition. *Manual Medicine*, **2**, 101–4.

Littlejohn, J.M. *Fundamentals of Osteopathic Technique*, Wernham J, Maidstone School of Osteopathy.

Magoun, H.I. (1966) *Osteopathy in the Cranial Field*, 2nd edn, Journal Printing Co., Kirksville, MO.

Maitland, G.D. (1980) *Vertebral Manipulation*, 4th edn, Butterworths, Stoneham, MA.

Middleton, H.C. (1970) Osteopathic Technique. *British Osteopathic Journal*, **4**(4), 21–6.

Mitchell, F.L. Jr, Moran, P.S. and Pruzzo, N.A. (1979) *An Evaluation and Treatment Manual of Osteopathic Muscle Energy Procedures*. Mitchell, Moran, and Pruzzo Associates, Valley Park, MO.

Nicholas, N.S. (1974) *Atlas of Osteopathic Techniques*, Philadelphia College of Osteopathic Medicine, Philadelphia.

Rahlmann, J.F. (1987) Mechanisms of intervertebral joint fixation: A literature review. *Journal of Manipulative and Physiological Therapeutics*. **10**, 177–8.

Stoddard, A. (1993) *Manual of Osteopathic Practice*, 2nd edn, Osteopathic Supplies, Hereford.

Stoddard, A. (1993) *Manual of Osteopathic Practice*, 3rd edn, Osteopathic Supplies, Hereford.

Terrett, A. (1994) Manipulation and pain tolerance. *American Journal of Physical Medicine*, **63** (5), 217–25.

Upleger, J.E. and Vredevoogd, J. D. (1983) *Craniosacral Therapy*. Eastland Press, Chicago.

Walton, W.J. (1970) *Osteopathic Diagnosis and Technique Procedures*, 2nd edn, American Academy of Osteopathy, Colorado Springs, CO.

Wernham, J. (1989) The Art and Science of Osteopathy. *British Osteopathic Journal*, **III**, 35–38.

INDEX